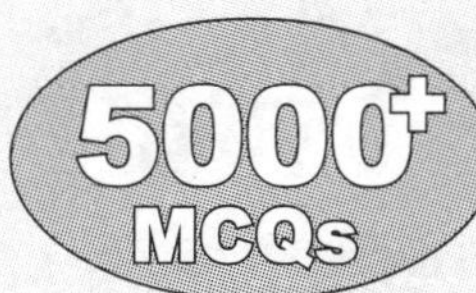

Aimed at
Diploma in Pharmacy Exit Examination (DPEE)

Pharma Success

An Excellent Key to Achieve Success

Multiple Choice Questions (MCQs)

Based on the latest PCI Syllabus ER 2020

- **Diploma in Pharmacy Exit Examination (DPEE)**
- **Sessional Examinations**
- **Board Examinations**
- **University Examinations**
- **Pharmacists Recruitment Examinations**
- **Competitive Examinations in Pharmacy Profession**

Salient Features

- Subject-wise and chapter-wise MCQs with Answer Keys
- Covers maximum MCQs as per PCI New Syllabus ER 2020
- Useful for all competitive examinations for getting better job opportunities in pharmacy profession such as pharmacists in PHCs, civil hospitals, railways, Indian Army, banking sector, corporate sector, pharmacists posts under Zila Parishads, etc.
- Infusing confidence in the reader to appear in the examinations with high-score results.

Other books by the same author under

CBS Confident Pharmacy Series

- *Social Pharmacy* for First Year Diploma in Pharmacy
- *Pharmaceutics, 4/e* for First Year Diploma in Pharmacy
- *Pharmacognosy, 4/e* for First Year Diploma in Pharmacy
- *Pharmaceutical Chemistry, 4/e* for First Year Diploma in Pharmacy
- *Human Anatomy and Physiology, 4/e* for First Year Diploma in Pharmacy
- *Pharmacy Law and Ethics* for Second Year Diploma in Pharmacy
- *Biochemistry and Clinical Pathology, 4/e* for Second Year Diploma in Pharmacy
- *Hospital and Clinical Pharmacy, 4/e* for Second Year Diploma in Pharmacy
- *Pharmacotherapeutics* for Second Year Diploma in Pharmacy
- *Community Pharmacy and Management* for Second Year Diploma in Pharmacy
- *Pharmacology* for Second Year Diploma in Pharmacy

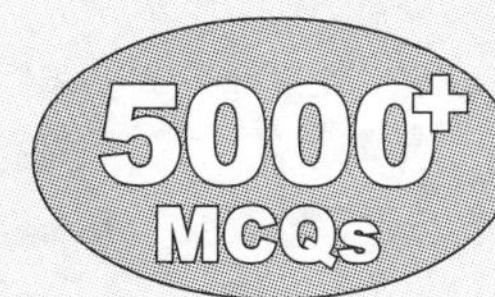

Aimed at
Diploma in Pharmacy Exit Examination (DPEE)

Pharma Success

An Excellent Key to Achieve Success

Multiple Choice Questions (MCQs)

Based on the latest PCI Syllabus ER 2020

Subjects Covered

First Year Diploma in Pharmacy
- Pharmaceutics
- Pharmaceutical Chemistry
- Pharmacognosy
- Human Anatomy and Physiology
- Social Pharmacy

Second Year Diploma in Pharmacy
- Pharmacology
- Community Pharmacy and Management
- Biochemistry and Clinical Pathology
- Pharmacotherapeutics
- Hospital and Clinical Pharmacy
- Pharmacy Law and Ethics

VN Raje M Pharm, MBA
Principal
Gourishankar Education Society's
GES College of Pharmacy (DPharm)
Limb, Satara, Maharashtra

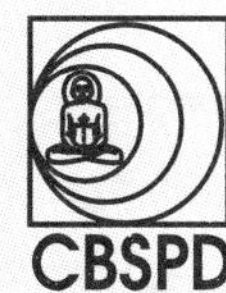

CBS Publishers & Distributors Pvt Ltd
New Delhi • Bengaluru • Chennai • Kochi • Kolkata • Lucknow • Mumbai
Hyderabad • Jharkhand • Nagpur • Patna • Pune • Uttarakhand

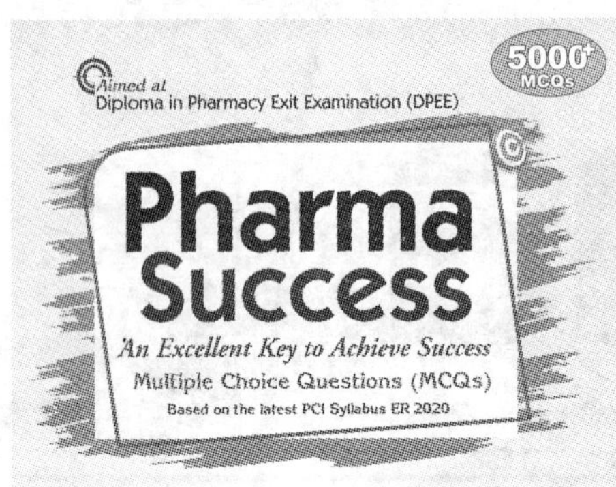

ISBN: 978-93-5466-841-8

First Edition: 2024

Published by **Satish Kumar Jain** and produced by **Varun Jain** for

CBS Publishers and Distributors Pvt Ltd

4819/XI Prahlad Street, 24 Ansari Road, Daryaganj, New Delhi 110 002, India.
Ph: 011-23266838, 23289259 Website: www.cbspd.com
e-mail: delhi@cbspd.com

Corporate Office: 204 FIE, Industrial Area, Patparganj, Delhi 110 092, India
Ph: 011-4934 4934 Fax: 011-4934 4935 e-mail: publishing@cbspd.com; publicity@cbspd.com

Branches

- **Bengaluru:** Seema House 2975, 17th Cross, K.R. Road, Banasankari 2nd Stage, Bengaluru 560 070, Karnataka, India
  Ph: +91-80-26771678/79 Fax: +91-80-26771680 e-mail: bangalore@cbspd.com
- **Chennai:** 7, Subbaraya Street, Shenoy Nagar, Chennai 600 030, Tamil Nadu, India
  Ph: +91-44-26680620, 26681266 Fax: +91-44-42032115 e-mail: chennai@cbspd.com
- **Kochi:** 42/1325, 1326, Power House Road, Opposite KSEB, Power House, Ernakulam 682 018, Kochi, Kerala, India
  Ph: +91-484-4059061–67 Fax: +91-484-4059065 e-mail: kochi@cbspd.com
- **Kolkata:** 147 Hind Ceramics Compound, 1st Floor, Nilgunj Road, Belghoria, Kolkata 700 056, West Bengal, India
  Ph: +033-25633055/56 e-mail: kolkata@cbspd.com
- **Lucknow:** Basement, Khushnuma Complex, 7-Meerabai Marg (Behind Jawahar Bhawan), Lucknow 226 001, Uttar Pradesh, India
  Ph: +91-522-4000032 e-mail:tiwari.lucknow@cbspd.com
- **Mumbai:** PWD Shed, Gala No. 25/26, Ramchandra Bhatt Marg, Next to JJ Hospital, Gate No. 2, Opp Union Bank of India, Noorbaug, Mumbai 400009, Maharashtra, India
  Ph: +91-22-66661880, 66661889 e-mail: mumbai@cbspd.com

Representatives

- **Hyderabad** 0-9885175004
- **Jharkhand** 0-9811541605
- **Nagpur** 0-8692091830
- **Patna** 0-9334159340
- **Pune** 0-9664372571
- **Uttarakhand** 0-9716462459

Printed at: Mudrak, Noida, Uttar Pradesh, India

Preface

The Pharmacy Council of India framed the "Diploma in Pharmacy Exit Examination (DPEE) Regulations, 2022" to boost the core competencies in pharmacy student while entering in profession of pharmacy.

Objective of Diploma in Pharmacy Exit Examination (DPEE)

The objective of the Diploma in Pharmacy Exit Examination (DPEE) is to ensure that a candidate applying for registration as pharmacist with the State Pharmacy Council has undergone pharmacy education and a comprehensive practical training programme in Diploma in Pharmacy (DPharm) course as provided in the Education Regulations, 2020 or the regulations that may be in force from time to time in an institution approved by Pharmacy Council of India under Section 12 of the Pharmacy Act, 1948 and acquired core competencies in dispensing of medicines and other areas of pharmacy practice and to reinforce his discipline, integrity, judgement, skills, knowledge and quest for learning so that after having passed the examination he is able to become a registered pharmacist who is able to exercise his professional skills in addition to carrying his duties and responsibilities professionally.

This exit examination for the registration of diploma in pharmacy holder is an excellent step which will build self-confidence in pharmacy students and able to exercise the professional skills in addition to carrying his duties and responsibilities professionally.

This book has been written to fulfil and face the forthcoming Diploma in Pharmacy Exit Examination as per PCI notification and includes 5000+ MCQs.

This book is mostly useful as reference for Multiple Choice Questions (MCQs) in regular sessional examinations, final board examinations, university examinations, pharmacist recruitment competitive examinations, etc. This book covers Multiple Choice Questions (MCQs) on all subjects of first year and second year Diploma in Pharmacy as per ER 2020 and questions are arranged chapter-wise with answer keys.

I have already published 23 books of Diploma in Pharmacy with CBS Publishers & Distributors, New Delhi, since 2008-09 and out of these 11 books are as per PCI new syllabus ER 2020 and I have received huge response from the teachers and students.

Hope this book will fulfil the dreams of students to qualify in Exit Examination and various competitive examinations of pharmacist recruitments.

VN Raje

Acknowledgements

I express my heartfelt thanks to Prof Madan Jagtap, Chairman, Gourishankar Education Society, Satara, Maharashtra, for consistent encouragement and inspiration for writing this book.

I wish to acknowledge the prompt and efficient help given by Prof Milind Jagtap, Mr Jaywant Salunkhe, Mr Appa Rajage, Mr Nitin Mudalgikar, and Mr Shrirang Katekar of Gourishankar Education Society, Satara.

I am grateful to Mr Ranjit Thavare, BPharm, MBA, Assistant Lecturer at GES College of Pharmacy (DPharm), Limb, Satara, for his valuable efforts in making this book successfully. His dedication and attention have improved the quality of our work, and I appreciate his contributions throughout the process.

I am also thankful to Mr Satish Kumar Jain, Chairman and Managing Director, and Mr Shantanu Sarkar, Assistant General Manager, Mumbai Branch, CBS Publishers & Distributors Pvt Ltd, for their sustained efforts and keen interest in the publication of this book.

I wish all my beloved students to have a great success in the Exit Examination as well as various competitive examinations in profession of pharmacy.

VN Raje

Contents

Sections IX: Pharmacotherapeutics

Sections X: Hospital and Clinical Pharmacy

Sections XI: Pharmacy Law and Ethics

Part 1

First Year Diploma in Pharmacy Subjects

I. Pharmaceutics

II. Pharmaceutical Chemistry

III. Pharmacognosy

IV. Human Anatomy and Physiology

V. Social Pharmacy

Section I

Pharmaceutics

1. History of the Profession of Pharmacy in India
2. Packaging Materials
3. Pharmaceutical Aids and Preservatives
4. Unit Operations
5. Tablets and Capsules
6. Liquid Oral Preparations
7. Topical Preparations
8. Sterile Formulations and Immunological Products
9. Quality Control and Quality Assurance
10. Novel Drug Delivery System

Syllabus (As Per ER 2020) Pharmaceutics

Chapter	Topics
1	History of the profession of pharmacy in India in relation to pharmacy education, industry, pharmacy practice, and various professional associations. Pharmacy as a career **Pharmacopoeia:** Introduction to IP, BP, USP, NF and extra pharmacopoeia. Salient features of Indian pharmacopoeia
2	**Packaging materials:** Types, selection criteria, advantages and disadvantages of glass, plastic, metal, rubber as packaging materials
3	**Pharmaceutical aids:** Organoleptic (colouring, flavouring, and sweetening) agents **Preservatives:** Definition, types with examples and uses
4	**Unit operations:** Definition, objectives/applications, principles, construction, and working of: ■ **Size reduction:** Hammer mill and ball mill ■ **Size separation:** Classification of powders according to IP, cyclone separator, sieves standards of sieves **Mixing:** Double cone blender, Turbine mixer, Triple roller mill and Silverson mixer homogenizer **Filtration:** Theory of filtration, membrane filter and sintered glass filter **Drying:** Working of fluidized bed dryer and process of freeze drying **Extraction:** Definition, Classification, method, and applications
5	Tablets—coated and uncoated, various modified tablets (sustained release, extended-release, fast dissolving, multi-layered, etc.) Capsules—hard and soft gelatine capsules Liquid oral preparations—solution, syrup, elixir, emulsion, suspension, dry powder for reconstitution Topical preparations—ointments, creams, pastes, gels, liniments and lotions, suppositories, and pessaries Nasal preparations, Ear preparations Powders and granules—Insufflations, dusting powders, effervescent powders, and effervescent granules Sterile formulations—Injectables, eye drops and eye ointments **Immunological products:** Sera, vaccines, toxoids, and their manufacturing methods.
6	Basic structure, Layout, sections, and activities of pharmaceutical manufacturing plants **Quality control and quality assurance:** Definition and concepts of quality control and quality assurance, current good manufacturing practice (cGMP) Introduction to the concept of calibration and validation
7	**Novel drug delivery systems:** Introduction, classification with examples, advantages, and challenges

CHAPTER 1.

History of the Profession of Pharmacy in India in Relation to Pharmacy Education, Industry, Pharmacy Practice and Various Professional Associations; Pharmacy as a Career; Pharmacopoeia

1. The Greek word *Poeio* means:

A. To cure **B.** To make
C. To diagnose **D.** To treat

2. In 1948 ___________ prepared the first edition of Indian pharmacopoeia.

A. Dr Mukherjee **B.** William Martindale
C. Dr BN Ghosh **D.** ML Schroff

3. The first British pharmacopoeia was published in _________.

A. 1890 **B.** 1864
C. 1870 **D.** 1895

4. In the year 2018 which edition of Indian pharmacopoeia was published?

A. 2nd edition **B.** 5th edition
C. 7th edition **D.** 8th edition

5. The British Pharmacopoeia is the National Pharmacopoeia of the __________.

A. Europe
B. United Kingdom
C. France
D. South Africa

6. DEC stands for __________.

A. Drug Education Committee
B. Drug Ethical Committee
C. Drug Enquiry Committee
D. None of the above

7. Who organizes the Indian Pharmaceutical Congress every year?

A. Indian Pharmaceutical Congress
B. Indian Pharmacy Graduates Association
C. Indian Pharmaceutical Congress Association
D. Indian Pharmaceutical Association

8. Earliest pharmacies were known as

A. Apothecary shops
B. Pharmacy
C. Medicine point
D. Drugstore

9. The architect of Indian pharmaceutical industry is _________.

A. Acharya SB Manikdas
B. Dr RC Subhedar
C. Dr APJ Abdul Kalam
D. Acharya PC Ray

10. At least ______________ is required to practice as a pharmacist in India.

A. Degree in Pharmacy
B. Masters in Pharmacy
C. Pharm D
D. Diploma in pharmacy

11. Pharmacy education in India as a university level programme started in 1937 at _________ .

A. Delhi University
B. University of Madras
C. Banaras Hindu University
D. Patna University

12. According to the reference, the commonly worshipped Hindu God of Medicine, "__________" is the original exponent of the Indian medicine.

A. Ganesh
B. Mahadev
C. Dhanvantari
D. Bramha

13. The ____________ was enacted as the nation's first minimum standard of educational qualification for pharmacy practice.

A. Drugs and Cosmetics Act 1940 (1945)
B. DPCO Act
C. Pharmacy Act 1948
D. All of the above

14. Pharmacy practice in India is governed by which of the following Act?

A. Pharmacy Act 1948
B. Drugs and Cosmetics Act 1940 (1945)
C. DPCO Act
D. All of the above

15. Key strengths of pharmaceutical industry are ______.

A. Strong manufacturing base
B. Cost competitiveness
C. Fast growing healthcare industry
D. All of the above

16. The word 'pharmacy' is derived from the Greek word __________.

A. Pharmaces **B.** Pharma
C. Pharmacisto **D.** Pharmakon

17. The present education regulations 2020 framed replaced __________.

A. Education Regulations 1981
B. Education Regulations 1991
C. Education Regulations 1982
D. Education Regulations 2014

18. ______________ is the federation of five national pharmaceutical associations as its constituents.

A. Indian Pharmaceutical Congress
B. Indian Pharmaceutical Congress Association
C. Indian Pharmacy Graduates Association
D. Indian Pharmaceutical Association

19. __________ is the premier professional association of pharmacists in India.

A. Indian Pharmaceutical Congress
B. Indian Pharmacy Graduates Association
C. Indian Pharmaceutical Association
D. Indian Pharmaceutical Congress Association

20. ____________ has the highest number of US FDA approved drug manufacturing units (outside USA) today.

A. India **B.** Russia
C. China **D.** America

21. _____________ were medical doctors as well as pharmacists.

A. Charaka and Chanakya
B. Chanakya and Sushruta
C. Charaka and Sushruta
D. Aryabhatta and Valmiki

22. The Drugs and Cosmetics Act was passed in the year __________.

A. 1940 **B.** 1945
C. 1948 **D.** 1955

23. Who is known as the "Father of Pharmacy Education in India"?

A. Acharya PC Ray
B. Prof Mahadev Lal Schroff
C. Sushruta
D. Charaka

24. Pharmacy education in India at the certificate level was started in 1842 in Goa by ___________.

A. Britishers **B.** Jews
C. Native businessmen **D.** Portuguese

25. __________ was the first pharmaceutical manufacturing facility establishment in India.

A. Indian Pharmaceutical Company Ltd.
B. Bengal Chemicals and Pharmaceutical Works Ltd.
C. Calcutta Chemicals
D. Ranbaxy Pharmaceuticals Ltd.

26. The first edition of IP was published in __________.

A. 1948 **B.** 1955
C. 1940 **D.** 1960

27. Extra pharmacopoeia is also termed __________.

A. Martindale: The Complete Drug Reference
B. Pharmacopoeia codex
C. National formulary
D. International pharmacopoeia

28. __________ is pharmacy as the minimum required qualification to enter into the pharmacy profession in India.

A. Degree **B.** Postgraduation
C. Diploma **D.** Pharm D

29. Dioscorides wrote __________

A. Merck Index
B. Indian Pharmacopoeia
C. Martindale
D. De Materia Medica

30. Which edition of Indian Pharmacopoeia was published in 2018?

A. 3rd B. 7th
C. 6th D. 8th

31. Who is the Father of Medicine?

A. Ebers B. Hippocrates
C. Egyptian D. Pontus

32. Drugs converted to suitable form are known as ______.

A. Excipient B. Source of drug
C. Dosage forms D. API

33. Every dosage form is a combination of drug and different kinds of non-drug components called _________.

A. Additives B. Non-additives
C. New chemical entity D. All of the above

34. The 7th edition of IP was published in _________.

A. 2007 B. 1996
C. 2014 D. 2012

35. USP first edition was published in _________.

A. Latin B. English
C. English and Latin D. French

36. The meaning of Pharmakon means _________.

A. Powder
B. Medicine or drug
C. Emulsion
D. None of the above

37. The fourth edition of IP was published in _________.

A. 1965 B. 1975
C. 1996 D. 1985

38. The content of pharmacopoeia includes _________.

A. Monograph of drug/substance
B. Standard test
C. Description, formulae
D. All of the above

39. The first chemist shop in India was opened by _______ in 1811 in Kolkata.

A. Scotch Bathgate
B. Acharya PC Ray
C. Cal RN Chopra
D. Haroon Zaffer

40. The first Pharmacy Council of India (PCI) was constituted by Central Government in _________.

A. 1947 B. 1949
C. 1948 D. 1950

41. Drug Enquiry Committee is known as _________.

A. Chopra committee
B. Bhor committee
C. Import of drug bill
D. Indian Pharmacopoeia Committee

42. The Pharmacy Education in India is regulated by Pharmacy Council of India under _________.

A. The Pharmacy Act 1948
B. Drugs And Cosmetics Act 1940
C. DPCO Act
D. The Industry Act

43. The first 2 years of professional course "Chemist and Druggist Diploma" was started in __________.

A. Banaras Hindu University
B. Bengal Chemical and Pharmaceuticals
C. Madras Medical College
D. Indian Pharmaceutical Association

44. The second edition of Indian pharmacopoeia was published in ___________.

A. 1985 B. 2007
C. 1955 D. 1966

45. All the following are official books *except* _________.

A. Merk Index
B. The Drug Bill
C. National Formulary
D. Indian Pharmaceutical Codex

46. The Indian Government appointed a 'Drug Inquiry Committee' under the Chairmanship of _________.

A. Dr BN Ghosh B. Dr Mukharji
C. William Martindale D. Lt Col RN Chopra

47. The long form of AIOCD is__________.

A. All India Organization of Chemist and Druggist
B. All India Organization of Chemistry and Discovery
C. All India Organization of Chemist and Distributor
D. None of the above

48. The current Education Regulations were framed by PCI are known as __________.

A. ER 1981 B. ER 1991
C. ER 2014 D. ER 2020

49. The 'Import of Drugs Bill' was introduced in __________ in legislative assembly to control import of drugs.

A. 1940 B. 1937
C. 1935 D. 1931

50. **__________ is an art and science of compounding and dispensing of medications.**
   A. Biotechnology
   B. Pharmacodynamics
   C. Pharmacy
   D. Pharmacovigilance

51. **The first of pharmacy shop was opened in __________.**
   A. France B. Italy
   C. Germany D. Bagdad

52. **USP means**
   A. United States Pharmacology
   B. United States Pharmacy
   C. United States Pharmacopoeia
   D. United States Pharmaceutical

53. **Alembic Chemical Works at Baroda was established by ________.**
   A. Prof TK Gujjar B. Acharya PC Ray
   C. RN Chopra D. Mr Bathgate

54. **Pharmacopoeia contains __________.**
   A. Monograph and drug substances
   B. Standard tests
   C. Description formulae
   D. All of the above

55. **Who organises the Indian Pharmaceutical Congress every year?**
   A. Indian Pharmaceutical Congress
   B. Indian Pharmaceutical Congress Association
   C. Indian Pharmacy Graduate Association
   D. Indian Pharmaceutical Association

56. **The Pharmacy Act was established in __________.**
   A. 1960
   B. 1952
   C. 1948
   D. 1949

57. **Long form of APTI is ___________.**
   A. Association of pharmaceutical teachers of India
   B. Association of pharmaceutical training in India
   C. Association of pharmaceutical theories in India
   D. Association of post teachers in India

58. **The Pharmacy Council of India is reconstituted after every __________ years.**
   A. 5 B. 4
   C. 3 D. 2

59. **IDMA stands for __________.**
   A. Indian Drug Manufacturer Association
   B. Import of Drug Manufacturer Association
   C. Indian Drug Management Association
   D. Indian Dosage Management Association

60. **In 1842, in India Portuguese started pharmacy education by providing a certificate course in __________.**
   A. Hyderabad
   B. Goa
   C. Bangalore
   D. Delhi

Answer Key

1 B	2 C	3 B	4 D	5 B	6 C	7 C	8 A	9 D	10 D
11 C	12 C	13 C	14 B	15 D	16 D	17 B	18 B	19 C	20 A
21 C	22 A	23 B	24 D	25 B	26 B	27 A	28 C	29 D	30 D
31 B	32 C	33 A	34 C	35 C	36 B	37 C	38 D	39 A	40 B
41 A	42 A	43 C	44 D	45 B	46 D	47 A	48 D	49 B	50 C
51 D	52 C	53 A	54 D	55 B	56 C	57 A	58 A	59 A	60 B

CHAPTER 2

Packaging Materials

1. **Which one of the following is not an official test for rubber closure?**
   A. Extractive test B. Pyrogen test
   C. Permeability test D. Compatibility test

2. **Following are the materials used for container *except* ___________.**
   A. Glass B. Plastic
   C. Rubber D. Metal

3. **PVC means __________.**
   A. Polyvinyl chloride B. Polyvinyl carbon
   C. Polyvinyl carbide D. Polyvinyl carbonate

4. **_______________ is a material of choice for a flexible packaging.**
   A. Metal B. Glass
   C. Cellulose D. Cellophane

5. **___________ is a device by means of which container can be closed and opened.**
   A. Aerosol B. Closure
   C. Container D. None of the above

6. **Which of the following materials are used in pharmaceutical packaging?**
   A. Glass B. Plastic
   C. Metal D. All of the above

7. **Major disadvantages of glass as a packaging material are**
   A. Fragility B. Weight
   C. Both A and B D. None of the above

8. **Composition of glass is __________.**
   A. Sand B. Soda ash
   C. Lime stone and cullet D. All of the above

9. **Which of the following packaging materials is used to protect the drug against the light?**
   A. Plastic containers
   B. Amber coloured glass containers
   C. Both A and B
   D. None of the above

10. **Type-I glass is also known as __________.**
    A. Borosilicate glass
    B. Regular soda-lime glass
    C. Treated soda-lime glass
    D. None of the above

11. **Which of the following methods are used in the production of glass?**
    A. Blowing B. Drawing
    C. Pressing and casting D. All of the above

12. **To protect the contents of a bottle from the effects of sunlight by UV rays, which glass is used?**
    A. Amber coloured glass B. Red coloured glass
    C. Both A and B D. None of the above

13. **Soda ash is also known as __________.**
    A. Pure silica B. Treated soda-lime
    C. Limestone D. Sodium carbonate

14. **Plastic containers are generally made from which of the following materials?**
    A. Polyethylene B. Polypropylene
    C. Polystyrene D. All of the above

15. **The package that is directly in contact with formulation is called __________.**
    A. Secondary package B. Tertiary package
    C. Primary package D. All of the above

16. The advantages of plastic containers over glass containers are __________.

A. Easy formation
B. Resistance to breakage
C. Freedom of design
D. All of the above

17. LDPE stands for ________.

A. Low density polyethylene
B. Light density polyethylene
C. Low density polypropylene
D. None of the above

18. Hermetic containers are also known as _________.

A. Air-tight containers
B. Multi-dose containers
C. Single dose containers
D. None of the above

19. Thermoplastics are ________.

A. Does not softened upon exposure to high temperature
B. Hard and brittle
C. Softened upon exposure to high temperature
D. None of the above

20. HDPE stands for __________.

A. High density polyethylene
B. High density polyethene
C. High density polypropylene
D. None of the above

21. Type-II glasses are __________.

A. Treated soda-lime glass
B. NP glass
C. Borosilicate glass
D. General soda-lime glass

22. Rubbers are used as material for construction of _________.

A. Container **B.** Closure
C. Both A and B **D.** None of the above

23. Plastic containers are sterilized using ___________.

A. Autoclave
B. Bleaching agent
C. Ethylene oxide
D. All of the above

24. The package composed of a layer having cavities that hold the pharmaceutical product and a lid is called _________.

A. Strip package
B. Child resistant package
C. Blister package
D. Well-closed package

25. A light-resistant container provides protection against __________.

A. Moisture **B.** Light
C. Both A and B **D.** None of the above

26. Glass containers are __________ in nature.

A. Fragile **B.** Light
C. Both A and B **D.** None of the above

27. Which is the most resistant type of glass?

A. Type I **B.** Type II
C. Type III **D.** Type IV

28. Which of the following is used as vulcanizing agent in the manufacture of rubber closures?

A. Activated carbon black
B. Sulphur
C. Talc
D. Stearic acid

29. __________ glass is a glass of highest pharmaceutical grade

A. Type I **B.** Type II
C. Type III **D.** Type IV

30. Soda-lime glass is also known as __________.

A. Hard glass **B.** Soft glass
C. Potash glass **D.** Lead glass

Answer Key

1 B	2 C	3 A	4 D	5 B	6 D	7 C	8 D	9 B	10 A
11 D	12 C	13 C	14 D	15 C	16 D	17 A	18 A	19 C	20 A
21 A	22 B	23 C	24 C	25 B	26 A	27 A	28 B	29 A	30 B

CHAPTER 3

Pharmaceutical Aids and Preservatives

1. Identify the artificial sweetener among the following:

A. Sucrose
B. Dextrose
C. Sucralose
D. Mannitol

2. To increase viscosity of liquid which of the following reagent is used?

A. PVP
B. Sodium carboxymethyl cellulose
C. Methyl cellulose
D. All of the above

3. Which of the following is not used as a diluent?

A. Lactose
B. Microcrystalline cellulose
C. Calcium carbonate
D. Polyvinyl Pyrrolidine

4. Which among the following is not an example for natural colors?

A. Annatto
B. Carotene
C. Saffron
D. Naphthalene blue

5. Chelating agents act by __________ mechanism.

A. Complexation
B. Hydration
C. Oxidation
D. None of the above

6. Diluents are used to __________.

A. Add cohesiveness to the powder blend
B. Make up the required bulk of the tablet
C. Both A and B
D. None of the above

7. Antioxidants act by inhibiting __________ mechanism.

A. Complexation
B. Hydration
C. Oxidation
D. None of the above

8. Preservatives improve __________ .

A. Shelf life of the product
B. Product stability
C. Appearance of the product
D. All of the above

9. Lakes are example for __________.

A. Colouring agent
B. Flavouring agent
C. Sweetening agent
D. None of the above

10. Which of the following is an example of a non-nutritive sweetening agent?

A. Sucralose
B. Sucrose
C. Mannitol
D. None of the above

11. EDTA is an example of __________.

A. Chelating agent
B. Antifungal preservative
C. Anti-oxidant
D. None of the above

12. A flavouring agent is used to enhance __________ of the product.

A. Smell
B. Appearance
C. Palatability
D. None of the above

13. Which of the following are widely used and excellent preservatives?

A. Quaternary ammonium compounds
B. Mercurials
C. Chelating agents
D. Chloroform

14. Benzalkonium chloride is categorized as _________.
A. Acidic preservative
B. Neutral preservative
C. Mercurial preservative
D. Quaternary ammonium compounds

15. Which of the following is an example of synthetic colouring agent?
A. Amaranth B. Curcumin
C. Cochineal D. None of the above

16. Which of the following sugar has bitter taste?
A. Glucose B. Sucrose
C. Saccharine D. None of the above

17. Which of the following is a synthetic sweetener?
A. Glucose B. Sucrose
C. Sorbitol D. Aspartame

18. At which concentration, phenol acts as preservative?
A. 0.2–0.5 B. 0.5–0.8
C. 0.05–0.1 D. None

19. Most widely used flavouring agent in food industry is
A. Menthol
B. Chloroform
C. Monosodium glutamate
D. None of the above

20. Ingredients used to enhance the elegance of pharmaceutical formulations are called _______.
A. Carminatives
B. Pharmaceutical aids
C. Astringent
D. None of the above

21. Cochineal is a ___________ agent.
A. Flavouring B. Colouring
C. Sweetening D. Thickening

22. Which of the following flavour is not responsible for sour taste?
A. Citrus flavour B. Liquorice
C. Raspberry D. Mint spice

23. Which of the following agents are used as flavouring agents?
A. Menthol B. Chloroform
C. Both A and B D. None of the above

24. Which of the following is a coal tar colour?
A. Amaranth B. Caramel
C. Titanium dioxide D. Cochineal

25. The colouring agents are permitted under the Act __________.
A. Pharmacy Act 1948 B. DMR Act 1954
C. NDPS Act 1985 D. D and C Act 1940

26. Which of the following is used as a colouring agent?
A. Lemon B. Sorbitol
C. Clove D. Caramel

27. Pharmaceutical aids are also known as __________.
A. Adjuvants B. Adjuncts
C. Excipients D. All of the above

28. Titanium dioxide is used as ___________.
A. Flavouring agent B. Colouring agent
C. Sweetening agent D. All of the above

29. BHA and BHT are used as ____________.
A. Buffers B. Antioxidants
C. Diluents D. Vehicles

30. _________ is a propellant for sprays and aerosols.
A. Benzalkonium chloride
B. Trichlorofluoromethane
C. Carbon tetrachloride
D. Propyl gallate

Answer Key

1 A	2 D	3 D	4 D	5 A	6 B	7 C	8 D	9 A	10 A
11 A	12 C	13 A	14 D	15 A	16 C	17 D	18 A	19 C	20 B
21 B	22 D	23 C	24 A	25 D	26 D	27 D	28 B	29 B	30 B

CHAPTER 4

Unit Operations

Size Reduction, Size Separation, Mixing, Filtration, Drying, Extraction

1. ___________ is a solvent for extraction of alkaloids, glycosides, volatile oils and resins.

A. Water B. Alcohol
C. Kerosene D. Light petroleum

2. Following are the processes of extraction *except* ___________.

A. Percolation B. Digestion
C. Drying D. Maceration

3. ___________ is used for drying of biological product like plasma, serum, vaccines, enzymes, etc.

A. Tray dryer B. Spray dryer
C. Rotary dryer D. Freeze dryer

4. Thermolabile material can be sterilised by using ___________.

A. Filter leaf B. Sintered glass filter
C. Filter press D. Filter paper

5. The efficiency of ball mill is maximum at _________.

A. Low speed
B. High speed
C. Very high speed
D. 2/3 speed (critical speed)

6. Most simple and most frequently used method for size separation is ___________.

A. Sieve Shaker
B. Cyclone separator
C. Air separator
D. Elutriation

7. Which type of mixtures is easily formed?

A. Positive B. Negative
C. Neutral D. Ampholytic

8. The process of separation of insoluble particle from suspension or slurry is called ___________.

A. Filtration B. Sieving
C. Distillation D. Drying

9. Which one of the following does not influence filtration?

A. Temperature B. Density
C. Viscosity D. pH

10. Metafilter is also known as ___________.

A. Filter press B. Filter candle
C. Edge filter D. Sintered filter

11. Filter aids are added to the liquid ___________.

A. To increase the porosity
B. To increase cake permeability
C. Both A and B
D. None of the above

12. Size reduction is also called __________.

A. Comminution
B. Continuation
C. Communication
D. Elutriation

13. Which of the following factor is not affecting on the process of size reduction?

A. Hardness B. Stickiness
C. Viscosity D. Abrasiveness

14. In the ball mill maximum size reduction occurs at __________ speed.

A. Low
B. High
C. Optimum/critical
D. None of the above

15. Gyration is the rotation of the wheel which makes the sieves to ___________.

A. Vibrate B. None
C. Oscillate D. Spin

16. The mechanisms of mixing are ___________.

A. Convection
B. Diffusion
C. Convection, shear, diffusion
D. Both A and B

17. Which of the following is NOT a method used for size reduction?

A. Cutting B. Impact
C. Burning D. Shear

18. A ball mill works on the principle of ___________.

A. Impact B. Attrition
C. Impact and attrition D. None of the above

19. Attrition is a mechanism of size reduction found in ___________.

A. Ball mill B. Plate mill
C. Roller mill D. All of the above

20. Size reduction helps in ___________.

A. Increase size
B. Decrease absorption
C. Decrease solubility
D. Decrease size and increase stability

21. For ease in reduction of size, material must be ______.

A. Hard, brittle B. Soft tough
C. Hard tough D. Soft brittle

22. Principle of hammer mill is ___________.

A. Cutting B. Crushing
C. Attrition D. Impact

23. The mechanism involved in the ball mill is ___________.

A. Compression
B. Impact
C. Attrition
D. Attrition and impact

24. ___________ of the space of the cylinder is occupied by the balls in ball mill.

A. 100% B. 30 to 50%
C. 80% D. 20%

25. The rate of filtration is expressed as ___________.

A. Mass
B. Volume in litres per unit time
C. Weight
D. Density

26. In cyclone separator, the separation depends on

A. Density in shape
B. Shape and surface area
C. Size and density
D. Surface texture and size

27. Which of the following is the type of size separation?

A. Sifting
B. Classifying and screening
C. Sieving
D. All of the above

28. A powder of which the entire particles pass through a Sieve No. 10 and not more than 40.0% through a Sieve No. 44?

A. Coarse powder
B. Moderately coarse powder
C. Fine powder
D. Very fine powder

29. The filtration which involves the separation of the intermicellar liquid from solid by semipermeable membrane under reduced pressure is ___________.

A. Surface B. Ultra filtration
C. Cross flow D. Depth

30. The main component of asbestos is ___________.

A. Aluminosilicate B. Carbon
C. Sodium D. Cellulose

31. Surface type cartridges are usually in the shape of candles made up of porcelain, and ___________.

A. Asbestos B. Cotton
C. Glass D. Kieselguhr

32. The freeze dryer works on the principle of ___________.

A. Freezing and sublimation
B. Freezing
C. Sublimation
D. Melting

33. The solid residue which is obtained after the completion of the extraction process is called ___________.

A. Solvent B. Marc
C. Filtrate D. Extract

34. Continuous hot percolation is called ___________.

A. Soxhlation B. Maceration
C. Infusion D. Decoction

35. Size classification is also known as ___________.

A. Size separation B. Size reduction
C. Size analysis D. Size filtration

36. **Which mechanism help in size separation by sieve shaker?**
A. Centrifugal force B. Sedimentation
C. Brushing D. Shearing forces

37. **Movement of particle can be enhanced during size separation by which one of the following modes?**
A. Agitation B. Attrition
C. Gravitation D. Mixing

38. **The solvent used for extraction is called __________.**
A. Menstruum B. Marc
C. Expression D. Galenical

39. **For __________ mixing each particle of one material lies as nearly adjacent as possible to a particle of other material.**
A. Positive B. Negative
C. Perfect D. Neutral

40. **The Pharmacopoeia has prescribed only the upper limit for the __________ fine grades of powder**
A. 2 B. 3
C. 5 D. 4

41. **The preparations which are made by using extraction method are called __________.**
A. Biologicals B. Botanicals
C. Galenicals D. All of the above

42. **__________ is not used for mixing, in dispensing.**
A. Sizing B. Spatulation
C. Trituration D. Tumbling

43. **Which type of the following is also known as twin shell blender?**
A. Double cone blender B. Tumbler mixer
C. Sigma blade mixer D. Paddle mixer

44. **Degree of mixing is also known as __________.**
A. Degree of homogeneity B. Extent of mixing
C. Random mixing D. None of the above

45. **Sieve through which all the particles must pass in case of moderately fine particles is __________**
A. 44 B. 85
C. 22 D. 10

46. **The principle behind cyclone separator is __________.**
A. Agitation B. Centrifugal force
C. Sieves D. None of the above

47. **Sintered glass filter is made from __________.**
A. Limestone B. Soda-lime glass
C. Sulphur glass D. Borosilicate glass

48. **Membrane filter works on the principle of __________.**
A. Physical separation B. Chemical separation
C. Shearing force D. Gravitational force

49. **'Kozeny-Carman equation' and 'Poiseulle's law' are the theories of __________.**
A. Extraction B. Separation
C. Filtration D. Mixing

50. **Final removal of liquid from the solid with the help of heat is called __________.**
A. Extraction B. Drying
C. Separation D. Mixing

51. **__________ is also known as freezer drying.**
A. Homogenization B. Lyophilization
C. Clarification D. Filtration

52. **In cyclone separator the powder is separated depending on its __________.**
A. Particle size B. Density
C. Particle size and density D. Shape of powder

53. **Which of the following equipment can be used for mixing of powder?**
A. Turbine mixer B. Double cone blender
C. Sigma blade mixer D. All of the above

54. **A clear liquid passing through the filter is called __________.**
A. Filtrate B. Slurry
C. Filter media D. Filter cake

55. **The separation process in which the amount of solid in liquid is not more than 1% w/v is called __________.**
A. Clarification B. Filtration
C. Centrifugation D. Evaporation

56. **Leaching means __________.**
A. Liquid–liquid extraction B. Solid–liquid extraction
C. Solid-phase extraction D. All of the above

57. **__________ is the process of removal of an active constituent from crude drug by using suitable solvent in which it is soluble.**
A. Filtration B. Size reduction
C. Drying D. Extraction

58. **Continuous hot percolation is also known as __________.**
A. Lyophilization B. Soxhalation
C. Homogenization D. None of the above

59. **Which of the following is standard for sieve?**
A. Sieve number B. Nominal aperture size
C. Nominal diameter of wire D. All of the above

60. Which materials are not used in drying in a freeze dryer?

A. Seafood B. Fruits
C. Pharmaceuticals D. Dyes

61. In drying process, the final product is in the form of ________.

A. Slurry B. Solution
C. Solid D. Solvent concentrate

62. Condition that is highly critical in drying process is ________.

A. Moisture B. Pressure
C. Temperature D. Volume

63. Advantage of fluidized bed dryer is ________.

A. No attrition
B. Entire material is continuously exposed to heat source
C. Fluppy mass is formed
D. Humidity can be increased

64. In sieving, sieves are arranged in ________ orders.

A. Ascending B. Random
C. Descending D. Horizontal

65. Mechanism of mixing in silverson mixer is ________.

A. Convective B. Laminar
C. Random D. Turbulent

66. A double cone mixer is used for mixing ________.

A. Solids B. Semi-solids
C. Liquids D. Suspensions

67. Triple roller mill works on the principle of ________

A. Diffusion mixing B. Convective mixing
C. Dry mixing D. Shear mixing

68. The rate of flow of the filtrate through the filter cake is ________ to the thickness of the cake.

A. Inversely proportional
B. Directly proportional
C. Remain constant
D. None of the above

69. Which of the following is not a filter aid?

A. Diatomaceous earth B. Perlite
C. Cellulose D. Cotton

70. Filter aids are added to the liquid ________.

A. To increase the porosity
B. To increase cake permeability
C. Both A and B
D. None of the above

71. Which of the following theory not describe rate of filtration?

A. Darcy Law
B. Poiseulle's equation
C. Kozeny-Carman equation
D. Noyes-Whitney equation

72. The slurry is ________.

A. A suspension to be filtered
B. A porous membrane used to retain the solids
C. The solids which are present on the filter
D. A clear liquid passing through the filter

73. Which of the following dryer is known as lyophilizer?

A. Fluidized bed dryer B. Spray dryer
C. Freeze dryer D. Vacuum dryer

74. ________ means extraction carried out by mechanical means.

A. Evaporation B. Expression
C. Galenicals D. Filtration

75. Proper drying can prevent ________ of the product.

A. Loss B. Weight
C. Deterioration D. Solubility

76. Drying involves ________ transfer operation.

A. Mass B. Heat
C. Mass and heat D. Either mass or heat

77. For extraction of thermolabile drugs which extraction process should be used?

A. Percolation B. Maceration
C. Decoction D. Both A and B

78. The solvent used for extraction is known as

A. Distillate B. Extract
C. Marc D. Menstruum

79. The inert insoluble material that remains after extraction is called ________

A. Distillate B. Extract
C. Marc D. Menstruum

80. Which of the following process is used for extraction?

A. Infusion B. Decoction
C. Digestion D. All of the above

81. Pouring water over the drugs and then allowing it to keep in contact with water usually for the 15 min is called ________.

A. Infusion B. Decoction
C. Percolation D. Digestion

82. Extraction does not involve one of the following components __________.

A. Active constituents
B. Solvent
C. Vapour
D. Crude solids

83. Which of the following is not a mechanism of size reduction?

A. Compression B. Impact
C. Attrition D. Elutriation

84. Following are the processes used for extraction *except* __________

A. Maceration B. Sublimation
C. Digestion D. Percolation

85. Preparations like infusions, decoctions, spirits, elixirs are commonly known as __________

A. Pharmaceuticals
B. Galenicals
C. Nutraceuticals
D. Cosmeceuticals

86. Solvent used for extraction is __________.

A. Water B. Alcohol
C. Ether D. All of the above

87. What is the disadvantage of alcohol as solvent for extraction?

A. Toxicity B. Stability
C. Cost D. Selectivity

88. Ball mill is based on principle of __________.

A. Cutting
B. Compression
C. Impact and attrition
D. Attrition

89. Hammer mill is based on the principle of __________.

A. Impact B. Attrition
C. Cutting D. Compression

90. Elutriation is a method of__________.

A. Size reduction B. Extraction
C. Size separation D. Filtration

91. In cyclone separator __________ force is used to separate solid from the fluid.

A. Fractional force
B. Centrifugal force
C. Electromagnetic force
D. Nuclear force

92. __________ is a unit operation in which two or more substance combined together in such a way that each particle of material looks similar to particles of other material.

A. Filtration B. Extraction
C. Mixing D. Drying

93. Following is the mechanism of mixing __________.

A. Shear mixing
B. Convective mixing
C. Diffusion mixing
D. All of the above

94. Propeller mixer and turbine mixer are used for mixing of __________.

A. Solids B. Liquids
C. Semi-solids D. Powders

95. Double cone blender works on the mechanism of __________.

A. Convective mixing
B. Diffusion mixing
C. Shearing mixing
D. All of the above

96. Silverson mixer is used for __________.

A. Homogenization B. Filtration
C. Extraction D. Separation

97. Clarification is used for the removal of small amount of suspended solids __________.

A. Not more than 2%
B. Not more than 0.15%
C. Not more than 1.5%
D. Not more than 2.5%

98. The deposited layer of solid on the filter medium is called __________ .

A. Filter cake B. Filter medium
C. Filtrate D. Slurry

99. Which of the following filters are used for sterile filtration?

A. Cotton wool and filter paper
B. Cotton wool and glass wool
C. Membrane filter and sintered glass filter
D. Muslin cloth and asbestos

100. __________ are the examples of filter aids.

A. Diatomic and Kieselguhr
B. Asbestos and cotton wool
C. Glass wool and cotton wool
D. Muslin cloth and asbestos

Answer Key

1 B	2 C	3 D	4 B	5 D	6 A	7 A	8 A	9 D	10 C
11 C	12 A	13 C	14 C	15 D	16 C	17 C	18 C	19 D	20 D
21 A	22 D	23 D	24 B	25 B	26 C	27 D	28 A	29 B	30 A
31 D	32 A	33 B	34 A	35 A	36 D	37 A	38 A	39 C	40 A
41 C	42 A	43 A	44 A	45 A	46 B	47 D	48 A	49 C	50 B
51 B	52 C	53 B	54 A	55 A	56 B	57 D	58 B	59 D	60 D
61 C	62 A	63 B	64 C	65 D	66 A	67 D	68 A	69 D	70 C
71 D	72 A	73 C	74 B	75 C	76 C	77 C	78 C	79 C	80 D
81 A	82 C	83 D	84 B	85 B	86 D	87 C	88 C	89 A	90 C
91 B	92 C	93 D	94 B	95 B	96 A	97 B	98 A	99 C	100 A

CHAPTER 5.

Tablets and Capsules

1. **The disintegration time limit for film coated tablet is __________.**
   - **A.** 15 minutes
   - **B.** 30 minutes
   - **C.** 45 minutes
   - **D.** 60 minutes

2. **Which of the following is used as glidant in tablet formulation?**
   - **A.** Cellulose acetate phthalate
   - **B.** Talc
   - **C.** Polyvinyl chloride
   - **D.** Carbowax

3. **Which type of coating is done to disintegrate the tablet in intestine?**
   - **A.** Sugar coating
   - **B.** Film coating
   - **C.** Enteric coating
   - **D.** None of the above

4. **Which of the following is a method of preparation of granules?**
   - **A.** Slugging
   - **B.** Dry granulation
   - **C.** Wet granulation
   - **D.** All of the above

5. **The partial or complete removal of top or bottom portion of tablet is known as ___________.**
   - **A.** Picking
   - **B.** Capping
   - **C.** Sticking
   - **D.** Mottling

6. **Shellac is the material used in ___________ of tablets**
   - **A.** Film coating
   - **B.** Enteric coating
   - **C.** Sugar coating
   - **D.** Control release shooting

7. **Disintegration time for enteric coated tablet as per IP is __________.**
   - **A.** 1 hour
   - **B.** 2 hours
   - **C.** 5 hours
   - **D.** 3 hours

8. **The strength of the tablet is measured by ___________.**
   - **A.** Thickness
   - **B.** Weight variation
   - **C.** Friability
   - **D.** None of the above

9. **How many tablets are required for content uniformity test?**
   - **A.** 10
   - **B.** 20
   - **C.** 30
   - **D.** 40

10. **The temperature of dissolution media is maintained at by the constant temperature is __________.**
    - **A.** 37 ± 0.5°C
    - **B.** 37 ± 1.0°C
    - **C.** 37 ± 1.5°C
    - **D.** 37 ± 2°C

11. **Weight variation for tablet weight ranging from 80–250 mg is __________.**
    - **A.** 10%
    - **B.** 7.5%
    - **C.** 5%
    - **D.** None of the above

12. **Lactose is used as ___________.**
    - **A.** Diluent
    - **B.** Glidant
    - **C.** Lubricant
    - **D.** Disintegrant

13. **To increase bulk of the tablet, which of the following excipients is often added to tablet formulation?**
    - **A.** Glidants
    - **B.** Lubricants
    - **C.** Diluents
    - **D.** Disintegrants

14. Which of the following excipients can be used as a binder in granulation?

A. Magnesium stearate
B. Starch mucilage
C. Kaolin
D. Fuller's earth

15. Unequal distribution of colour in tablet is known as __________.

A. Capping
B. Picking
C. Mottling
D. Lamination

16. __________ is performed to determine the ability of tablet withstand wear and tear during packing, handling and transportation.

A. Disintegration test
B. Friability test
C. Dissolution test
D. All of the above

17. __________ means formation of film surface like orange peel due to rapid drying.

A. Wrinkling
B. Blistering
C. Sweating
D. Orange peel

18. Disintegration time of effervescent tablet is ________.

A. 3 minutes
B. 5 minutes
C. 15 minutes
D. 30 minutes

19. Separation of tablet in two or more distinct layers is called __________.

A. Picking
B. Capping
C. Lamination
D. Broken

20. Appearance of uneven spot on a film surface of the tablet is known as __________.

A. Splitting
B. Pitting
C. Blistering
D. Flaking

21. Disintegration time for hard gelatin capsule is __________.

A. 30 minutes
B. 50 minutes
C. 60 minutes
D. 70 minutes

22. __________ are solid dosage form in which drugs or inert substances are enclosed in small water-soluble shell of gelatin.

A. Tablet
B. Pills
C. Capsule
D. Granules

23. __________ is an ingredient of opaque hard gelatin capsule.

A. Glycerine
B. Titanium dioxide
C. Polyhydric alcohol
D. Sorbitol

24. __________ should be stored at temperature not exceeding 30°C.

A. Tablet
B. Capsule
C. Sustained release tablet
D. Sublingual tablet

25. The disintegration time for soft gelatin capsule is __________.

A. 45 minutes
B. 60 minutes
C. 20 minutes
D. 10 minutes

26. Gelatin is a hydrolysed product of ________.

A. Pectin
B. Tannin
C. Alkaloid
D. Collagen

27. The elasticity of the soft gelatin capsule shell is improved with the addition of __________.

A. Lubricant
B. Increasing water content
C. Plasticizer
D. None of the above

28. Rotary die process is used for __________ filling into capsules.

A. Powders
B. Liquids
C. Pellets
D. Granules

29. The moisture content of a soft gelatin capsule is __________

A. <10%
B. 9–13%
C. >16%
D. 20–26%

30. Capsules normally fall into two main categories as __________.

A. Hard gelatin capsules and soft gelatin capsules
B. Hard gelatin capsules and layered capsules
C. Soft gelatin capsules and compressed capsules
D. Compressed and layered capsules

31. The largest size of capsule is denoted by which number?

A. 000
B. 1
C. 2
D. 5

32. Which of the following steps NOT involved in manufacturing of "hard gelatine capsule shells"?

A. Dipping
B. Spinning
C. Trimming
D. Roughing

33. The plasticiser used in manufacturing of soft gelatin capsule is __________.

A. Sorbitol
B. Povidone
C. Polyethylene glycol
D. Hydroxypropyl methylcellulose

34. Which step is involved in hard gelatin capsule shells production?

A. Dipping
B. Spinning
C. Trimming
D. All of the above

35. The moisture content of a hard gelatin capsule is ___________.

A. <10%
B. 10–13%
C. 12–16%
D. >16%

36. Which capsule size has the smallest capacity?

A. 0
B. 1
C. 3
D. 5

37. Capsules are

A. Unit solid dosage forms
B. Liquid dosage form
C. Gas dosage form
D. All of the above

38. Empty gelatine capsule shell can be made from ___________.

A. Gelatine
B. HPMC
C. Carragenan
D. All of the above

39. Empty capsule has moisture content in the range of ___________.

A. 60%
B. 12–15%
C. 50–70%
D. 30–64%

40. The capsule size number for the capacity of 300 milligram powdered drug is ___________.

A. 00
B. 1
C. 2
D. 3

Answer Key

1 B	2 B	3 C	4 D	5 B	6 B	7 D	8 C	9 A	10 A
11 C	12 A	13 C	14 B	15 C	16 B	17 D	18 B	19 C	20 C
21 A	22 C	23 B	24 B	25 B	26 D	27 C	28 B	29 B	30 A
31 A	32 D	33 A	34 D	35 C	36 D	37 A	38 A	39 B	40 B

CHAPTER 6

Liquid Oral Preparations

Solutions, syrups, Elixirs, Emulsion, Suspensions

1. __________ is a formulation of relatively concentrated layer of emulsion from the original.
A. Cracking
B. Flocculation
C. Creaming
D. Disintegration

2. Which of the following is instability in the emulsion?
A. Phase inversion
B. Cracking
C. Creaming
D. All of the above

3. HLB means __________.
A. Hydrolytic lipolytic balance
B. Hydrophilic lipophilic balance
C. Hydrogen lipid balance
D. High lipid balance

4. HLB plays an important role in __________ of emulsion
A. Dissolution and disintegration
B. Formation and solubility
C. Formulation and stability
D. None of the above

5. __________ in 1949 discovered HLB method.
A. Griffin
B. Darcy
C. Poiseulle
D. Kozeny-Carman

6. A wetting agent is included in the formulation of a suspension, particularly when the suspended particles __________.
A. Are hydrophobic
B. Are denser than the vehicle
C. Are water soluble
D. Have lesser interfacial tension

7. For an ideal suspension, the sedimentation volume should be __________.
A. Equal to one
B. Less than one
C. More than one
D. Zero.

8. The size of dispersed particles in coarse dispersion ranges from __________.
A. 1 μm to 100 μm
B. 1 nm to 100 nm
C. 1 mm to 100 cm
D. Less than 1 μm

9. The primary emulsion formula for fixed oils is ______.
A. 4:2:1
B. 3:2:1
C. 2:2:1
D. 1:2:1

10. In suspensions __________ are added to suspend the insoluble drug in the vehicle.
A. Suspending agents
B. Emulsifying agents
C. Surfactants
D. Electrolytes

11. In suspensions, the stability of suspension depends upon __________.
A. Sedimentation volume
B. Zeta potential
C. Particle size
D. All of the above

12. Simple syrup contains __________ amount of sucrose.
A. 50% w/v
B. 60% w/v
C. 66.7% w/v
D. 85% w/v

13. Elixir contains __________ amount of alcohol.
A. 10–50%
B. 5–15%
C. 4–40%
D. 100%

14. A __________ is a mixture in which one substance of microscopically dispersed insoluble particles is suspended through another substance.
A. Suspension B. Emulsion
C. Colloid D. None of the above

15. The primary emulsion formula for volatile oil is ________.
A. 1:2:1 B. 2:2:1
C. 3:2:1 D. 1:1:2

16. Dry syrups are _________.
A. Suspensions B. Emulsions
C. Solutions D. None of the above

17. Monophasic liquid dosage forms include ________.
A. Aromatic waters B. Tinctures
C. Solutions D. All of the above

18. Simple syrup is a saturated solution of _________.
A. Sucrose B. Fructose
C. Dextrose D. None of the above

19. HLB value of SLS is _________.
A. 10 B. 12
C. 40 D. None of the above

20. The component present in solution in small quantity is known as __________.
A. Solvent B. Solution
C. Solute D. Liquid

21. Which of the following is not monophasic liquid dosage form?
A. Solution B. Gargles
C. Suspension D. Enemas

22. Elixirs are __________.
A. Hydro-alcoholic liquids B. Aqueous
C. Viscous D. Semi-solids

23. Mandl's paint is also known as _________.
A. Compound iodine throat paint
B. Aqueous iodine solution
C. Strong iodine solution
D. Lugol's solution

24. Syrups containing lesser concentration of sucrose require _________.
A. Diluents B. Preservative
C. Binders D. Adjuvants

25. Tween and spans are ________.
A. Diluents B. Wetting agents
C. Flocculating agents D. Colouring agents

26. Which method is used for evaluation or stability of suspension?
A. Sedimentation method B. Electrokinetic method
C. Rheological method D. All of the above

27. Liniments must not be applied on the _________ skin.
A. Swelled B. Broken
C. Painful D. Normal

28. Immiscibility of oil and water can be overcome by ______________.
A. Formulating an emulsion
B. Formulating suspension
C. Formulating an insufflation
D. Formulating an elixir

29. Gargles must be ________ before use.
A. Concentrated B. Warmed
C. Diluted D. Cooled

30. All are the tests used for identification of emulsion *except* _________.
A. Fluorescence test B. Staining test
C. Electric conductivity test D. LAL test

Answer Key

1 C	2 D	3 B	4 C	5 A	6 A	7 A	8 D	9 A	10 A
11 D	12 C	13 C	14 A	15 B	16 A	17 D	18 A	19 C	20 C
21 C	22 A	23 A	24 B	25 C	26 D	27 B	28 A	29 C	30 D

CHAPTER

7

Topical Preparations

Ointments, Creams, Pastes, Topical Gels, Liniments, Lotions, Suppositories, Pessaries, Nasal Preparations, Ear Preparations, Powders, Granules

1. __________ disintegrate or melt at body temperature.
   A. Powders B. Suppository
   C. Tablet D. Capsule

2. Suppositories intended for the vagina are called __________.
   A. Cone B. Suppositories
   C. Bougies D. Pessaries

3. Weight of rectal suppository is generally _____ grams.
   A. 5–6 B. 1–2
   C. 3–4 D. 6–7

4. Suppositories intended for the nose and urethra are called __________.
   A. Bougies B. Pessaries
   C. Suppositories D. None of the above

5. Theobroma oil is also known as __________.
   A. Bees wax B. Lanolin
   C. Coca butter D. Macrogols

6. Witepsol and Massupol are suppository bases belongs to type __________.
   A. Fat bases
   B. Water soluble bases
   C. Emulsifying bases
   D. None of the above

7. __________ of suppository mould is necessary to avoid sticking of suppository to the mould.
   A. Lubrication B. Purification
   C. Calibration D. Washing

8. Weight of pessaries varies from __________ gm.
   A. 1–2 B. 2–3
   C. 4–8 D. 8–10

9. Suppositories are generally evaluated by __________.
   A. Melting range test B. Breaking test
   C. Liquefaction D. All of the above

10. The intracellular absorption of the drugs through skin in which the drugs diffuse through the __________ present in the stratum corneum.
    A. Lipids B. Proteins
    C. Minerals D. None of the above

11. Toothpastes are __________ type of pastes.
    A. Fatty B. Aqueous
    C. Non-aqueous D. Hydrocolloids

12. Agents which prevent products from drying are called __________.
    A. Astringent B. Antiseptic
    C. Humectants D. Antimicrobial

13. Bentonite is an example of __________.
    A. Hydrogel B. Organogel
    C. Xerogel D. Non-aqueous gel

14. Gels are prepared by __________ method.
    A. Fusion B. Dispersion
    C. Cold D. All of the above

15. Liniments are applied with __________.
    A. Without friction B. With friction
    C. Without massage D. None of the above

16. Calamine lotion is used as __________.
    A. Topical protectant B. Abrasive
    C. Antidote D. Antipyretic

17. Macrogols are __________.
    A. Hydroalcohols B. Polyethylene glycols
    C. Ethylene dioxides D. Methylsalicylate

18. The number of parts by weight of medicament that displaces one part by weight of base is __________.

A. Density value B. Saponification value
C. Iodine value D. Displacement value

19. Petrolatum are example of ___________.

A. Water-soluble bases B. Water removable
C. Emulsion bases D. Hydrocarbon bases

20. Sulphur ointment is prepared by ___________.

A. Emulsification method
B. Fusion method
C. Levigation method
D. Chemical reaction method

21. Pastes consists of __________% of solids.

A. 0–10 B. 20–50
C. 100 D. 0

22. Pastes should contain ___________ solids to allow perspiration.

A. Porous B. Larger
C. Smaller D. Fine

23. The length of urethral bougies is ___________.

A. 100–150 mm B. 20–30 mm
C. 10–20 mm D. 10–50 mm

24. Which of the following mechanical equipment can be used for emulsification?

A. Homogenizers B. Mechanical stirrers
C. Ultrasonifiers D. All of the above

25. Which of the following is not used as an emulsifying agent?

A. Surfactant B. Hydrophilic colloids
C. Electrolytes D. Finely divided solids

26. Most widely used hydrocarbon in semisolid dosage forms is ___________

A. Petrolatum B. Mineral oil
C. Both A and B D. None of the above

27. A suppository is generally intended for use in _______.

A. Rectum B. Vagina
C. Urethra D. All of the above

28. Vaginal suppositories also called ___________.

A. Pessaries B. Simple suppositories
C. Bougies D. None of the above

29. Which of the following is not a vegetable oil?

A. Peanut oil B. Almond oil
C. Olive oil D. Petrolatum

30. ___________ are water-soluble ointment basis.

A. Cetrimide B. Macrogols
C. Wool fat D. YSP

31. YSP stands for __________.

A. Yellow soft polymer
B. Yellow soft polycarbon
C. Yellow soft paraffin
D. Yellow soft polyhalide

32. Wool fat is also called __________.

A. Anhydrous lanolin B. Lanolin
C. Petrolatum D. Vaseline

33. Paste usually contains ___________.

A. Beewax B. Glycerin
C. Wool alcohol D. Cetrimide

34. Liniments usually contain counter irritants like ______.

A. Almond oil
B. Beewax
C. Lanolin
D. Methyl salicylate

35. Gum Arabic is a ___________.

A. Anionic polysaccharide
B. Cationic polysaccharide
C. Neutral polysaccharide
D. None of the above

36. Which of the following is not a semisolid dosage form?

A. Paste B. Creams
C. Ointments D. Suspensions

37. Generally, pastes contain ___________.

A. High percentage of insoluble solids
B. Low percentage of insoluble solids
C. Both A and B
D. None of the above

38. Lotion is fluid preparation applied to skin ________.

A. Without friction
B. With friction
C. With massage
D. None of the above

39. _______________ are used for soothing, cooling and softening effect on the skin.

A. Liniment B. Paste
C. Lotion D. Gargles

40. The most common vehicle for nasal preparation is __________.

A. Water B. Glycerine
C. Ethyl alcohol D. Propylene glycol

41. Nasal drops must be ____________ with nasal fluid.
A. Hypertonic B. Hypotonic
C. Isotonic D. Paratonic

42. __________ are also called otic or aural preparations.
A. Nasal drop B. Ear drop
C. Eye drop D. None of the above

43. Nasal drop must not interfere with the __________ action of epithelial cilia of nasal mucosa.
A. Smoothening action
B. Cleansing action
C. Relieving action
D. All of the above

44. Ear drop solution is generally prepared by using __________.
A. Water
B. Glycerine and propylene glycol
C. Dil alcohol
D. All of the above

45. __________ is used for to instilling the nasal drops in nasal cavity.
A. Soft containers
B. Sifters
C. Dropper
D. None of the above

46. Nasal drop should be isotonic with __________.
A. 0.3% Sodium chloride
B. 0.4% Sodium chloride
C. 0.5% Sodium chloride
D. 0.9 % Sodium chloride

47. Ear drops are generally used for __________ .
A. Cleaning
B. Softening the wax
C. Treating the mild infections
D. All of the above

48. Most preferred vehicles for ear drop is __________.
A. Glycerin
B. Propylene glycol
C. Both A and B
D. None of the above

49. The ear drop label should be stated as __________.
A. For external use only
B. For internal use only
C. Dilute before use
D. None of the above

50. __________ is most effective ingredients for relief from itching and hard wax of ear.
A. Sodium bicarbonate B. Glycerine
C. Both A and B D. None of the above

51. One of the common uses of nasal solution is for the relief of __________.
A. Cough B. Congestion
C. Throat infection D. Body pain

52. Ear drops and nasal drops should be __________ .
A. Sterile solutions B. Non-toxic
C. Non-irritant D. All of the above

53. The wrapping of powder in two papers (packing) covering is called __________.
A. Flexible packing
B. Blister packing
C. Double wrapping
D. Strip packing

54. Double wrapping is essential for __________ drugs
A. Hydrophilic
B. Hygroscopic
C. Lipophilic
D. None of the above

55. Which of the following powders are applied on umbilical cord of infants?
A. Dusting powders
B. Surgical dusting powders
C. Cosmetic dusting powders
D. All of the above

56. Effervescent granules usually contain __________.
A. Sodium bicarbonate, citric acid, tartaric acid
B. Sodium sulphate, citric acid, tartaric acid
C. Calcium carbonate, citric acid, tartaric acid
D. Sodium chloride, citric acid, tartaric acid

57. __________ are very fine medicated powders which are inhaled into nostrils for nasal decongestant action
A. Dusting powders
B. Tooth powders
C. Snuffs
D. Medicated dusting powders

58. __________ must be sterile.
A. Face powder
B. Surgical powder
C. Both A and B
D. None of the above

59. __________ is a finely divided powder meant for introduction into the body cavities
A. Inhalation
B. Dusting powders
C. Medical powder
D. Insufflation

60. ________________ powder contains more than one ingredient.
A. Simple powder
B. Compound powders
C. Both A and B
D. None of the above

61. Method of granule formulation is __________.
A. Spatulation
B. Fusion method
C. Wet method
D. Both B and C

62. Dusting powders are dispensed in ______________ containers.
A. Plastic
B. Sifter top container
C. Cardboard box
D. None of the above

63. Medicated dusting powders are mainly used for _________.
A. Superficial skin conditions
B. In body cavities
C. During surgery
D. In major wounds

64. Liquefaction of some solid substances when mixed in a dry form due to adsorption of moisture from environment is due to _________.
A. Immiscibility
B. Insolubility
C. Hygroscopicity
D. None of the above

65. _________ Containers are labelled with direction, immerse in water for a few seconds and then swallow with draught of water.
A. Dusting powder
B. Cachets
C. Insufflations
D. Snuffs

66. Powders consisting of more than one ingredient are called __________ .
A. Compound powders
B. Simple powders
C. Both A and B
D. None of the above

67. __________ is supplied in a sterile form.
A. Tooth powder
B. Surgical powder
C. Both A and B
D. None of the above

68. The method used when potent substances are to be mixed with a large amount of diluents is _________.
A. Solubility
B. Salvation
C. Geometric dilution
D. Complexation

69. Abrasive agents used in dentifrices are _________.
A. Calcium sulphate
B. Magnesium carbonate
C. Sodium carbonate
D. All of the above

70. Advantage of powders is _________.
A. Easy to adjust the dose
B. Rapid onset of action
C. No difficulty in swallowing
D. All of the above

71. ____________ are powders consisting of fine particles which are supplied in cylindrical or flat metal boxes with hinge lid meant for inhaling through the nostrils for decongestion.
A. Snuffs
B. Dentifrices
C. Eutectic powder
D. Explosive powder

72. __________ are intended for cleaning the teeth or other parts of oral cavity using a toothbrush.
A. Snuffs
B. Dentifrices
C. Eutectic powder
D. Explosive powder

73. Powders are meant for cleansing or irrigation of body cavity with a suitable liquid especially for cleansing vaginal cavity are _________.
A. Douches
B. Snuffs
C. Insufflations
D. Eutectic

74. Powder containing mixture of powdered ingredients which produces explosion on trituration is _________.
A. Snuffs
B. Dentifrices
C. Eutectic powder
D. Explosive powder

75. __________ consists of one water molecule which acts as binder in fusion method for making effervescent granules.

A. Citric acid
B. Tartaric acid
C. Benzoic acid
D. All of the above

76. Powders for internal use can be classified as ________.

A. Divided powders
B. Bulk powders
C. Both A and B
D. Dusting powders

77. Cachets contain dry powder enclosed in a shell commonly prepared from a mixture of _________ .

A. Rice flour and water
B. Gram flour and water
C. Polymer
D. All of the above

78. The substance that tends to liquefy on mixing_______.

A. Camphor
B. Thymol
C. Menthol
D. All of the above

79. Powders that absorb moisture from the atmosphere but retain its solid form are termed ___________.

A. Efflorescent powders
B. Deliquescent powders
C. Hygroscopic powders
D. Explosive powders

80. Tablet triturates are also called ___________.

A. Moulded tablets
B. Multilayer tablets
C. Sublingual tablets
D. Chewable tablets

Answer Key

1 B	2 D	3 B	4 A	5 C	6 C	7 A	8 C	9 D	10 A
11 D	12 C	13 A	14 D	15 B	16 A	17 B	18 D	19 C	20 C
21 B	22 A	23 A	24 D	25 C	26 C	27 A	28 A	29 D	30 B
31 C	32 A	33 B	34 D	35 C	36 D	37 A	38 A	39 C	40 A
41 C	42 B	43 B	44 D	45 C	46 D	47 D	48 C	49 A	50 C
51 B	52 D	53 C	54 B	55 B	56 A	57 C	58 B	59 D	60 B
61 D	62 B	63 A	64 C	65 B	66 A	67 B	68 C	69 D	70 D
71 A	72 B	73 A	74 D	75 A	76 C	77 A	78 D	79 C	80 A

CHAPTER 8

Sterile Formulations and Immunological Products

1. **TPN means __________.**
   A. Total pure nutrition
   B. Total polymer nutrition
   C. Total parenteral nutrition
   D. Total paratonic nutrition

2. **SVPs means ___________ .**
   A. Slow volume parenterals
   B. Small value parenterals
   C. Small volume parenterals
   D. Small viscous parentals

3. **The volume of small volume parenteral is less than ___________.**
   A. 100 ml B. 200 ml
   C. 300 ml D. 500 ml

4. **SVPs are manufactured as ____________.**
   A. Multidose containers
   B. Single dose containers
   C. Both A and B
   D. None of the above

5. **_____________ is used to detect presence of particulate matter in parental products**
   A. Pyrogen test B. Leaker test
   C. Sterility test D. Clarity test

6. **Bacterial endotoxin test is also known as __________.**
   A. Clarity test B. LAL test
   C. Leaker test D. Sterility test

7. **Drugs are injected between first and second cervical nerve is called ___________ route.**
   A. Intracisternal B. Intrathecal
   C. Intra-articular D. Peridural

8. **LAL stands for ___________.**
   A. Limulus acyte lysate
   B. Limulus amoebocyte lysate
   C. Left auricular lymphocyte
   D. Lipo acrylic lysate

9. **pH of tear fluid is ____________.**
   A. 2.1 B. 4.5
   C. 9.2 D. 7.4

10. **Which of the following is gelling agent?**
    A. EDTA B. Lanolin
    C. Paraben D. Sodium alginate

11. **Injections are ___________ preparations.**
    A. Conventional B. Non-sterile
    C. Sterile D. Traditional

12. **Drugs are injected into subarachnoid space is called __________ route.**
    A. Intravenous B. Intrathecal
    C. Intra-articular D. Peridural

13. **Viscosity enhancer in ophthalmic preparation is __________.**
    A. Poly vinyl alcohol B. Povidone
    C. Dextran D. Macrogol

14. **Ophthalmic solution is sterilized by ___________ .**
    A. Autoclave B. Hot air oven
    C. Membrane filter D. Bacterial filters

15. **Drugs are injected into bone is called ___________ __________ route.**
    A. Intravenous B. Intrathecal
    C. Intra-articular D. Peridural

16. Which of the following is antibacterial agent?

A. Methylcellulose
B. Paraffins
C. Benzalkonium chloride
D. Tween

17. Which one of the following is used to adjust the isotonicity?

A. Dextrose B. Boric acid
C. NaCl D. All of the above

18. To increase contact time of preparation to eye which of the following additives are added?

A. Carboxy methyl cellulose
B. Polyethylene glycol
C. Methyl cellulose
D. All of the above

19. Polysorbate 80 is used in ophthalmic preparations as a __________.

A. Preservative
B. Antioxidants
C. Wetting agents
D. All of the above

20. Thermolabile drug containing ophthalmic solution is sterilized by __________.

A. Oven B. Autoclave
C. Membrane filtration D. All of the above

21. Which of the following wax is used to prepare eye ointment?

A. Bees wax B. White soft wax
C. Carnauba wax D. None of the above

22. Optimum viscosity of ophthalmic solution ranges between __________

A. 15 and 25 cps B. 10 and 15 cps
C. 25 and 30 cps D. 30 and 40 cps

23. __________% bioavailability is given by IV route.

A. 50 B. 80
C. 100 D. 70

24. LVPs are administered in volume of __________ ml per day by slow IV drip.

A. 1–10 B. 20–50
C. 50–100 D. 250–1000

25. __________ is a non-aqueous oily vehicle used in parenterals.

A. BHT B. BHA
C. WFI D. Arachis oil

26. LVPs mean __________.

A. Less volume parenterals
B. Large volume parenterals
C. Large vacuum parenterals
D. Large volume polymers

27. LVPs are packed in large __________.

A. Multi dose containers
B. Single dose containers
C. Both A and B
D. None of the above

28. __________ is performed to test degree of immunity of an individual against diphtheria.

A. Killer test B. Tuberculin test
C. Schick test D. Bacillus test

29. The smallpox vaccines are stored at temperature between __________.

A. 8° and 10°C B. 2° and 8°C
C. 5° and 7°C D. 10° and 12°C

30. The following are endotoxins *except* __________.

A. Precipitins B. Opsonins
C. Agglutinins D. Virulence

31. The immunity developed after the body has recovered from a disease is called __________.

A. Passive immunity B. Active immunity
C. Both A and B D. None of the above

32. Vaccines are prepared from immune __________.

A. Vitamins B. Blood
C. Serum D. Plasma

33. BCG vaccine is used for __________.

A. Tuberculosis B. Measles
C. Both A and B D. None of the above

34. Which of the following provides the long-term immunity against pathogens?

A. Naturally acquired passive immunity
B. Artificially acquired passive immunity
C. Naturally acquired active immunity
D. All of the above

35. The branch of biology which involves immune systems in all organisms is known as __________.

A. Zoology B. Microbiology
C. Immunology D. Biotechnology

36. The first vaccine was developed by __________.

A. Louis Pasteur B. Edward Jenner
C. Carl Landsteiner D. Joseph Miester

37. **Which of the following immunity is obtained during a lifetime?**
A. Acquired immunity
B. Active immunity
C. Passive immunity
D. None of the above

38. **__________ are the preparations which are meant for the prevention of diseases such as vaccines or for treatment of disease such as antitoxin and antiserum for diagnostic purpose.**
A. Immunity
B. Immunological products
C. Lotions
D. None of the above

39. **A vaccine can be __________.**
A. An antigenic protein
B. Weakened pathogen
C. Live attenuated pathogen
D. All of the above

40. **Which of the following protects our body against disease-causing pathogens?**
A. Digestive system
B. Respiratory system
C. Excretory system
D. Immune system

41. **Hepatitis is an example of __________.**
A. Recombinant vaccine
B. Subunit vaccine
C. Toxoids vaccine
D. Killer vaccine

42. **Which of the following cells of the immune system do not perform phagocytosis?**
A. Eosinophil
B. Basophil
C. Neutrophil
D. Macrophage

43. **Newborns get their antibodies from mother's milk. This is an example of __________.**
A. Naturally acquired active immunity
B. Artificially acquired active immunity
C. Naturally acquired passive immunity
D. Artificially acquired passive immunity

44. **Vaccination is an example of __________.**
A. Naturally acquired active immunity
B. Artificially acquired active immunity
C. Naturally acquired passive immunity
D. Artificially acquired passive immunity

45. **Which of the following immune mechanisms is responsible for protecting us from diseases of other species?**
A. Active immunity
B. Passive immunity
C. Innate immunity
D. Adaptive immunity

46. **BCG is __________.**
A. Bacterial Colony Guerin
B. Bacillus Cox Calmette
C. Bacillus Calmette-Guérin
D. Bacterial Centric Guerin

47. **Whooping cough is caused by __________.**
A. *Mycobacterium tuberculosis*
B. *Vibrio cholerae*
C. *Pseudomonas aeruginosa*
D. *Bordetella pertussis*

48. **Sera contain __________.**
A. Live antigen
B. Attenuated antigen
C. Antibodies
D. None of the above

49. **Typhus vaccine is __________.**
A. Killed Rickettsia
B. Killed bacillus
C. Live Rickettsia
D. Live bacillus

50. **Mantoux test is __________.**
A. Tuberculin test
B. Schick test
C. Keller test
D. Bacillus test

Answer Key

1 C	2 C	3 A	4 A	5 D	6 B	7 A	8 B	9 C	10 D
11 C	12 B	13 D	14 A	15 C	16 C	17 D	18 D	19 C	20 C
21 B	22 A	23 C	24 D	25 D	26 B	27 B	28 C	29 D	30 D
31 B	32 C	33 A	34 C	35 C	36 B	37 A	38 B	39 D	40 D
41 A	42 B	43 C	44 B	45 C	46 C	47 D	48 C	49 A	50 A

CHAPTER 9

Quality Control and Quality Assurance

1. **SOP means __________.**
   A. Sample operating procedures
   B. Standard operating procedures
   C. Some operating procedures
   D. Standard ongoing procedures

2. **cGMP means __________.**
   A. Current Goal Manufacturing Practices
   B. Current Good Manufacturing Practices
   C. Current Good Maintenance Practices
   D. Current Good Managing Practices

3. **__________ explains the GMP and requirement of premises, plants, equipments for pharmaceutical products.**
   A. Schedule N B. Schedule M
   C. Schedule W D. Schedule Y

4. **cGMP regulations are established by __________.**
   A. FDA B. PCI
   C. IDMA D. IPA

5. **__________ is the documented act of proving that any procedure process, equipment, material, activity or system actually leads to the expected results.**
   A. Quality control B. Quality assurance
   C. Validation D. GMP

6. **The soft gelatine capsule involves the process of encapsulation of medicaments with the sizes of __________ ml.**
   A. 0.1–30 B. 40–50
   C. 60–70 D. 80–90

7. **Which of the following is a type of validation?**
   A. Process validation
   B. Cleaning validation
   C. Equipment validation
   D. All of the above

8. **__________ of an instrument of the process of determining its accuracy.**
   A. Validation B. Calibration
   C. Documentation D. Quality control

9. **LAFH is __________.**
   A. Light air and fluid homogenizer
   B. Left air flow heat
   C. Laminar attributes of air humidity
   D. Laminar air flow hood

10. **BMR is __________.**
   A. Batch manufacturing record
   B. Bilayer manufacture register
   C. Batch multilayer record
   D. Bilayer multilayer register

11. **The dispensing area has the pressure of __________.**
   A. 80 Pascal B. 50 Pascal
   C. 20 Pascal D. 10 Pascal

12. **__________ is the document evidence for the equipment tested at the manufacturers place and operated by end-user.**
   A. Site acceptance test (SAT)
   B. Factory acceptance test (FAT)
   C. Both A and B
   D. None of the above

13. **Lower the class number, __________ the cleansing of air.**
   A. Higher B. Lower
   C. Neutralizes D. Stabilizes

14. Quality control is a __________.

A. Destructive tool

B. Managerial tool

C. Corrective tool

D. Constructive tool

15. __________________ is the document evidence for the equipment that it is not damaged during transport and have undergone sufficient testing at end user's facility and operated as per the expectations of end user.

A. Site acceptance test (SAT)

B. Factory acceptance test (FAT)

C. Both A and B

D. None of the above

16. Validation of new product is _________.

A. Prospective validation

B. Retrospective validation

C. Concurrent validation

D. All of the above

17. The measure of capacity to remain unaffected by small variations indicating the reliability during normal use is __________.

A. Accuracy B. Robustness

C. Precision D. Linearity

18. Process validation includes _________.

A. Prospective validation

B. Retrospective validation

C. Concurrent validation

D. All of the above

19. The interval between lower and higher concentration of an analyte is __________.

A. Range B. Linearity

C. Accuracy D. Precision

20. FDA stands for __________

A. Food and Dose Administration

B. Food and Distribution Administration

C. Food and Drug Administration

D. Food and Dental Administration

Answer Key

1 B	2 B	3 B	4 A	5 C	6 A	7 D	8 B	9 D	10 A
11 C	12 B	13 A	14 B	15 A	16 A	17 B	18 D	19 A	20 C

CHAPTER 10

Novel Drug Delivery System

1. **Liposomes consist of bilayer of __________.**
   A. Hydrophilic molecule
   B. Hydrophobic molecule
   C. Both A and B
   D. None of the above

2. **Liposomes have __________ half life.**
   A. Longer
   B. Shorter
   C. Intermediate
   D. Both A and B

3. **________ is a method of preparation of nanoparticle.**
   A. Pan coating
   B. Filtration
   C. Solubilization
   D. Precipitation

4. **Which among the following is limitation associated with conventional drug delivery system?**
   A. Lower effectiveness
   B. Easy of manufacturing
   C. Decrease side effect
   D. Septal and temporal control

5. **Drug release from the feedback regulated drug delivery systems depends upon __________.**
   A. Concentration of biochemical substance
   B. Physicochemical properties of the drug
   C. Thickness of the polymer coating
   D. None of the above.

6. **NDDS improves __________.**
   A. Solubility properties of drug
   B. Pharmacokinetics
   C. Pharmacodynamics
   D. All of the above

7. **Osmotic drug delivery systems have __________.**
   A. A membrane that is soluble at intestinal pH
   B. The membrane is impermeable to GI fluids
   C. The membrane is permeable to water
   D. The membrane must swell

8. **__________ is the disadvantage of the NDDS.**
   A. Higher cost
   B. Dose dumping
   C. Poor *in-vitro–in-vivo* correlation
   D. All of the above

9. **Hydration activated drug delivery systems depends on __________.**
   A. Hydration of polymer
   B. Ionic strength within the reservoir
   C. Osmotic pressure and ionic strength
   D. Osmotic pressure and environment in GIT

10. **Which statement is correct with respect to Novel Drug Delivery Systems?**
    A. It causes fluctuation of blood levels
    B. It cannot be target specific
    C. It increases toxicity of the drug
    D. It reduces side effects of the drug

11. **Drug release from osmotic drug delivery systems depends on __________.**
    A. Ionic strength
    B. Osmotic pressure
    C. Osmotic pressure and ionic strength
    D. Osmotic pressure and environment in GIT

12. **NDDS means __________.**
    A. Non-Drug Delivery System
    B. Novel Drug Discovery System
    C. Novel Drug Delivery System
    D. Novel Dose Delivery System

13. Nanoparticles have a particle size range from ______.

A. 50–100 nm
B. 200–500 nm
C. 300–700 nm
D. 100–200 nm

14. Drug release from the activation modulated drug delivery systems depends upon __________.

A. External/internal stimuli
B. Physicochemical properties of the drug
C. Thickness of the polymer coating
D. None of the above

15. Bio-responsive activated drug delivery systems release rate depends on __________.

A. Hydration of polymer
B. Concentration of biochemical substance
C. Osmotic pressure and ionic strength
D. Osmotic pressure and environment in GIT

16. The size of microsphere ranges from __________ μm

A. 1–1000
B. 1000–1500
C. 1500–2000
D. None of the above

17. CDDM means __________.

A. Controlled Drug Delivery Molecules
B. Control Drug Dissolution Modules
C. Controlled Drug Delivery Modules
D. Constant Drug Delivery Modules

18. Which of the following are 'films and strips' as a Novel Drug Delivery system?

A. Spray bandages
B. Buccal strips
C. Zero order release film
D. All of the above

19. __________ are small sterile hypodermic tablets which are placed under skin by minor surgery.

A. Liposomes
B. Implants
C. Nanoparticles
D. Microspheres

20. Liposomes are spherical structures usually between in a diameter _________ nm

A. 80–100 B. 60–100
C. 55–1000 D. 15–1000

Answer Key

1 C	2 B	3 D	4 A	5 A	6 D	7 C	8 D	9 A	10 D
11 B	12 C	13 B	14 A	15 A	16 A	17 C	18 D	19 B	20 D

Section II

Pharmaceutical Chemistry

1. Introduction to Pharmaceutical Chemistry
2. Volumetric Analysis
3. Inorganic Pharmaceuticals
4. Introduction to Nomenclature of Organic Chemical Systems
5. Drugs Acting on Central Nervous System
6. Drugs Acting on Autonomic Nervous System
7. Drugs Acting on Cardiovascular System
8. Diuretics
9. Hypoglycemic Agents
10. Analgesic and Anti-inflammatory Agents
11. Anti-infective Agents
12. Antibiotics
13. Anti-neoplastic Agents

Syllabus (As Per ER 2020) Pharmaceutical Chemistry

Chapter	Topics
1	**Introduction to Pharmaceutical chemistry:** Scope and objectives **Sources and types of errors:** Accuracy, precision, significant figures **Impurities in Pharmaceuticals:** Source and effect of impurities in Pharmacopoeial substances, importance of limit test, Principle and procedures of Limit tests for chlorides, sulphates, iron, heavy metals and arsenic.
2	**Volumetric analysis:** Fundamentals of volumetric analysis, acid–base titration, non-aqueous titration, precipitation titration, complexometric titration, redox titration. **Gravimetric analysis:** Principle and method.
3	**Inorganic Pharmaceuticals:** Pharmaceutical formulations, market preparations, storage conditions and uses of ■ **Haematinics:** Ferrous sulphate, Ferrous fumarate, Ferric ammonium citrate, Ferrous ascorbate, Carbonyl iron ■ **Gastro-intestinal Agents:** Antacids: Aluminium hydroxide gel, Magnesium hydroxide, Magaldrate, Sodium bicarbonate, Calcium Carbonate, Acidifying agents, Adsorbents, Protectives, Cathartics ■ **Topical agents:** Silver Nitrate, Ionic Silver, Chlorhexidine Gluconate, Hydrogen peroxide, Boric acid, Bleaching powder, Potassium permanganate ■ **Dental products:** Calcium carbonate, Sodium fluoride, Denture cleaners, Denture adhesives, Mouth washes ■ **Medicinal gases:** Carbon dioxide, nitrous oxide, oxygen
4	**Introduction to Nomenclature of Organic Chemical Systems** with particular reference to heterocyclic compounds containing up to three rings
5	**Drugs Acting on Central Nervous System** ■ **Anaesthetics:** Thiopental Sodium*, Ketamine Hydrochloride*, Propofol ■ **Sedatives and Hypnotics:** Diazepam*, Alprazolam*, Nitrazepam, Phenobarbital* ■ **Antipsychotics:** Chlorpromazine Hydrochloride*, Haloperidol*, Risperidone*, Sulpiride*, Olanzapine, Quetiapine, Lurasidone ■ **Anticonvulsants:** Phenytoin*, Carbamazepine*, Clonazepam, Valproic Acid*, Gabapentin*, Topiramate, Vigabatrin, Lamotrigine ■ **Anti-Depressants:** Amitriptyline Hydrochloride*, Imipramine Hydrochloride*, Fluoxetine*, Venlafaxine, Duloxetine, Sertraline, Citalopram, Escitalopram, Fluvoxamine, Paroxetine
6	Drugs Acting on Autonomic Nervous System ■ **Sympathomimetic Agents:** • ***Direct Acting:*** Nor-Epinephrine*, Epinephrine, Phenylephrine, Dopamine*, Terbutaline, Salbutamol (Albuterol), Naphazoline*, Tetrahydrozoline. • ***Indirect Acting Agents:*** Hydroxy Amphetamine, Pseudoephedrine. Agents With Mixed Mechanism: Ephedrine, Metaraminol • ***Adrenergic Antagonists:*** *Alpha Adrenergic Blockers:* Tolazoline, Phentolamine, Phenoxybenzamine, Prazosin. *Beta Adrenergic Blockers:* Propranolol*, Atenolol*, Carvedilol • ***Cholinergic Drugs and Related Agents:*** *Direct Acting Agents:* Acetylcholine*, Carbachol, and Pilocarpine. • ***Cholinesterase Inhibitors:*** Neostigmine*, Edrophonium Chloride, Tacrine Hydrochloride, Pralidoxime Chloride, Echothiopate Iodide • ***Cholinergic Blocking Agents:*** Atropine Sulphate*, Ipratropium Bromide ■ **Synthetic Cholinergic Blocking Agents:** Tropicamide, Cyclopentolate Hydrochloride, Clidinium Bromide, Dicyclomine Hydrochloride*
7	**Drugs Acting on Cardiovascular System** ■ **Anti-arrhythmic Drugs:** Quinidine Sulphate, Procainamide Hydrochloride, Verapamil, Phenytoin Sodium*, Lidocaine Hydrochloride, Lorcainide Hydrochloride, Amiodarone and Sotalol ■ **Anti-hypertensive Agents:** Propranolol*, Captopril*, Ramipril, Methyldopate Hydrochloride, Clonidine Hydrochloride, Hydralazine Hydrochloride, Nifedipine, ■ **Antianginal agents:** Isosorbide Dinitrate

Contd...

8	**Diuretics:** Acetazolamide, Frusemide*, Bumetanide, Chlorthalidone, Benzthiazide, Metolazone, Xipamide, Spironolactone
9	**Hypoglycemic Agents:** Insulin and its Preparations, Metformin*, Glibenclamide*, Glimepiride, Pioglitazone, Repaglinide, Gliflozins, Gliptins
10	**Analgesic and Anti-inflammatory Agents:** Morphine Analogues, Narcotic Antagonists; Nonsteroidal Anti-inflammatory Agents (NSAIDs) - Aspirin*, Diclofenac, Ibuprofen*, Piroxicam, Celecoxib, Mefenamic Acid, Paracetamol*, Aceclofenac
11	**Anti-Infective agents** ■ **Antifungal agents:** Amphotericin-B, Griseofulvin, Miconazole, Ketoconazole*, Itraconazole, Fluconazole*, Naftifine Hydrochloride ■ **Urinary Tract Anti-infective agents:** Norfloxacin, Ciprofloxacin, Ofloxacin*, Moxifloxacin ■ **Anti-Tubercular agents:** INH*, Ethambutol, Para Amino Salicylic Acid, Pyrazinamide, Rifampicin, Bedaquiline, Delamanid, Pretomanid* ■ **Antiviral agents:** Amantadine Hydrochloride, Idoxuridine, Acyclovir*, Foscarnet, Zidovudine, Ribavirin, Remdesivir, Favipiravir ■ **Antimalarials:** Quinine Sulphate, Chloroquine Phosphate*, Primaquine Phosphate, Mefloquine*, Cycloguanil, Pyrimethamine, Artemisinin ■ **Sulfonamides:** Sulfanilamide, Sulfadiazine, Sulfamethoxazole, Sulfacetamide*, Mafenide Acetate, Cotrimoxazole, Dapsone*
12	**Antibiotics:** Penicillin G, Amoxicillin*, Cloxacillin, Streptomycin, Tetracyclines: Doxycycline, Minocycline, **Macrolides:** Erythromycin, Azithromycin, Miscellaneous: Chloramphenicol* Clindamycin
13	**Anti-neoplastic agents:** Cyclophosphamide*, Busulfan, Mercaptopurine, Fluorouracil*, Methotrexate, Dactinomycin, Doxorubicin Hydrochloride, Vinblastine Sulphate, Cisplatin*, Dromostanolone Propionate

CHAPTER 1

Introduction to Pharmaceutical Chemistry

1. **Limit tests are ___________ tests used to identify and control small quantities of impurities present in the substances.**
   A. Quantitative B. Qualitative
   C. Assay D. None of the above

2. **Impurities in pharmaceutical preparation may be due to the following sources __________.**
   A. Raw material
   B. Manufacturing process
   C. Chemical instability
   D. All of the above

3. **Limit tests are performed in __________.**
   A. Measuring cylinder
   B. Kipp's apparatus
   C. Iodine flask
   D. Nessler's cylinder

4. **In limit test for iron IP, iron impurity react with ________.**
   A. Hydrofluoric acid B. Acetic acid
   C. Thioglycolic acid D. Nitric acid

5. **Barium sulphate reagent (BSR) is used in _________.**
   A. Limit test for arsenic
   B. Limit test for chloride
   C. Limit test for iron
   D. Limit test for sulphate IP

6. **Limit test for arsenic is based on which test?**
   A. Gutzeit test B. Fehling's test
   C. Benedict's test D. None of the above

7. **In the limit test of sulphate alcohol not allowed due to ___________.**
   A. Saturation
   B. Supersaturation
   C. Less saturation
   D. Precipitation

8. **Limit test for iron purple colour is due to formation of ___________.**
   A. Ferrous sulphate
   B. Ferrous mercaptoacetate
   C. Citric acid
   D. None of the above

9. **Limit test of iron is based upon the reaction of Fe with __________ solution buffered with ammonium citrate.**
   A. Thioglycollic acid
   B. Acetic acid
   C. Sodium hydroxide
   D. Thioglyconate

10. **Limit test for lead is based upon reaction between ___________ and ___________ to form complex.**
    A. Pb, dithizone
    B. Pb, ammonia
    C. Both A and B
    D. None of the above

11. **In limit test for iron, ferrous thioglycolate has stable pink to reddish purple colour in which medium?**
    A. Acidic
    B. Alkaline
    C. Neutral
    D. None of the above

12. **In limit test for arsenic _________ is evolved.**
    A. Arsine gas
    B. Arsenide
    C. Both A and B
    D. None of the above

13. Gutzeit apparatus is used for the ________.

A. Limit test of arsenic
B. Limit test of sulphate
C. Limit test of lead
D. Limit test for heavy metals

14. Cool storage condition means temperature range ________.

A. Between 2°C and 8°C
B. Between 8°C and 25°C
C. Between 30°C and 40°C
D. Any temperature above 40°C

15. The difference between measured value and true value is called ________.

A. Precision
B. Error
C. Accuracy
D. Deviation

16. The residue left after complete agitation of the drug is called ________.

A. Anions
B. Precipitate
C. Ash
D. Turbidity

17. LOD means ________.

A. Loss of drug
B. Loss on drying
C. Length of drug
D. Loss on degradation

18. LOI means ________.

A. Loss of intensity
B. Loss of indicator
C. Loss on ignition
D. None of the above

19. Determinant errors are ________.

A. Random errors
B. Systematic errors
C. Significant errors
D. Absolute errors

20. The concentration of standard iron solution in the limit test for iron is ________.

A. 10 ppm
B. 15 ppm
C. 20 ppm
D. 25 ppm

21. Arsine gas is carried and comes in contact with ________ produces a yellow or brown stain.

A. Mercuric chloride paper
B. Zinc
C. Both A and B
D. None of the above

22. The sources of impurities in pharmaceuticals arises due to ________.

A. Raw materials
B. Chemical or physical instability during the storage
C. Degradation due to temperature
D. All of the above

23. Dil. HNO_3 and silver nitrate is used as reagents in ________.

A. Limit test of chloride
B. Limit test of sulphate
C. Limit test of lead
D. Limit test for heavy metals

24. Barium chloride in presence of dil. HCl is used as reagent in ________.

A. Limit test of chloride
B. Limit test of sulphate
C. Limit test of lead
D. Limit test for heavy metals

25. Identify the correct use of lead acetate cotton plug in limit test of arsenic.

A. To trap the lead impurity
B. To trap the moisture
C. To trap the sulphides
D. To trap the acetate impurity

26. In which of the following limit tests hydrogen sulphide solution is required?

A. Limit test for chloride
B. Limit test for arsenic
C. Limit test for heavy metals
D. Limit test for lead

27. 0.1N H_2SO_4 solution is prepared by dissolving 4.904 gm in ________.

A. 1000 ml of water
B. 10 L of water
C. 1000 L of water
D. None of the above

28. Silver nitrate is used in the limit test of ________.

A. Arsenic
B. Iron
C. Sulphate
D. Chloride

29. Temporary hardness of water is removed by ________.

A. Boiling
B. Lime process
C. Deionized water
D. All of the above

30. Permanent hard water is softened by ________.

A. Addition of soluble carbonate
B. Polyphosphate chelation
C. Zeolite
D. All of the above

31. In the limit test of chloride, standard solution is a ________.

A. 0.0824% w/v sodium chloride solution
B. 5.85% w/v sodium chloride solution
C. 1% w/v sodium chloride solution
D. None of the above

32. The parameter used in limit test is __________.

A. Opalescence
B. Turbidity
C. Colour intensity
D. All of the above

33. Limit test is a quantitative test designed to identify __________.

A. Purity B. Impurity
C. Acidity D. Basicity

34. Buffer system resist changes in __________ of solution.

A. Oxidation **B.** Reduction
C. pH **D.** None of the above

35. The assay of compound is done to identify __________.

A. Impurity **B.** Purity
C. Both **D.** None of the above

36. Silver nitrate reagent is used to identify __________ impurity.

A. Sulphate **B.** Chloride
C. Iron **D.** Lead

37. Barium sulphate reagent does not contain __________.

A. Alcohol
B. Sodium sulphate
C. Barium chloride
D. Potassium sulphate

38. Limit test of heavy metal is based on reaction with __________.

A. Na_2S **B.** H_2S
C. Both A and B **D.** None of the above

39. The limit test for arsenic is based on __________ test.

A. Turbidity
B. Stain
C. Colour solution
D. None of the above

40. Assay of sodium chloride is based on __________ titration

A. acid–base **B.** Redox
C. Precipitation **D.** Complexometric

Answer Key

1 A	2 D	3 D	4 C	5 D	6 A	7 B	8 B	9 A	10 B
11 B	12 A	13 A	14 B	15 B	16 C	17 B	18 C	19 B	20 C
21 A	22 D	23 A	24 B	25 C	26 C	27 A	28 D	29 D	30 D
31 A	32 D	33 B	34 C	35 B	36 B	37 B	38 C	39 B	40 C

CHAPTER

2

Volumetric Analysis

1. __________ it is a volumetric analysis which involves titration with standardized solution of iodine (free iodine solution).

A. Iodometry
B. Iodimetry
C. Gravimetry
D. Precipitation titration

2. A solution of known concentration is the definition of a __________.

A. Standard solution
B. Substandard solution
C. Weak solution
D. Strong solution

3. Which of the following is the strongest Bronsted-Lowry base?

A. NH_3
B. CO_3^{2+}
C. HSO^{3+}
D. $H_2BO_3^+$

4. An Arrhenius acid is defined as a chemical species that __________.

A. Produces hydrogen ions in solution
B. Reduces hydrogen ions
C. Produces CO_2 ions
D. None of the above

5. Which of the following indicators is yellow at a pH of 10.0?

A. Methyl red
B. Phenol red
C. Thymol blue
D. Methyl violet

6. AgCl has to be filtered of before titration using __________.

A. Modified Volhard's method
B. Mohr's method
C. Fajan's method
D. None of the above

7. Titrations based on the use of silver nitrate are called __________ titration.

A. Argentometric
B. Complexometric
C. Amperometric
D. Conductometric

8. Which method follows the principle of formation of coloured precipitate at the end point?

A. Fajan's method
B. Volhard's method
C. Modified Volhard's method
D. All of the above

9. In which method, Ferric ammonium sulphate is used as an indicator?

A. Fajan's method
B. Mohr's method
C. Volhard's method
D. None of the above

10. Potassium chromate (K_2CrO_4) is used as an indicator in __________.

A. Mohr's method
B. Volhard's method
C. Fajan's method
D. None of the above

11. Which of the following is an example of adsorption indicators?

A. Eosin
B. Phenolphthalein
C. Methyl red
D. Ninhydrin

12. EDTA has __________ binding sites and therefore it is also called multidentate ligand.

A. Six
B. Five
C. Four
D. Seven

13. The endpoint for an EDTA titration is usually found by using a __________ indicator.

A. Metallochromic
B. Redox
C. Acid–base
D. All of the above

14. Which one is sequestering agent?

A. Salicylaldimine
B. 8-hydroxy quinoline
C. EDTA
D. All of the above

15. Which is used as masking agent for lead in complexometric titration?

A. Sodium sulphide
B. Oxalate
C. Thioacetamide
D. All of the above

16. Dimercaprol is used as complexing agent for complexion of __________.

A. Mercury
B. Arsenic
C. Lead
D. All of the above

17. Indicator used in complexometric titration is _______.

A. Erichrome black T
B. Xylenol orange
C. Mordant black II
D. All of the above

18. Name the assay method for the drug calcium gluconate __________.

A. Non-aqueous titration
B. Acid–base titration
C. Complexometric titration
D. Iodometric titration

19. Oxidation involves __________.

A. Loss of hydrogen
B. Loss of oxygen
C. Gain in hydrogen
D. Gain in electrons

20. Oxidizing agents __________.

A. Are mostly non-metals
B. Are mostly metals
C. Decrease in oxidation state
D. Are mostly transition metals

21. Hydrogen acts as a reducing agent __________.

A. By taking oxygen
B. By giving electrons
C. By taking hydrogen
D. Both A and B

22. Reduction involves __________.

A. Loss of oxygen
B. Gain in hydrogen
C. Gain in oxygen
D. Loss of electrons

23. Which one of the following substances is a good oxidising agent?

A. Hydrogen peroxide
B. Water
C. Sulphur dioxide
D. Coke (carbon)

24. Volumetric analysis is applied to determine the concentration of the __________.

A. Solvent
B. Analyte
C. Titrant
D. None of the above

25. A substance or chemical that changes its colour in acidic and basic medium during titration called __________.

A. Indicator
B. Titrant
C. Equivalency
D. Buffer solution

26. In formula-N1V1 the N1 stands for __________.

A. Volume of acid
B. Normality of acid
C. Normality of base
D. Volume of base

27. Acetic acid (CH_3COOH) and sodium hydroxide (NaOH) is the __________.

A. Strong and strong base
B. Weak acid–weak base
C. Strong acid–weak base
D. Weak acid–strong base

28. Acetic acid and alcohols are the __________.

A. Aprotic solvents
B. Protophilic solvents
C. Amphiprotic solvents
D. Protogenic solvents

29. __________ is the method involving the titration of halides (bromides, iodides, and chlorides), in an acidic medium.

A. Fajan's method
B. Volhard's method
C. Mohr's method
D. None of the above

30. EDTA is used as titrant in __________.

A. Complexometric titration
B. Acid–base titration
C. Non-aqueous titration
D. Gravimetry analysis

31. A reduction–oxidation reaction between an oxidizing agent and a reducing agent occurs in __________.

A. Mohr's method
B. Gravimetry analysis
C. Precipitation titration
D. Redox titration

32. Precipitation, digestion of the precipitate, washing and filtering along with drying and ignition steps involve in __________.

A. Gravimetry analysis
B. Redox titration
C. Precipitation titration
D. Acid–base titration

33. The term "precision" refers to __________.

A. The level of measurement and exactness of description in a database
B. Measurements that are within (1 mm)
C. Logical accuracy
D. Highly accurate data

34. The degree to which information matches true or accepted values are referred to as __________.

A. Precision and accuracy B. Precision
C. Accuracy D. Average correct data

35. Standard deviation of a sampling distribution is __________.

A. Standard error B. Random error
C. Sampling error D. Potential error

36. Personal errors can be corrected by __________.

A. Taking more observations
B. Proper reading the observation
C. Proper recording the reading
D. All of the above

37. A measured variation from the mean in a sample is the __________.

A. Coefficient of variation B. Variable mean
C. Mode D. Standard deviation

38. Which of the following is false in case of determinate errors?

A. Personal but non-operational
B. Reagent and instrumental
C. Methodic and instrumental
D. Nonsystematic

39. Which of the following is not true in relation to rules for significant figures?

A. All non-zero digits are significant
B. Leading zeros are never significant
C. Zeros between non-zero digits are not significant
D. All of the above

40. How can systematic instrumental error be eliminated?

A. Frequent observations and calculations
B. Replacement or repair of instrument
C. Rearrangements in instrument
D. Finding mean of readings

41. Replacement of water with other non-aqueous solvent is known as __________.

A. Acid–base titration
B. Precipitation titration
C. Non-aqueous titration
D. None of the above

42. Which solvent can be used in non-aqueous titration?

A. Acetic acid
B. Sulphuric acid
C. Glacial acetic acid
D. None of the above

43. The basic solvents which are used to enhance the acidity of weak acid are called __________.

A. Proteogenic solvent B. Protophilic solvent
C. Amphoteric solvent D. Aprotic solvent

44. The formation of a solid in solution and solid form is called __________.

A. Solvent B. Solute
C. Precipitation D. Product

45. The end point detection in Volhard method involve __________.

A. Common ion effect B. Demasking
C. Masking D. Fractional ppt

46. Which indicator is used in Mohr's Method?

A. Ferric ammonium sulphate B. Fluorescein
C. Phenolphthalein D. Potassium chromate

47. Adsorption indicators are used in __________.

A. Fajan's method B. Mohr's method
C. Volhard's Method D. All of the above

48. When 1 mole of the substance is dissolved in 1000 ml of solution, it is called __________.

A. Normal solution B. Molar solution
C. Formal solution D. None of the above

49. pH of neutral solution is __________.

A. 10 B. 15
C. 7 D. 1

50. Which is not a strong acid?

A. Acetic acid B. Hydrochloric acid
C. Sulphuric acid D. Nitric acid

51. Which one of the following is not titration?

A. Acid–base B. Oxidation–reduction
C. Gravimetric D. Complexometric

52. pH is defined as __________.

A. + log of $[H^+]$ B. – log of $[H^+]$
C. only log of $[H^+]$ D. None of the above

53. Solvents which can accept as well as donate proton is known as __________.

A. Inert solvent B. Photophilic solvent
C. Amphiprotic D. Proteogenic solvent

54. Which indicator is used in Mohr's method?

A. $KMnO_4$
B. K_2CrO_4
C. $NH_4Fe(SO_4)_2$ (ferric ammonium sulphate)
D. Nitric acid

55. Ferric ammonium sulphate is used as indicator in which method?

A. Volhard method
B. Mohr method
C. Fajan's method
D. None of the above

56. The point at which the reaction is complete is called as __________.

A. Initial point
B. End point
C. Middle point
D. None of the above

57. The substance to be determined is called ________.

A. Titration
B. Indicator
C. Titrate
D. Normality

58. __________ is a substance of known concentration.

A. Indicator
B. Titrate
C. End point
D. Titrant

59. Assay of sodium chloride is based on ____________ titration.

A. Acid–base
B. Redox
C. Precipitation
D. Complexometric

60. Assay of calcium gluconate is __________ type.

A. Complexometric
B. Acidimetry
C. Iodimetry
D. Gravimetric

Answer Key

1 B	2 A	3 B	4 A	5 A	6 A	7 A	8 D	9 B	10 A
11 A	12 C	13 A	14 C	15 C	16 D	17 D	18 C	19 A	20 A
21 D	22 A	23 A	24 B	25 A	26 B	27 D	28 C	29 B	30 A
31 D	32 A	33 A	34 C	35 A	36 D	37 D	38 D	39 C	40 C
41 C	42 C	43 B	44 C	45 D	46 D	47 A	48 B	49 C	50 A
51 C	52 B	53 C	54 B	55 A	56 B	57 C	58 D	59 C	60 A

CHAPTER

3

Inorganic Pharmaceuticals

Haematinics, GIT Agents, Topical Agents, Dental Products, Medicinal Gases

1. **Anaemia means ___________.**
   A. Decrease in percentage of Hb
   B. Increase in percentage of Hb
   C. Decrease in WBC
   D. Increase in WBC

2. **The substance in which increase the amount of haemoglobin in the blood is called ___________ .**
   A. Cardiotonics B. Carminatives
   C. Haematinics D. Haemostatics

3. **Green vitriol is synonym of __________.**
   A. Ferrous sulphate
   B. Magnesium sulphate
   C. Calcium sulphate
   D. Ferric sulphate

4. **The molecular formula of carbonyl iron is _________.**
   A. $C_4H_2FeO_4$ B. $FeSO_4$
   C. $Fe(CO)_5$ D. $FePO_4$

5. **Which one of the following is acidifying agent?**
   A. Magnesium sulphate B. Calcium carbonate
   C. Dil. H_2SO_4 D. Dil. HCl

6. **Magnesium sulphate is used as ___________.**
   A. Antacid B. Protective adsorbent
   C. Saline cathartic D. Astringent

7. **Absence of gastric secretion, the condition is termed __________.**
   A. Insomnia B. Achlorhydria
   C. Constipation D. Purgation

8. **China clay is a synonym of __________.**
   A. Milk of Bismuth B. Kaolin
   C. Talc D. Activated charcoal

9. **'Soap stone and fresh chalk' are synonyms of ______.**
   A. Talc B. Kaolin
   C. Bismuth subgallate D. Zinc oxide

10. **'Muriatic acid and spirit of salt' are the synonyms of ___________.**
    A. Copper sulphate B. Magnesium sulphate
    C. Dil. HCl D. Zinc oxide

11. **Which of the following one is water soluble antacid?**
    A. Calcium carbonate
    B. Magnesium hydroxide
    C. Magnesium trisilicate
    D. Sodium bicarbonate

12. **___________ it called prepared chalk.**
    A. Magnesium carbonate B. Calcium carbonate
    C. Calcium gluconate D. Aluminium hydroxide

13. **Which one of the following is aluminium containing antacid?**
    A. Magnesium oxide B. Calcium carbonate
    C. Magnesium hydroxide D. Magaldrate

14. **Liquid paraffin is an example of**
    A. Saline purgative B. Emollient purgative
    C. Stimulant purgative D. Bulk purgative

15. **Synonym of magnesium sulphate is ___________ .**
    A. Spirit of salt B. French chalk
    C. Epsom salt D. Rochelle's salt

16. **Rochelle's salt is a synonym of a ___________.**
    A. Antimony potassium tartarate
    B. Calcium carbonate
    C. Magnesium sulphate
    D. Sodium potassium tartarate

17. **Titanium dioxide is a __________.**
A. Topical protective B. Anti-microbial agent
C. Purgative D. Astringent

18. **Bacteriostatic means __________.**
A. Inhibit the growth of bacteria
B. Kills the bacteria
C. Increase growth of bacteria
D. None of these

19. **Mild silver protein is an example of __________.**
A. Antacid B. Anti-microbial
C. Acidifier D. Astringent

20. **Which one of the following is not a mechanism of action of antimicrobials?**
A. Dissolution B. Halogenation
C. Oxidation D. Precipitation

21. **__________ is called "oxygenated water".**
A. Hydrogen peroxide
B. Bleaching powder
C. Boric acid
D. Potassium permanganate

22. **Synonym of bleaching powder is __________.**
A. Baking soda B. Mitha soda
C. Chlorinated lime D. Caustic soda

23. **Stannous fluoride and calcium carbonate are used as __________.**
A. Sweetening agent B. Polishing agent
C. Cleaning agent D. Flavouring agent

24. **Example of desensitizing agent is __________.**
A. Strontium Chloride B. Calcium phosphate
C. Calcium carbonate D. Sodium phosphate

25. **Deposition of fluorine produces mottled enamel which is known as __________.**
A. Dental fluorosis B. Tooth decay
C. Pigmentation of teeth D. Yellowing of teeth

26. **__________ is a removable replacement for missing teeth and surrounding tissue.**
A. Toothpaste B. Suture
C. Culture D. Denture

27. **Which one of the following is not a type of denture adhesive?**
A. Denture adhesive cream
B. Denture adhesive powder
C. Denture cleaner
D. Denture adhesive strips

28. **Oxygen cylinder are painted by __________.**
A. Black and white B. Green and white
C. Blue colour D. Red colour

29. **Which of the following is known as 'laughing gas' or 'Happy gas'?**
A. Oxygen B. Carbon dioxide
C. Nitrous oxide D. Sulphur dioxide

30. **The gas which is used in preparation of soft drinks and dry ice is __________**
A. CO_2 B. N_2O
C. O_2 D. S_2O

31. **Causes of anaemia are __________.**
A. Decreased RBC production
B. Increased RBC destruction
C. Stem cell proliferation disturbance
D. All of the above

32. **Hydrogen peroxide is used as __________.**
A. Antiseptic B. Acidifying agent
C. Antioxidant D. Protective

33. **Requirement of folic acid in pregnant woman is ________.**
A. 0.5 mg/day B. 1 mg/day
C. 0.1 mg/day D. 0.3 mg/day

34. **$KMnO_4$ solutions are used as __________.**
A. Astringent B. Antifungal
C. Both A and B D. None of the above

35. **Formula for ferrous sulphate is __________.**
A. $FeSO_4$ B. $CusO_4$
C. $SeSO_4$ D. $MgSO_4$

36. **Adult dose for ferrous fumarate is __________.**
A. 360 mg/day B. 100 mg/day
C. 50 mg/day D. 500 mg/day

37. **Which of the following are haematinics?**
A. Ferrous sulphate B. Ferrous gluconate
C. Both A and B D. None of the above

38. **Which of the following are antacids?**
A. Aluminium hydroxide gel
B. Magnesium hydroxide
C. Magaldrate
D. All of the above

39. **Which of the following are brand names of aluminium hydroxide?**
A. Acidel B. Abicid
C. Both A and B D. None of the above

40. **Chemically, boric acid is ________.**
A. H_3PO_4 B. H_3BO_3
C. H_2SO_4 D. None of the above

41. **Which of the following are anti-microbial agents?**
A. Silver Nitrate
B. Hydrogen peroxide
C. Potassium permanganate
D. All of the above

42. **Sodium fluoride is used in the treatment of ________.**
A. Cavities B. Dental caries
C. Both A and B D. None of the above

43. **Which of the following are dental products?**
A. Calcium carbonate B. Sodium fluoride
C. Denture cleaners D. All of the above

44. **Which of the following are medicinal gases?**
A. Carbon dioxide B. Nitrous oxide
C. Oxygen D. All of the above

45. **Chemical formula of bleaching powder is ________.**
A. $Ca(ClO)_2$ B. $Ca(ClO)_4$
C. $CaCO_2$ D. H_2SO_4

46. **Which of the following dental products are used as mouthwash?**
A. Chlorhexidine
B. Potassium permanganate
C. Both A and B
D. None of the above

47. **The increased level of carbon dioxide in blood leads to ________.**
A. Acidosis B. Alkalosis
C. Both A and B D. None of the above

48. **What is pH range of gastric juices?**
A. 4.5–7 B. 1.5–3.5
C. 7.3–8 D. 6–8

49. **If blood pH is higher than 7.3, it is termed ________.**
A. Alkalosis
B. Acidosis
C. Both A and B
D. None of the above

50. **Which property of antacids is responsible for systemic alkalosis?**
A. Due to formation of non-absorbable ions
B. Due to formation of absorbable ions
C. Both A and B
D. None of the above

51. **Which antacid is water soluble in nature?**
A. $Al(OH)_3$ B. $Mg(OH)_2$
C. $NaHCO_3$ D. $Ca(OH)_2$

52. **Which gas is liberated by neutralization of the antacids?**
A. N_2 B. O_2
C. CO_2 D. NH_3

53. **In which term the neutralization capacity of an antacid is expressed?**
A. Meq B. MEq
C. mEq D. None of the above

54. **Which acid is used to protect against irritating effect of HCl?**
A. Alginic acid B. Citric acid
C. Glutamic acid D. Lactic acid

55. **Which surface active agent is used to dispense foam?**
A. Simethicone B. Amethicone
C. Both A and B D. None of the above

56. **Which compound is produced if $Al(OH)_3$ gel reacts with gastric HCl?**
A. Al_3O_3 B. $AlCl_3$
C. Al_3Cl_3 D. Al_3Cl

57. **Which of the following antacid absorbs CO_2 from atmosphere?**
A. Aluminium hydroxide B. Sodium bicarbonate
C. Magnesium hydroxide D. Bismuth subnitrate

58. **Which water is used for washing the precipitate of $Al(OH)_3$?**
A. Boiling Water B. Hot Water
C. Both A and B D. Cold Water

59. **Why the calcium and magnesium combination is preferred for antacid preparation not a single one?**
A. To overcome laxative effect
B. To overcome constipative effect
C. Both A and B
D. None of the above

60. **The example of systemic antacids is ________.**
A. Calcium carbonate B. Sodium bicarbonate
C. Magnesium hydroxide D. Aluminium salts

61. **Acidifiers are the drugs which ________**
A. Decrease the acidity
B. Increase the acidity
C. First increase then decrease
D. No effect on acidity

62. **Systemic antacids are __________.**
A. Readily absorbable B. Soluble in water
C. Both A and B D. None of the above

63. **Antacids are the __________.**
A. Acidic substance B. Neutral substance
C. Alkaline substance D. Slightly acidic

64. **Which of the following are antacids?**
A. Aluminium hydroxide gel
B. Magnesium hydroxide
C. Magaldrate
D. All of the above

65. **Which of the following are anti-microbial agents?**
A. Silver nitrate B. Hydrogen peroxide
C. Potassium permanganate D. All of the above

66. **Gastric acidifier is the drug which is used to ________ the acidity.**
A. Increase B. Decrease
C. Neutralise D. None of the above

67. **HCl is also known as __________.**
A. Epsom salt B. Spirit of salt
C. White vitriol D. None of the above

68. **The neutralizing capacity of an antacid is expressed in _________.**
A. Milliequivalence of HCl B. ppm
C. Milliliter D. Mg

69. **Sodium bicarbonate is also known as __________.**
A. Baking soda
B. Meetha soda
C. Sodium hydrogen carbonate
D. All of the above

70. **Which GIT agent is used in treatment of diarrhoea?**
A. Protective and adsorbent
B. Saline cathartics
C. Antacid
D. None of the above

71. **Nitrous oxide is __________.**
A. Analgesic B. Anaesthetic
C. Both A and B D. None of the above

72. **Which one of the gas is not used as inhalants?**
A. Argon B. Carbon dioxide
C. Helium D. Nitrous oxide

73. **Inhalants are dependent upon the __________.**
A. Nature of the gas B. Concentration
C. Both A and B D. None of the above

74. **The laughing gas is a synonym of __________.**
A. Nitrous oxide B. Nitric oxide
C. Nitrogen D. None of the above

75. **Which inhalant is most widely used in "fire extinguishers"?**
A. Oxygen B. Nitrous oxide
C. Argon D. Carbon dioxide

76. **At a higher temperature (500°C) nitrous oxide gets decomposed into __________.**
A. H_2N_2O and H_2O B. N_2O and H_2O
C. N_2 and O_2 D. H_2O and O_2

77. **The colour of CO_2 gas cylinder is __________.**
A. Red B. Brown
C. Blue D. Green

78. **Which inorganic gas is used as anaesthetic?**
A. Nitrous oxide
B. Helium
C. Carbon dioxide
D. A mixture of carbon dioxide and nitrous oxide

79. **Carbon dioxide has ________ odour and ________ taste.**
A. Faint, sweet B. Pungent, salty
C. Bitter almond, acrid D. Faint, sour

80. **Fluoride inhibits carries formation via __________.**
A. Downward acid solubility of enamel
B. Bacterial inhibition
C. Both A and B
D. None of the above

81. **Dental caries is a medical term of __________.**
A. Cleaning action
B. Polishing action
C. Tooth decay or cavities
D. None of the above

82. **Fluoride can be administered either __________.**
A. Orally B. Topically
C. Both A and B D. None of the above

83. **Sodium metaphosphate is also known as __________.**
A. Precipitated chalk B. Maddrell's salt
C. Both A and B D. None of the above

84. **Desensitizers tend to __________.**
A. Downward the hypersensitivity of the teeth
B. Hypersensitivity of the teeth
C. Bacterial inhibition
D. None of the above

85. Following one is example of desensitizing agent ________.
A. Zinc chloride
B. Sodium fluoride
C. Stannous fluoride
D. Calcium carbonate

86. Which vitamin is necessary for tooth formation?
A. Vitamin A
B. Vitamin C
C. Vitamin D
D. All of the above

87. Calcium phosphate is used as ________.
A. Cleansing agent
B. Polishing agent
C. Removing stains
D. None of the above

88. How do astringents act?
A. Lipid precipitant
B. Bacterial inhibition
C. Protein precipitant
D. Enzymatic catalysis

89. Antacids are ________ in nature.
A. Acidic
B. Alkaline
C. Buffer
D. None of the above

90. The agents which inhibit the growth of microorganisms are called ________ agents.
A. Dentifrice
B. Anti-inflammatory
C. Anti-microbial
D. Anticaries

91. Antimicrobial agents act by ________ mechanism.
A. Oxidation
B. Halogenation
C. Protein precipitation
D. All of the above

92. Disinfectants inhibit microbial growth on ________.
A. Living cells
B. Objects
C. Both A and B
D. None of the above

93. Agents that have cleaning action on teeth are ________.
A. Dentifrice
B. Anti-inflammatory
C. Anti-microbial
D. Anticaries

94. The compound that prevents dental caries is ________.
A. NaF
B. $CaCO_3$
C. $SnCl_2$
D. $ZnCl_2$

95. The compound that neutralises gastric hydrochloric acid is called ________.
A. Emetics
B. Expectorants
C. Astringents
D. Antacids

96. The compounds that are used in treatment of iron deficiency are called ________.
A. Emetics
B. Expectorants
C. Haematinics
D. Antacids

97. Antacids act by ________ the gastric pH.
A. Increasing
B. Decreasing
C. Both A and B
D. None of the above

98. The agents that prevent tooth decay are called ________.
A. Dentifrice
B. Anticaries
C. Anti-microbial
D. Mouthwash

99. Absence of oxygen in the tissues is called ________.
A. Hypoxia
B. Asphyxia
C. Anoxia
D. None of the above

100. Which of the following is used to remove stain from the teeth?
A. Abrasives
B. Polishing agents
C. Desensitizing agents
D. Flavouring agents

Answer Key

1 A	2 C	3 A	4 C	5 D	6 C	7 B	8 B	9 A	10 C
11 D	12 B	13 D	14 B	15 C	16 D	17 A	18 A	19 B	20 A
21 A	22 C	23 B	24 A	25 A	26 D	27 C	28 A	29 C	30 A
31 D	32 A	33 A	34 B	35 A	36 A	37 C	38 D	39 C	40 B
41 D	42 C	43 D	44 D	45 A	46 A	47 A	48 B	49 A	50 B
51 B	52 C	53 C	54 A	55 A	56 B	57 C	58 B	59 C	60 B
61 B	62 C	63 C	64 D	65 D	66 A	67 B	68 A	69 D	70 A
71 C	72 A	73 C	74 A	75 D	76 C	77 D	78 A	79 D	80 C
81 C	82 C	83 B	84 A	85 A	86 C	87 A	88 C	89 B	90 C
91 D	92 B	93 A	94 A	95 D	96 C	97 A	98 B	99 C	100 A

CHAPTER 4

Introduction to Nomenclature of Organic Chemical Systems

1. **__________ is a 3 membered heterocyclic ring.**
   A. Azepine B. Benzazepine
   C. Dibenzoazepine D. Aziridine

2. **5 membered unsaturated heterocyclic rings with oxygen as a heteroatom is __________.**
   A. Furan B. Thiophene
   C. Oxazole D. Isothiazole

3. **_______ contains four nitrogen atoms.**
   A. Pyrazole B. Imidazole
   C. Thiazole D. Tetrazole

4. **Metronidazole contains heterocyclic ring ________.**
   A. Pyrazole B. Pyrrole
   C. Imidazole D. Imidazolidine

5. **Imidazolidine 2,4 dione means ________.**
   A. Hydantoin B. Indole
   C. Pyrazolidine D. Leptazole

6. **Saturated 5 membered heterocyclic ring with nitrogen as a heteroatom is _________.**
   A. Pyrrole B. Pyrrolidine
   C. Imidazole D. Imidazolidine

7. **Caffeine contains heterocyclic ring __________.**
   A. Acridine B. Phenothiazine
   C. Xanthine D. Imidazolidine

8. **Which of the following is piperidine ring?**
   A. 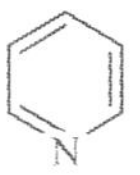 N
   B. 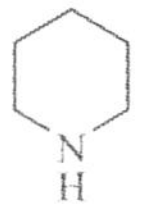 N H
   C. 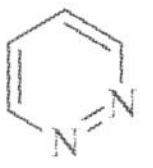 N=N
   D. 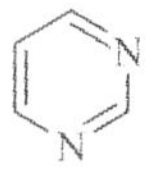 N N

9. **Which of the following is pyrazole heterocycle?**
   A. 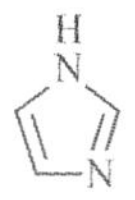 H N N
   B. 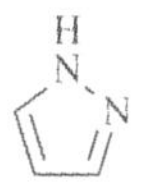 H N N
   C. 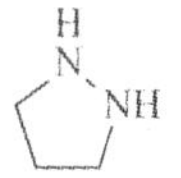 H N NH
   D. 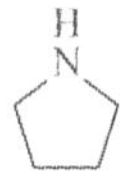 H N

10. **Two benzene rings attached to azepine nucleus is______.**
    A. 1,4-Diazepine
    B. 1,4-Benzodiazepine
    C. Dibenzoazepine
    D. Azepine

1 . **Structure of ethyl amino group is __________.**
    A. $-NH-C_2H_5$ B. $-NH-CH_3$
    C. $-NH-(C_2H_5)_2$ D. $-NH-C_3H_8$

12. **Acetamido group is __________.**
    A. $CH_3COONH-$ B. CH_3CONH-
    C. CH_3CO-CH_2-NH- D. CH_3NH-

13. **–CN means __________.**
    A. Carbonyl group
    B. Cyano/Nitrile group
    C. Carbamoyl group
    D. Nitrogen group

14. **Following one is halogen group __________.**
    A. Vinyl B. Thio
    C. Fluoro D. Nitro

15. **Structure of mercapto group is ___________.**
    A. –CHO B. –SH
    C. $-NH_2$ D. $-CONH_2$

16. Name of $-CH_2-CH=CH_2$ group is __________.

A. Allyl
B. Vinyl
C. Vinyloxy
D. Allyloxy

17. Structure of anilino group is __________.

A. $-O-C_6H_5$
B. $-NH-C_6H_5$
C. $-C_6H_5$
D. $-CH_2-C_6H_5$

18. Which of the following is not an example of hetero-atom?

A. Carbon
B. Oxygen
C. Nitrogen
D. Sulphur

19. Example for five membered heterocyclic compounds with nitrogen heteroatom is __________.

A. Pyrrole
B. Pyridine
C. Aziridine
D. Acridine

20. Which of the following is six membered heterocyclic compounds?

A. Pyridine
B. Benzene
C. Phenol
D. None of the above

21. Which of the following are heteroatoms?

A. O
B. N
C. S
D. All of the above

22. Aza represents the presence of __________.

A. O
B. S
C. N
D. All of the above

23. Which of the following possess polycyclic aromatic ring?

A. Naphthalene
B. Anthracene
C. Phenanthrene
D. All of the above

24. General formula for alkene __________.

A. C_nH_{2n+2}
B. C_nH_{2n}
C. C_nH_{2n-2}
D. All of the above

25. Bicyclic heterocyclic compounds are __________.

A. Quinoline
B. Isoquinoline
C. Indole
D. All of the above

26. Halogen compounds possess __________.

A. F
B. Cl
C. Br
D. All of the above

27. Five membered heterocyclic rings present in which of the following?

A. Furan
B. Thiophene
C. Pyrrole
D. All of the above

28. Which of the following solvents is a heterocyclic compound?

A. Pyridine
B. THF
C. DMF
D. DMSO

29. Which of the following statements is correct?

A. Pyridine is a tertiary amine
B. Pyrrole is a strong base
C. Pyrrole has less aromatic character than furan
D. Pyridine is 6-membered heterocycle

30. Pyridine on reduction gives __________.

A. Piperidine
B. Pyrimidine
C. Pyrrole
D. Pyrazine

31. Heterocyclic compounds are classified based on their __________.

A. Electronic structure
B. Number of rings
C. Resonance
D. Internal energy

32. The unsaturated heterocyclic compounds of 5 and 6 member rings is __________.

A. Quinoline
B. Isoquinoline
C. Indole
D. All of the above

33. "N" as a heteroatom is suffixed by __________.

A. Azo
B. Oxo
C. Nitro
D. All of the above

34. "S" as a heteroatom is suffixed by __________.

A. Thio
B. Sulpho
C. Sulpha
D. Sulfonyl

35. "O" as a heteroatom is suffixed by __________.

A. Oxo
B. Hydro
C. Oxy
D. None of the above

36. __________ are the compounds containing one or more heteroatoms in ring along with carbon atoms forming the ring".

A. Polycyclic compounds
B. Heterocyclic compounds
C. Inorganic compounds
D. Hydrophilic compounds

37. Furan is also named ___________.

A. Oxole

B. Isoxazole

C. Oxirane

D. All of the above

38. The trivial name of ethylene oxide is ___________.

A. Ethylene oxide

B. Oxirane

C. Oxirene

D. Oxo

39. The name of given structure (S) is ___________.

A. Thiolol

B. Thiophene

C. Pyrrole

D. Furan

40. $-O-CH_2-CH_3$ is a structure of ___________ group.

A. Methoxy-

B. Propoxy-

C. Butoxy-

D. Ethoxy-

Answer Key

1 D	2 A	3 D	4 C	5 A	6 B	7 C	8 B	9 B	10 C
11 A	12 B	13 B	14 C	15 B	16 A	17 B	18 A	19 A	20 A
21 D	22 C	23 D	24 B	25 D	26 D	27 D	28 A	29 D	30 A
31 A	32 D	33 A	34 A	35 A	36 B	37 A	38 B	39 B	40 D

CHAPTER

5

Drugs Acting on Central Nervous System

Anaesthetics, Sedatives and Hypnotics, Antipsychotics, Anticonvulsants, Anti-depressants

1. **At which stage of anaesthesia the patient passes through four plans __________.**
   A. Stage of analgesia
   B. Stage of delirium
   C. Stage of surgical anesthesia
   D. Stage of a respiratory paralysis

2. **Following are gaseous anaesthetics __________.**
   A. Propofol and methohexital
   B. Nitrous oxide and cyclopropane
   C. Ketamine and propanidid
   D. Thiopentone and althesin

3. **Insomnia means __________.**
   A. Lack of sleep B. Excessive sleep
   C. Lack of appetite D. None of the above

4. **__________ is a derivative of barbituric acid.**
   A. Alprazolam
   B. Meprobamate
   C. Paraldehyde
   D. Phenobarbitone

5. **5-ethyl, 5-phenyl barbituric acid is a chemical name of __________.**
   A. Butobarbital B. Secobarbitone
   C. Phenobarbitone D. Barbital

6. **Calmpose and Valium are popular brand names of __________.**
   A. Paracetamol B. Diazepam
   C. Alprazolam D. Phenobarbitone

7. **Which of the following is not a psychiatric disorder?**
   A. Schizophrenia B. Depression
   C. Angina pectoris D. Mania

8. **Imipramine and Amitriptyline are __________.**
   A. Anticonvulsants B. Mood elevators
   C. Acidifiers D. Antiemetics

9. **Chlorpromazine is a derivative of __________.**
   A. Azepine B. Dibenzoazepine
   C. Phenothiazine D. Pyrazolidine

10. **Which drug is popularly called "Largactil"?**
    A. Clonazepam
    B. Chlorpromazine
    C. Chlorpheniramine
    D. Chlorambucil

11. **Risperidone is a member of the class __________.**
    A. Pyridopyrimidine
    B. Pyrazolidine
    C. Imidazolidine
    D. P-amino Phenol

12. **__________ is a second generation a typical anti-psychotic used in schizophrenia.**
    A. Fluphenazine B. Haloperidol
    C. Thiothixene D. Quetiapine

13. **Which of the following is chemical name of phenytoin?**
    A. 2,2-diphenyl hydantoin
    B. 4,4-diphenyl hydantoin
    C. 5,5-diphenyl hydantoin
    D. 3,3-diphenyl hydantoin

14. **__________ is a carbonic anhydrase inhibitor.**
    A. Gabapentin
    B. Topiramate
    C. Lamotrigine
    D. Vigabatrin

15. MAOIs stands for __________.

A. Major amino oxidase inhibitors
B. Mono amino oxidase inhibitors
C. Minor amino oxidase inhibitors
D. Mono anti-oxidase inhibitors

16. Venlafaxine, Duloxetine, Citalopram, Escitalopram are the drugs used in the treatment of __________.

A. Angina pectoris B. CHF
C. Depression D. Constipation

17. Ketamine is __________.

A. Anaesthetic agent
B. Antidiabetic agent
C. Anticonvulsant
D. Antianginal agent

18. __________ is a tricyclic antidepressant.

A. Amitriptyline B. Phenelzine
C. Bupropion D. Fluoxetine

19. ______________ is a mental illness characterized by pathological changes in mood.

A. Angina B. Anorexia
C. Depression D. Epilepsy

20. Olanzapine is a __________ derivative.

A. Benzodiazepine B. Imidazole
C. Acridine D. Phenothiazine

21. ____________ is a common neurological disorder characterized by paroxysmal cerebral dysrhythmia.

A. Depression B. Epilepsy
C. Obesity D. Gout

22. Which of the following is a psychic disorder?

A. Mania B. Depression
C. Neurosis D. All of the above

23. ___________ are the drugs which produce calming and quietening effects on the individuals.

A. Tranquilizers
B. Cardiotonics
C. Diuretics
D. Analgesics

24. The central nervous system (CNS) controls the functions of __________.

A. Brain and bones
B. All tissues of the body
C. Spinal cord and bones
D. None of the above

25. The important features of general anaesthesia are __________.

A. Loss of all sensation, especially pain
B. Sleep (unconsciousness) and amnesia
C. Immobility and muscle relaxation
D. All of the above

26. Halothane is the _______ form of general anaesthetic.

A. Inhalation B. Intravenous
C. Both A and B D. None of the above

27. Neuroleptics also known as _________.

A. Antipsychotics B. Anticonvulsants
C. Cholinergics D. None of the above

28. The drug used to treat epilepsy is known as _________.

A. Adrenergic drug B. Cholinergic drug
C. Anticonvulsant drug D. Antipsychotic drug

29. 5,5-diphenylimidazolidine-2,4-dione is the name of __________.

A. Diazepam B. Thiopental sodium
C. Mephenytoin D. Phenytoin

30. For the treatment of mania and depression which drugs are used?

A. Anti-depressants B. Antipsychotics
C. Antiepileptics D. None of the above

31. Carbamazepine is a tricyclic antidepressant. It is classified as __________.

A. Benzodiazepine B. Aryl alkanolamine
C. Iminostilbenes D. Benzimidazole

32. Drug used in day care anaesthesia is __________.

A. Propofol B. Enflurane
C. Xenon D. Thiopentone

33. The compound 1-Methyl 5,5 diethyl barbituric acid is __________.

A. short acting barbiturates
B. Long-acting barbiturates
C. Intermediate acting barbiturates
D. Ultra short acting barbiturates

34. The precursor of barbituric acid is __________.

A. Diethylmalonate B. Ethylacetoacetate
C. Chloro acetyl chloride D. None of the above

35. Which of the following drugs not comes under sedative hypnotic class?

A. Diazepam B. Alprazolam
C. Nitrazepam D. Aspirin

36. **Which of the following is not a benzazepine derivative?**
A. Olanzapine B. Clozapine
C. Quetipine D. Fluspiriline

37. **Antipsychotic drugs block the receptor in brain is __________.**
A. Dopamine D_2 receptor
B. Muscarinic receptor
C. Nicotinic receptor
D. None of the above

38. **General anesthesia usually uses a combination of __________.**
A. Intravenous drugs B. Inhaled gases
C. Both A and B D. None of the above

39. **Example of ultra short acting barbiturate is ________.**
A. Halothane
B. Thiopental sodium
C. Ketamine
D. None of the above

40. **$C_{12}H_{18}O$ is the molecular formula of __________.**
A. Ketamine B. Phenobarbital
C. Diazepam D. Propofol

41. **The agent or drugs which reduce the excitement and calm to the patient without inducing sleep called __________.**
A. Hypnotics B. Sedatives
C. General anaesthetics D. Tranquilizers

42. **Which of the following are examples of atypical antipsychotic drug __________.**
A. Clozapine B. Haloperidol
C. Risperidone D. Both A and C

43. **Which of the following drugs are used to treat convulsions?**
A. Phenytoin B. Carbamazepine
C. Olanzapine D. Both A and B

44. **Which of the following antidepressant drug is also used to treat allergic conjunctivitis?**
A. Amitriptyline B. Amphetamine
C. Fluoxetine D. Imipramine

45. **Which of the following drugs is used as muscle relaxant?**
A. Clonazepam B. Nitrazepam
C. Diazepam D. Meprobamate

46. **Thiopentone is given by IV as __________**
A. Sedative B. Anaesthetic
C. Analgesic D. Antidepressant

47. **Antidepressants are also called __________**
A. Temperature elevators
B. Blood pressure elevators
C. Mood elevators
D. None of the above

48. **Which of the following antipsychotic drugs is butyrophenone derivative?**
A. Chlorpromazine B. Reserpine
C. Thiothixene D. Haloperidol

49. **Valproic acid is used as __________**
A. Antipsychotic B. Anticonvulsant
C. Antihypertensive D. Antimalignant

50. **Which one of the following is a tricyclic antidepressant?**
A. Venlaflaxine B. Fluoxamine
C. Imipramine D. Phenelzine

Answer Key

1 C	2 B	3 A	4 D	5 C	6 B	7 C	8 B	9 C	10 B
11 A	12 D	13 C	14 B	15 B	16 C	17 A	18 A	19 C	20 A
21 B	22 D	23 A	24 B	25 D	26 A	27 A	28 C	29 D	30 A
31 C	32 A	33 B	34 A	35 D	36 D	37 A	38 C	39 B	40 D
41 B	42 D	43 D	44 D	45 D	46 B	47 C	48 D	49 B	50 C

CHAPTER 6

Drugs Acting on Autonomic Nervous System
Sympathomimetics, Sympatholytics, Parasympathomimetics, Parasympatholytics

1. **Chemical name of Adrenaline is ___________.**
   A. 1(3,4 dihydroxyphenyl) 2-methyl amino ethanol
   B. 4(2-amino-1-hydroxy methyl) benzene-1,2 diol
   C. 4(2-aminoethyl) benzene-1,2 diol
   D. None of the above

2. **2-methyl amino, 1-phenyl 1-propanol is a chemical name of ___________.**
   A. Adrenaline
   B. Ephedrine
   C. Isoprenaline
   D. Salbutamol

3. **Chemical transmitter of PNS is ___________.**
   A. Adrenaline B. Ephedrine
   C. Acetylcholine D. Dopamine

4. **Chemical transmitter of SNS is ___________.**
   A. Dopamine B. Acetylcholine
   C. Adrenaline D. Ephedrine

5. **Pilocarpine is a ___________.**
   A. Cholinergic antagonist
   B. Cholinergic agonist
   C. Adrenergic agonist
   D. None of the above

6. **__________ is a drug of choice in myasthenia gravis.**
   A. Physostigmine
   B. Acetylcholine
   C. Neostigmine
   D. None of the above

7. **Acetylcholine is an ester of choline with __________.**
   A. Hydrochloric acid B. Acetic acid
   C. Nitric acid D. Sulphuric acid

8. **Acetylcholine produces stimulation of skeletal muscles by its ___________.**
   A. Anticholinergic action
   B. Muscarinic action
   C. Nicotinic action
   D. Cardiotonic action

9. **___________ is used in Alzheimer's disease.**
   A. Edrophonium
   B. Pralidoxime
   C. Tacrine hydrochloride
   D. None of the above

10. **(1R, 3R, 5S) tropan-3-yl (+–) tropate is a chemical name of ___________.**
    A. Homatropine
    B. Atropine
    C. Benztropine
    D. Ipratropium bromide

11. **Which of the following drugs are not alpha-adrenergic blockers?**
    A. Propranolol B. Prazosin
    C. Tolazoline D. Phenoxybenzamine

12. **(2-Acetoxy-N, N, N-trimethylethanaminium) is a chemical name of which compound?**
    A. Carbachol B. Acetylcholine
    C. Neostigmine D. Pilocarpine

13. **How do the two divisions of ANS work?**
    A. Works with similar effects
    B. Works with opposite effect
    C. Does not work together
    D. Both A and B

14. Adrenergic drugs or adrenergic amines also known as __________.

A. Sympathomimetic agents
B. Parasympathetic agents
C. Adrenergic antagonist
D. None of the above

15. Which of the following drugs is imidazolidine derivative?

A. Naphazoline B. Ephedrine
C. Dopamine D. Metaraminol

16. Propranolol is a __________.

A. Beta adrenergic blockers
B. Alpha blocker
C. Cholinergic antagonist
D. None of the above

17. The agents which can reproduce the action of the acetylcholine by directly interacting with the receptors or by stimulating parasympathetic nervous system by inhibiting anticholinesterase enzyme are called __________.

A. Cholinergic blocking agents
B. Cholinergic agents
C. Adrenergic antagonist
D. None of the above

18. Pralidoxime is the __________.

A. Irreversible drug
B. Reversible drug
C. Direct acting agent
D. Cholinesterase reactivator

19. Cholinergic agents are also known as __________.

A. Parasympathomimetic agent
B. Parasympatholytics drugs
C. Both A and B
D. None of the above

20. Which of the following substances is the first precursor of adrenaline formation?

A. Tyrosine
B. DOPA
C. Dopamine
D. Non-adrenaline

21. Which of the following organs is activated by sympathetic system?

A. Hairs stimulation
B. Sweat gland
C. Heart
D. All of the above

22. The catechol ring contains (–OH) groups on which position?

A. Second and fourth B. Third and fourth
C. First and second D. Second and third

23. Which of the following adrenergic drug belongs to category of vasoconstrictors?

A. Metaraminol B. Isoprenaline
C. Amrinone D. Naphazoline

24. Which of the following is the selective antagonist of alpha-1 receptor?

A. Prazosin B. Yohimbine
C. Rauwolscine D. Clonidine

25. COMT stands for __________.

A. Catechol-o-methyl-transferase
B. Catechol-oxy-methyl-transferase
C. Catecholamine-o-methyl-transferase
D. Catecholamine-oxy-methyl-transferase

26. Ephedrine alkaloid is obtained from __________.

A. *Ephedra sinica* B. *Ephedra vulgaris*
C. *Ephedra fragilis* D. *Ephedra intermedia*

27. Beta-2 receptors are predominantly found in which system?

A. CNS B. Respiratory system
C. Endocrine system D. Vascular system

28. Alpha-1 receptors increase the intracellular level of __________.

A. K^+ B. Ca^{2+}
C. Na^+ D. Cl^-

29. Alpha-2 receptors activate G protein gated channels.

A. Ca^2 B. K^+
C. Na^+ D. Cl^-

30. Tyramine is __________type of agonist.

A. Direct acting B. Indirect acting
C. Dual acting D. None of the above

31. Dopamine comes under the category __________.

A. Catecholamines
B. Non-catecholamines
C. Both A and B
D. None of the above

32. DOMA is __________.

A. Dihydroxy mandelic acid
B. Dihydroxymandelonic acid
C. Decahydroxy maleic acid
D. Dihydroxy mandolic acid

33. Adrenergic blocking agent prevents the response of adrenergic drug at which adrenergic receptor?

A. Alpha
B. Beta
C. Both A and B
D. None of the above

34. Selective beta-1 antagonist drugs are used to act on which part?

A. Heart
B. Brain
C. Kidney
D. Respiratory system

35. Selective beta-2 antagonist drugs are used to act on which part?

A. Kidney
B. Brain
C. Heart
D. Respiratory system

36. Beta-2 mediated vasodilation is called __________.

A. Coronary atherosclerosis
B. Raynaud's syndrome
C. Mydriasis
D. Dale vasomotor reversal

37. Phenoxybenzaime inhibits the uptake of __________.

A. Histamine
B. Catecholamines
C. Prazosin
D. Carvedial

38. How much carbon chains are essential for activity of propranolol?

A. 1 carbon chain
B. 2 carbon chain
C. 3 carbon chain
D. 4 carbon chain

39. Beta blockers are structurally similar to __________.

A. Beta agonist
B. Beta antagonist
C. Alpha antagonist
D. Alpha agonist

40. Characteristics of atenolol is __________.

A. β_1 selective drug with low lipid solubility
B. β_1 non-selective drug with low lipid solubility
C. β_1 non-selective drug with high lipid solubility
D. β_1 selective drug with high lipid solubility

41. Which group of Acetylcholine contributes to the binding of compound to the muscarinic receptor?

A. Ammonium group
B. Methyl group
C. Ester group
D. All of the above

42. Muscarinic subreceptors are __________ types.

A. 3
B. 4
C. 5
D. 2

43. Drug is used as insecticide in agriculture is __________.

A. Parathion
B. Edrophonium
C. Neostigmine
D. Tacrine

44. __________ are synthetic analogues of atropine.

A. Homatropine
B. Propantheline
C. Both A and B
D. None of the above

45. Pilocarpine is a drug of choice in __________.

A. Xeropthalmia
B. Photophobia
C. Glaucoma
D. None of the above

46. Acetylcholine produces stimulation of skeletal muscles by its __________.

A. Muscarinic action
B. Nicotinic action
C. Vasoconstriction
D. Gastric action

47. __________ is used in Alzheimer's disease.

A. Edrophonium
B. Pralidoxime
C. Tacrine hydrochloride
D. None of the above

48. Anticholinergic used as spasmolytic is __________.

A. Pyridostigmine
B. Dicyclomine
C. Tropicamide
D. Neostigmine

49. Dopamine is a monoamine compound with __________ ionotropic effect.

A. Negative
B. Positive
C. Neutral
D. None of the above

50. Salbutamol is used in __________.

A. Epilepsy
B. Anxiety
C. Bronchial asthma
D. Anorexia

Answer Key

1 A	2 B	3 C	4 C	5 B	6 C	7 B	8 C	9 C	10 B
11 A	12 B	13 B	14 A	15 A	16 A	17 B	18 D	19 A	20 A
21 C	22 D	23 D	24 A	25 A	26 A	27 B	28 B	29 A	30 B
31 A	32 A	33 C	34 A	35 D	36 D	37 B	38 B	39 A	40 A
41 C	42 C	43 A	44 C	45 C	46 B	47 C	48 B	49 B	50 C

CHAPTER 7

Drugs Acting on Cardiovascular System

Antiarrhythmic drugs, Antihypertensive drugs, Antianginal drugs

1. **__________ is cardiotonic drug.**
   A. Procainamide B. Frusemide
   C. Digitoxin D. Quinidine

2. **Calciguard is a popular brand name of __________.**
   A. Diazepam
   B. Nifedipine
   C. Lignocaine
   D. Verapamil

3. **Verapamil and nifedipine are __________.**
   A. Adrenergic blockers
   B. Cholinergic blockers
   C. MAO inhibitors
   D. Calcium channel blockers

4. **Xylocaine is a brand name of __________.**
   A. Procaine B. Cinchocaine
   C. Lignocaine D. Amethocaine

5. **Amiodarone hydrochloride is __________.**
   A. Potassium channel blocker
   B. Calcium channel blocker
   C. Adrenergic blocker
   D. Cholinergic blocker

6. **Which of the following drugs is angiotensin converting enzyme inhibitor?**
   A. Verapamil B. Enalapril
   C. Guanethidine D. Spironolactone

7. **Mecamylamine is a __________.**
   A. Catecholamine depleter
   B. Cholinergic blocker
   C. Beta blocker
   D. Ganglionic blocker

8. **__________ is ACE inhibitor**
   A. Ramipril B. Propranolol
   C. Clonidine D. Methyl dopa

9. **__________ is a central acting alpha-adrenergic agonist.**
   A. Hydralazine B. Clonidine
   C. Captopril D. Propranolol

10. **Isosorbide dinitrate is __________.**
    A. Hypoglycemic B. Diuretic
    C. Antianginal drug D. Antimicrobial

11. **Lasix is a popular brand name of __________.**
    A. Mannitol B. Triamterene
    C. Frusemide D. Mersalyl

12. **Which one of the following is a derivative of anthranilic acid?**
    A. Acetazolamide B. Chlorpropamide
    C. Frusemide D. None of the above

13. **__________ is a potassium sparing diuretics.**
    A. Chlorthalidone B. Metolazone
    C. Ethacrynic acid D. Spironolactone

14. **Spironolactone is __________.**
    A. Cholinergic antagonist
    B. Adrenergic antagonist
    C. Aldosterone receptor antagonist
    D. Muscarinic blocker

15. **Which is correct about propranolol?**
    A. Is a β_1 specific blocker
    B. Causes prominent postural hypotension
    C. Used in angina (chest pain)
    D. Has a half-life of 12 hours

16. Which drug is used to reduce oedema (excess fluid retention)?
- **A.** Acetazolamide
- **B.** Isosorbide dinitrate
- **C.** Nifedipine
- **D.** Clonidine hydrochloride

17. Which one of the following drugs should be taken before meals?
- **A.** Glimepiride
- **B.** Repaglinide
- **C.** Benzthiazide
- **D.** Pioglitazone

18. Which of the following is antianginal agents?
- **A.** Isosorbide dinitrate
- **B.** Nitro-glycerine
- **C.** Both A and B
- **D.** None of the above

19. Which of the following drugs is beta-blocker class?
- **A.** Spironolactone **B.** Atenolol
- **C.** Frusemide **D.** All of the above

20. Emdopa is the brand name of __________.
- **A.** Methyldopate hydrochloride
- **B.** Bumetanide
- **C.** Nifedipine
- **D.** Amlodipine

21. Captopril is used for the treatment of __________.
- **A.** Hypertension
- **B.** Congestive heart failure
- **C.** Both A and B
- **D.** None of the above

22. Prazosin is used exclusively in the treatment _______.
- **A.** Cancer **B.** Brain tumour
- **C.** Diarrhoea **D.** Hypertension

23. Brand name cyclopam contains the molecule ______.
- **A.** Propranolol
- **B.** Atenolol
- **C.** Ephedrine
- **D.** Dicyclomine hydrochloride

24. The antianginal drug that inhibits phosphodiesterase is ___________.
- **A.** Phenylbutazone
- **B.** Isosorbide dinitrate
- **C.** Nifedipine
- **D.** Aspirin

25. Which of the following is a prodrug?
- **A.** Minoxidil
- **B.** Losartan
- **C.** Sodium nitroprusside
- **D.** Verapamil

26. The antihypertensive drugs inhibit the ACE is ______.
- **A.** Analpril **B.** Captopril
- **C.** Ramipril **D.** All of the above

27. The most common diuretics used as an antihypertensive agent is/are ___________.
- **A.** Loop diuretics
- **B.** Thiazide diuretics
- **C.** Aldosterone antagonist
- **D.** Both A and B

28. Which of the following is an example of beta-adrenergic blocker?
- **A.** Propranolol **B.** Sotalol
- **C.** Atenolol **D.** All of the above

29. Which of the following is an example of alpha-blocker?
- **A.** Prazosin
- **B.** Ergotamine
- **C.** Both A and B
- **D.** None of the above

30. _________ is a lipid lowering agent.
- **A.** Clonidine **B.** Guanethidine
- **C.** Captopril **D.** Clofibrate

31. Heart rate above 100 beats/minute is called _______.
- **A.** Tachycardia **B.** Atrial flutter
- **C.** Bradycardia **D.** Atrial fibrillation

32. Which of the following drug is a ganglionic blocker?
- **A.** Verapamil **B.** Mecamylamine
- **C.** Spironolactone **D.** Reserpine

33. Hydralazine is __________.
- **A.** Diuretic **B.** Antidiuretic
- **C.** Peripheral vasodilator **D.** Antiarrhythmic

34. _________ refers to pains in the chest.
- **A.** Angina pectoris **B.** Anaemia
- **C.** Anxiety **D.** Anorexia

35. CHF stands for ___________.
- **A.** Coronary heart failure
- **B.** Congestive heart failure
- **C.** Congenital heart force
- **D.** Common heart failure

36. **Glyceryl trinitrate is given by __________.**
A. Topical B. Rectal
C. Sublingual D. Intramuscular

37. **Clonidine is used as__________.**
A. Antihypertensive B. Anorexiants
C. Antidiuretic D. Antimalarial

38. **All of the following drugs may increase the effect of digoxin *except* __________.**
A. Carbamazepine B. Frusemide
C. Verapamil D. Amiodorone

39. **Which of the following calcium channel blocker has rapid onset of action?**
A. Verapamil
B. Diltiazem
C. Felodopine
D. Nifedipine

40. **Which of the following disorders is generally considered as silent killer?**
A. Hypertension B. Angina
C. Arrhythmia D. All of the above

Answer Key

1 C	2 B	3 D	4 C	5 A	6 B	7 D	8 A	9 B	10 C
11 C	12 C	13 D	14 C	15 C	16 A	17 B	18 C	19 B	20 A
21 C	22 D	23 D	24 C	25 A	26 D	27 B	28 D	29 C	30 D
31 A	32 B	33 C	34 A	35 B	36 C	37 A	38 A	39 D	40 A

CHAPTER 8

Diuretics

1. __________ are agents that accelerate rate of urine formation.
   A. Antigout B. Antidiuretics
   C. Diuretics D. Cardiotonic

2. Diuretic belongs to anthranilic acid derivative is __________.
   A. Acetazolamide B. Chlorthiazide
   C. Frusemide D. Spironolactone

3. Spironolactone is __________.
   A. Aldosterone antagonist
   B. Adrenergic antagonist
   C. Cholinergic antagonist
   D. Carbonic anhydrase inhibitor

4. Which drug used to reduce oedema (excess fluid retention)?
   A. Acetazolamide
   B. Isosorbide dinitrate
   C. Nifedipine
   D. Clonidine hydrochloride

5. Class of bumetanide is __________.
   A. Carbonic anhydrase inhibitor
   B. Osmotic diuretic
   C. Loop diuretic
   D. Potassium sparing diuretic

6. The frequency of dosing for Benzthiazide is __________.
   A. Thrice a day B. Once daily
   C. Twice daily D. 4 times a day

7. Which of the following is a loop diuretic?
   A. Frusemide B. Bumetanide
   C. Both A and B D. None of the above

8. One of the following diuretics acts on loop of Henle?
   A. Theophylline
   B. Ethacrynic acid
   C. Amiloride
   D. Mersalyl

9. Which of the following is a diuretic of carbonic anhydrase inhibitor class?
   A. Acetazolamide B. Frusemide
   C. Bumetanide D. None of the above

10. Which of the following are brand names of Spironolactone?
    A. Aldactone B. CaroSpir
    C. Both A and B D. None of the above

11. Reabsorption of which of the following substance is inhibited by most diuretics and causes diuresis?
    A. Magnesium B. Potassium
    C. Sodium D. Calcium

12. Chemically, benzthiazide is __________.
    A. 7-sulfamoyl-1,2,4-benzothiadiazine 1,1-dioxide
    B. 6-sulfamoyl-1,2,4-benzothiadiazine 1,1-dioxide
    C. 4-sulfamoyl-1,2,4-benzothiadiazine 1,1-dioxide
    D. None of the above

13. Which of the following is potassium sparing diuretic?
    A. Spironolactone B. Bumetanide
    C. Frusemide D. All of the above

14. The diuretic used to treat glaucoma by reducing intraocular pressure is __________.
    A. Mannitol B. Urea
    C. Acetazolamide D. Ethacrynic acid

15. **Which of the following is a long-acting thiazide diuretic?**
   A. Metformin
   B. Chlorthalidone
   C. Pioglitazone
   D. Repaglinide

16. **Which of the following is brand name of frusemide?**
   A. Lasix
   B. Frisix
   C. Frusenex
   D. All of the above

17. **Benzthiazide is used for the treatment of __________.**
   A. Hypertension
   B. Edema
   C. Both A and B
   D. None of the above

18. **Which of the following is not a loop diuretic?**
   A. Frusemide
   B. Torsemide
   C. Ethacrynic acid
   D. Chlorthalidone

19. **Bumetanide belongs to which class?**
   A. Carbonic anhydrase inhibitors
   B. Osmotic diuretics
   C. Potassium sparing diuretics
   D. Loop diuretics

20. **Which of the following diuretic competes with aldosterone?**
   A. Amiloride
   B. Frusemide
   C. Spironolactone
   D. Isosorbide

21. **Thiazide diuretics act on __________.**
   A. Loop of Henle
   B. Proximal tubule
   C. Collecting tubule
   D. Distal tubule

22. **Which one of the following acts on loop of Henle?**
   A. Spironolactone
   B. Dichlorophenamide
   C. Ethacrynic acid
   D. Acetazolamide

23. **The most appropriate diuretic for treatment of acute pulmonary oedema is __________.**
   A. Loop diuretic
   B. Thiazide diuretic
   C. Potassium sparing diuretic
   D. Osmotic diuretic

24. **Which one of the following is osmotic diuretics?**
   A. Glycerol
   B. Mannitol
   C. Isosorbide
   D. All of the above

25. **Which of the following is carbonic anhydrase inhibitor?**
   A. Triamterene
   B. Chlorothiazide
   C. Acetazolamide
   D. Amiloride

26. **The following diuretics are used in treatment of glaucoma *except* __________.**
   A. Glycerol
   B. Methazolamide
   C. Acetazolamide
   D. Furosemide

27. **Among the following which is having furfural moiety?**
   A. Acetazolamide
   B. Furosemide
   C. Bumetanide
   D. Spironolactone

28. **Potassium sparing diuretics inhibits the __________.**
   A. Chloride reabsorption
   B. Potassium reabsorption
   C. Sodium reabsorption
   D. Calcium reabsorption

29. **Which of the following is pteridine derivative?**
   A. Amiloride
   B. Isosorbide
   C. Mannitol
   D. Triamterene

30. **Diuretic containing furan heterocycle is __________.**
   A. Frusemide
   B. Acetazolamide
   C. Mannitol
   D. Amiloride

Answer Key

1 C	2 C	3 A	4 A	5 C	6 C	7 C	8 B	9 A	10 C
11 C	12 A	13 A	14 C	15 B	16 D	17 B	18 D	19 D	20 C
21 D	22 C	23 A	24 D	25 C	26 D	27 B	28 C	29 D	30 A

CHAPTER 9

Hypoglycemic Agents

1. **Hypoglycaemia is a condition in which blood sugar levels is ____________.**
   A. Higher than normal   B. Lower than normal
   C. Normal   D. None of the above

2. **IDDM and NIDDM are the types of __________.**
   A. Hypertension   B. Sleep
   C. Diabetes   D. Cancer

3. **-The hormone insulin is secreted by cells _________ of islets of Langerhans.**
   A. Beta   B. Alpha
   C. Gamma   D. Delta

4. **Which one of the following is parenteral hypoglycaemic agent?**
   A. Phenformin   B. Metformin
   C. Tolbutamide   D. Insulin

5. **__________ is a hypoglycaemic agent obtained from plant source.**
   A. Insulin   B. Gaur gum
   C. Tolbutamide   D. Phenformin

6. **Insulin should be stored at temperature ranges between __________.**
   A. 8°C and 10°C   B. 10°C and 20°C
   C. 2°C and 8°C   D. 20°C and 25°C

7. **1,1-dimethyl biguanide is a chemical name of_______.**
   A. Chlorpropamide   B. Tolbutamide
   C. Glibenclamide   D. Metformin

8. **Which of the following are gliptins?**
   A. Sitagliptin   B. Vildagliptin
   C. Sitagliptins   D. All of the above

9. **Which of the following are sulfonylurea derivative of hypoglycaemic agents?**
   A. Glibenclamide   B. Glimepiride
   C. Both A and B   D. None of these

10. **Chemically, metformin is __________.**
    A. 1,1-dimethylguanidine   B. 1,1-diethylguanidine
    C. 1.2-dimethylguanidine   D. None of the above

11. **Which of the following is a meglitinide class of hypoglycaemic agents?**
    A. Glibenclamide   B. Repaglinide
    C. Glimepiride   D. All of the above

12. **Which of the following is first-line medication for the treatment of type 2 diabetes?**
    A. Metformin   B. Glimepiride
    C. Pioglitazone   D. Repaglinide

13. **Which of the followings are DPP-4 inhibitors?**
    A. Sitagliptin   B. Vildagliptin
    C. Saxagliptin   D. All of the above

14. **Which of the following is thiazolidinediones class of orally active hypoglycaemic agent?**
    A. Glibenclamide   B. Glimepiride
    C. Pioglitazone   D. Repaglinide

15. **Which of the following drug is second generation hypoglycaemic agent of sulfonylureas class?**
    A. Glibenclamide   B. Pioglitazone
    C. Repaglinide   D. Metformin

16. **__________ is loop diuretic.**
    A. Frusemide   B. Spironolactone
    C. Chlorthalidone   D. None of the above

17. __________ is an aldosterone receptor antagonist.

A. Acetazolamide B. Bumetanide
C. Chlorthalidone D. Spironolactone

18. __________ is potassium sparing diuretic.

A. Acetazolamide B. Bumetanide
C. Spironolactone D. Chlorthalidone

19. __________ is used in treatment of petit mal epilepsy (absence seizures).

A. Acetazolamide B. Bumetanide
C. Spironolactone D. Chlorthalidone

20. __________ is given intravenously in treatment of acute left ventricular failure.

A. Frusemide B. Spironolactone
C. Chlorthalidone D. Acetazolamide

21. Bumetanide is __________ times more potent than Frusemide.

A. 10 B. 20
C. 30 D. 40

22. Diabetes is an __________ diseases

A. Endocrinochronic B. Infectious
C. Bacterial D. Microbial

23. Type 1 diabetes is also known as __________.

A. Insulin-dependent diabetes mellitus
B. Non-insulin-dependent diabetes mellitus
C. Juvenile-onset diabetes mellitus
D. A and C both

24. Chlorpropamide is an example of __________.

A. Biguanides
B. Thiazolidinediones
C. Meglitinides
D. Sulfonylureas

25. A chain of insulin is composed of __________.

A. 21-amino acids B. 31-amino acids
C. 20-amino acids D. 30-amino acids

26. __________ inhibit potassium ion channel, thus blocking the efflux of potassium.

A. Biguanides B. Thiazolidinediones
C. Meglitinides D. Sulfonylurea

27. AMPK is __________.

A. 2-adenosine monophosphate-activated protein kinase
B. 4-adenosine monophosphate-activated protein kinase
C. 5-adenosine monophosphate-activated protein kinase
D. 6-adenosine monophosphate-activated protein kinase

28. Name of scientists who identified insulin first time is __________.

A. Banting and Best
B. Laurence Brunton
C. Pamala A Jacobson
D. Michael E Ernst

29. Insulin was prepared from cow is also named __________.

A. Porcine B. Bovine
C. Both A and B D. None of the above

30. The drugs which lower the elevated blood sugar level to the normal level are called __________.

A. Antianginal agents
B. Hypoglycaemic agents
C. Antiarrhythmic agents
D. Vasodilators

Answer Key

1 B	2 C	3 A	4 D	5 B	6 C	7 D	8 D	9 C	10 A
11 B	12 A	13 D	14 C	15 A	16 A	17 D	18 C	19 C	20 A
21 D	22 A	23 B	24 D	25 A	26 A	27 D	28 C	29 A	30 B

CHAPTER 10

Analgesic and Anti-inflammatory Agents

1. **The drugs which relieve pain are called**
   A. Antipyretics B. Carminative
   C. Analgesics D. Purgative

2. **The drugs which reduce elevated body temperature to normal level are called**
   A. Analgesics B. Purgative
   C. Antipyretics D. Carminative

3. **__________ is a principal alkaloid obtained from opium.**
   A. Ephedrine B. Morphine
   C. Vinca D. Reserpine

4. **Heroin is also known as __________.**
   A. Triacetyl morphine
   B. Diacetyl morphine
   C. Tetra acetyl morphine
   D. Acetyl morphine

5. **Ethyl, 1-methyl, 4-phenyl-piperidine 4-carboxylate is a chemical name of __________.**
   A. Pethidine B. Methadone
   C. Morphine D. Heroin

6. **Nalorphine and Naloxone are __________.**
   A. Adrenergic antagonists
   B. Cholinergic antagonist
   C. Narcotic antagonists
   D. Muscarinic blockers

7. **Nalorphine and naloxone are used in __________.**
   A. Morphine poisoning
   B. Salicylate poisoning
   C. Barbiturate poisoning
   D. Organophosphorus poisoning

8. **The NSAIDs act by inhibiting of the __________.**
   A. CO-X enzyme B. Microsomal enzyme
   C. Catecholamines D. Peptides

9. **Ortho-acetoxy benzoic acid is a chemical name of __________.**
   A. Paracetamol B. Aspirin
   C. Phenacetin D. Indomethacin

10. **Which of the following drugs is a propionic acid derivative?**
    A. Ibuprofen B. Indomethacin
    C. Aspirin D. Paracetamol

11. **Which of the following are non-steroidal anti-inflammatory agents?**
    A. Aspirin B. Diclofenac
    C. Ibuprofen D. All of the above

12. **Which of the followings are aryl acetic acid derivative?**
    A. Diclofenac B. Aceclofenac
    C. Both A and B D. Ibuprofen

13. **Which of the following are brand names of paracetamol?**
    A. Calpol B. Cipmol
    C. Cofamol D. All of the above

14. **Which of the following is a phenylacetic acid derivative?**
    A. Diclofenac B. Ibuprofen
    C. Aspirin D. All of the above

15. **Mefenamic acid is the inhibitor of __________.**
    A. COX-1
    B. COX-2
    C. COX-1 and COX-2
    D. None of the above

16. Celecoxib is the inhibitor of __________.

A. COX-1 B. COX-2
C. COX-1 and COX-2 D. None of the above

17. Which of the following is propionic acid derivative?

A. Ibuprofen B. Diclofenac
C. Aceclofenac D. Both A and B

18. Voveran is the brand name of __________.

A. Ibuprofen B. Diclofenac
C. Aceclofenac D. Aspirin

19. Which of the following drug possesses antipyretic activity?

A. Paracetamol B. Celecoxib
C. Piroxicam D. All of the above

20. Aspirin is __________.

A. Salicylic acid derivative
B. p-aminophenol derivatives
C. Pyrazolid inedione derivatives
D. Anthranilic acid derivatives

21. Which of the following is not as selective COX-2 inhibitor?

A. Celecoxib B. Rolecoxib
C. Valedocoxib D. Aspirin

22. Salicylates are useful in treatment of __________.

A. Anorexia B. Peptic ulcer
C. Rheumatoid arthritis D. None of the above

23. Other name of aspirin is __________.

A. Emipirin B. Bufferin
C. Acetyl salicylic acid D. All of the above

24. Salsalate is __________.

A. Dimer of salicylic acid B. Trimer of salicylic acid
C. Both A and B D. None of the above

25. Sulphasalazine is used in treatment of __________.

A. Peptic ulcer B. Crohn's disease
C. Ulcerative colitis D. Both B and C

26. PG (Prostaglandin) is naturally occurring fatty acid derivative of __________.

A. 20°C cyclopentanone
B. 25°C cyclopentanone
C. 30°C cyclopentanone
D. 35°C cyclopentanone

27. Dolokind is a popular brand name of __________.

A. Paracetamol B. Aceclofenac
C. Aspirin D. Phenylbutazone

28. Narcotic analgesics are used __________.

A. To relieve moderate to severe pain
B. To suppress non-productive cough
C. To control diarrhoea
D. All of the above

29. __________ is also known as Acetaminophen.

A. Aspirin B. Aceclofenac
C. Paracetamol D. Piroxicam

30. Mefenamic acid is __________.

A. Salicylic acid derivative
B. Anthranillic acid derivative
C. Oxicam derivative
D. Indole acetic acid derivative

Answer Key

1 C	2 C	3 B	4 B	5 A	6 C	7 A	8 A	9 B	10 A
11 D	12 C	13 D	14 A	15 C	16 B	17 A	18 B	19 D	20 A
21 D	22 C	23 C	24 A	25 D	26 A	27 B	28 D	29 C	30 B

CHAPTER 11

Anti-infective Agents

Antifungal Agents, Urinary Tract Anti-infective Agents, Anti-tubercular Agents, Antiviral Agents, Antimalarial Agents, Sulphonamides

1. Ketoconazole is ___________.

A. Antitubercular drug
B. Antifungal drug
C. Antiviral drug
D. Antiamobeic drug

2. Unsaturated fatty acid used as antifungal is_______.

A. Undecylenic acid   B. Palmitic acid
C. Ricinoelic acid   D. Arachidonic acid

3. Norfloxacin is a __________ derivative.

A. Pyrazolone   B. Quinolone
C. Pyrazolidine   D. Imidazoline

4. PAS stands for ___________.

A. Para amino sulphonamide
B. Para amino salicylic acid
C. Para acetamido sulphone
D. Para amino sulphuric acid

5. The pyridine containing antitubercular drug is_______.

A. PAS   B. Pteromalid
C. Isoniazid   D. Ethambutol

6. Pyrazine-2-carboxamide is a chemical name of_______.

A. Isoniazid   B. Pyrimethamine
C. Pyrazinamide   D. Rifampicin

7. Idoxuridine is __________.

A. Antiamoebic drug   B. Antiviral drug
C. Anthelmintic   D. Antifungal

8. Which of the following drug is effective against HIV-1, HIV-2, HTLV-1 infections?

A. Ribavirin   B. Zidovudine
C. Amatidine   D. Idoxyridine

9. _______________ is a drug used for the treatment of COVID-19 infection.

A. Amantadine   B. Idoxyridine
C. Remdesivir   D. Ribavirin

10. The dose of Favipiravir tab is __________ orally twice daily for COVID-19.

A. 500 mg   B. 1000 mg
C. 1800 mg   D. 1400 mg

11. __________ is a 4-amino quinoline derivative.

A. Proguanil   B. Primaquine
C. Chloroquine   D. Mepacrine

12. Which drug belongs to 2,4-diaminopyrimidine derivative?

A. Chloroquine   B. Quinine
C. Pyrimethamine   D. Phenylbutazone

13. Artemisinin is used as __________.

A. Antifungal   B. Antimalarial
C. Antiviral   D. Antiamobeic

14. Chemical structure of sulphonamide group is________.

A. $-NH-C(N_2H_3)$
B. $-CONH_2$
C. $-SO_2NH_2$
D. $-NHCOCH_3$

15. Father of chemotherapy is ___________.

A. Alexander Fleming   B. Paul Ehrlich
C. Heman Helmholtz   D. Hippocrates

16. Sulphonamides completes with ______________ in bacterial metabolism.

A. GABA   B. PABA
C. PAS   D. MAO

17. The sulphonamide useful to treat eye infection is __________.

A. Sulphaguanidine
B. Succinyl sulphathiazole
C. Pthalylsulphathiazole
D. Sulphacetamide

18. Diaminodiphenylsulphone (DDS) means __________.

A. Solapsone B. Dapsone
C. Sulpiride D. Foscamet

19. Co-trimoxazole is a combination of __________.

A. 5 parts of sulphamethoxazole and 1 part of trimethoprim
B. 1 part of sulphamethoxazole and 5 parts of trimethoprim
C. 5 parts of sulphamethoxazole and 5 parts of trimethoprim
D. 1 part of sulphamethoxazole and 1 part of trimethoprim

20. __________ was synthesized for first time in 1908 by American chemist Paul Josef Jakob Gelmo.

A. Sulphacetamide B. Sulphanilamide
C. Sulphaguanidine D. PABA

21. N-1-(Pyrimidin-2-yl) sulphanilamide is a chemical name of __________.

A. Sulphaguanidine B. Sulphacetamide
C. Sulphadimidine D. Sulphadiazine

22. Which anti-infective agent used to treat infections such as athlete's foot?

A. Itraconazole B. Ketoconazole
C. Miconazole D. Griseofulvin

23. Diflucan is the brand name for which drug?

A. Naftifine Hydrochloride B. Fluconazole
C. Itraconazole D. Ketoconazole

24. Zovirax is the brand name for which drug __________.

A. Acyclovir
B. Idoxuridine
C. Amantadine hydrochloride
D. Favipiravir

25. Which drug is used to treat corona virus infection?

A. Remdesivir B. Ribavirin
C. Zidovudine D. Foscarnet

26. Idoxuridine is used as __________.

A. Nasal sprays B. Eye drops
C. Ear drops D. Suppositories

27. Which drug is used in 'travelers' diarrhoea?

A. Cotrimoxazole B. Dapsone
C. Mafenide acetate D. Sulfacetamide

28. Which of the following is the most common adverse effect of amphotericin B?

A. Bone marrow suppression
B. Hypokalemia
C. Hypomagnesemia
D. Nephrotoxicity

29. Which of the following is an imidazole antifungal?

A. Miconazole B. Ketoconazole
C. Both A and B D. None of the above

30. Griseofulvin is used in the treatment of __________.

A. Athlete's foot B. Ringworm
C. Both A and B D. None of the above

31. Itraconazole is used in the treatment of fungal infections such as __________.

A. Aspergillosis B. Blastomycosis
C. Coccidioidomycosis D. All of the above

32. Which of the following antiviral medication used for treatment of HIV?

A. Ribavirin B. Zidovudine
C. Both A and B D. None of the above

33. Ribavirin is used in the treatment of __________.

A. Hepatitis C B. HIV
C. Both A and B D. None of the above

34. The brand names of Remdesivir in India __________.

A. Cipremi B. Remdac
C. Redyx D. All of the above

35. Griseofulvin is obtained from the mold __________.

A. Penicillium notatum
B. Penicillium chrysogenum
C. Penicillium griseofulvum
D. None of the above

36. PAS stands for __________.

A. Pure amino salicylic acid
B. Para-amino salicylic acid
C. Pyridine amino salicylic acid
D. Polor amino salicylic acid

37. Pretomanid is __________.

A. Antifungal
B. Antiviral
C. Antitubercular
D. Antimalarial

38. 2-Carbamoyl pyrazine is a chemical name of________.
A. Isoniazid **B.** Pyrazinamide
C. Ethambutol **D.** Rifampicin

39. __________ is used as antiviral agent against herpes viruses.
A. Ribavirin **B.** Amantidine
C. Acyclovir **D.** Zidovudine

40. The following drug is a radical curative in vivax malaria __________.
A. Quinine **B.** Primaquine
C. Mefloquine **D.** Chloroquine

41. Chloroquine acts as __________.
A. Pre-erythrocytic schizontocide for both *P. falciparum* and *P. vivax*
B. Erythrocytic schizontocide for both *P. falciparum* and *P. vivax*
C. Exoerythrocytic schizontocide for *P. vivax*
D. Gametocidal for *P. falciparum*

42. Which of the following drugs is suitable for treatment of malaria during pregnancy?
A. Quinine **B.** Chloroquine
C. Pyrimethamine **D.** Primaquine

43. Idoxuridine is indicated in __________.
A. Herpes simplex keratitis
B. Herpes zoster
C. Chickenpox
D. All of the above

44. Which of the following virus is most susceptible to acyclovir?
A. Herpes simplex type I virus
B. Herpes simplex type II virus
C. Varicella-zoster virus
D. Epstein-Barr virus

45. Zidovudine inhibits the following virus/viruses_______.
A. Human immunodeficiency virus
B. Cytomegalovirus
C. Hepatitis B virus
D. Both A and B

46. The virus directed reverse transcriptase enzyme is inhibited by __________.
A. Amantadine
B. Zidovudine
C. Vidarabine
D. Acyclovir

47. Select drug that is active against both HIV and hepatitis B virus.
A. Lamivudine **B.** Indinavir
C. Didanosine **D.** Efavirenz

48. Which sulphonamide have both N1 and N4 substituents?
A. Phthalylsulphathiazole
B. Succinylsulphathaizole
C. Sulfacetamide
D. Both A and B

49. Which anti-malarial drug comes in 4-aminoquinoline group?
A. Mefloquine
B. Mepacrine
C. Chloroquine phosphate
D. Primaquine phosphate

50. Quinine is the chief alkaloid of _________.
A. Cinchona bark
B. Arjuna bark
C. Cinnamon bark
D. Ashoka bark

Answer Key

1 B	2 A	3 B	4 B	5 C	6 A	7 B	8 B	9 C	10 C
11 C	12 C	13 B	14 C	15 B	16 B	17 D	18 B	19 A	20 B
21 D	22 B	23 B	24 A	25 A	26 B	27 A	28 D	29 C	30 C
31 D	32 B	33 A	34 D	35 C	36 B	37 C	38 B	39 C	40 A
41 B	42 A	43 B	44 A	45 C	46 B	47 A	48 D	49 C	50 A

CHAPTER 12

Antibiotics

1. **Which of the following is not β-lactam antibiotics?**
   A. Benzyl penicillin B. Ampicillin
   C. Erythromycin D. Amoxicillin

2. **__________ is an aminoglycoside antibiotic.**
   A. Penicillin B. Streptomycin
   C. Rapamycin D. Nystatin

3. **Penicillin is the first antibiotic discovered by ________.**
   A. Joseph Lister
   B. Paul Elrich
   C. Alexander Fleming
   D. Laborit and Fluguenard

4. **6-(2-phenoxy acetamido) penicillanic acid is a chemical name of ____________.**
   A. Ampicillin B. Amoxicillin
   C. Penicillin G D. Penicillin V

5. **__________ was the first aminoglycoside antibiotic introduced in chemotherapy in 1944 by Waksman.**
   A. Streptomycin B. Neomycin
   C. Gentamicin D. Kenamycin

6. **__________ contains octahydrotetracene-2- carboxamide skeleton as structural unit.**
   A. Penicillins B. Sulphonamides
   C. Cephalosporins D. Tetracyclines

7. **Chlortetracycline was discovered by __________.**
   A. Alexander Fleming B. Dr Waston
   C. Dr Benjamin D. Paul Ehrlich

8. **Erythromycin and Azithromycin are ______________ antibiotics.**
   A. Aminoglycoside
   B. β-lactam
   C. Macrolide
   D. Peptide

9. **The drug effective in pharyngitis and tonsilitis is _______.**
   A. Streptomycin B. Azithromycin
   C. Kanamycin D. Nystatin

10. **________________ is a drug of choice in typhoid and parathyroid.**
    A. Streptomycin B. Azithromycin
    C. Nystatin D. Chromphenicol

11. **Erythromycin belongs to which category?**
    A. β-lactam B. Aminoglycosides
    C. Tetracyclines D. Macrolides

12. **β-lactam consists of how many membered cyclic amides?**
    A. 2 B. 3
    C. 4 D. 5

13. **Alexander Fleming discovered the first antibiotic, penicillin in which year?**
    A. 1922 B. 1928
    C. 1935 D. 1947

14. **Cephalosporins belong to the category of __________.**
    A. Aminoglycoside B. Tetracyclines
    C. Miscellaneous D. β-lactams

15. **Streptomycin acts by binding the bacterial ________ ribosomal subunit.**
    A. 20S B. 30S
    C. 10S D. 50S

16. **Which of the following species is used for producing streptomycin?**
    A. *S. ramosus* B. *S. griseus*
    C. *S. aureofaciens* D. *S. griseoflavus*

17. Which of the following species is used for producing erythromycin?
A. *S. erythreus* B. *S. griseus*
C. *S. aureofaciens* D. *S. griseoflavus*

18. Benzylpenicillin is the chemical name for which of the following penicillin?
A. Penicillin G B. Penicillin V
C. Penicillin F D. Phenethicillin

19. Structurally, all penicillins are __________.
A. β-lactam B. Fluoroquinolone
C. Oxazolidinone D. Monobactam

20. What type of side effect is most commonly observed in β-lactam antibiotics?
A. Hearing loss
B. Aplastic anaemia
C. Allergic reaction
D. Yellowing of teeth

21. Azithromycin belongs to which class of antibiotic?
A. Aminoglycosides
B. Fluoroquinolones
C. Tetracycline
D. Macrolides

22. Which of the following is an aminoglycoside?
A. Penicillin
B. Streptomycin
C. Clindamycin
D. Chloramphenicol

23. Chloramphenicol is used for the treatment of _______.
A. Meningitis B. Plague
C. Typhoid fever D. All of the above

24. ____________ is a fungal infection of nails.
A. Ringworm
B. Onychomycosis
C. Candidiasis
D. Dandruff

25. Candidiasis is caused by _________.
A. *Malassezia furfur*
B. Phialophora spp
C. *C. albicans*
D. *Aspergillus fumigatus*

26. ________ is a gold standard of anti-fungal treatment.
A. Amphotericin B B. Ketoconazole
C. Griseofulvin D. Naftifine HCl

27. UTIs are most commonly caused by ________ bacteria
A. Streptococci B. Staphylococci
C. *H. pylori* D. *E. coli*

28. __________ is the drug of choice for the treatment of typhoid fever.
A. Ampicillin
B. Cotrimoxazole
C. Ciprofloxacin
D. Doxycycline

29. ___________ are first line drugs for chemotherapy of TB.
A. Isoniazid, Rifampicin, Ethambutol
B. Isoniazid, Streptomycin, Thiacetazone
C. Thiacetazone, Para Amino Salicylic (PAS) acid, Amikacin
D. Bedaquiline, Ciprofloxacin, Rifampicin.

30. Rifampicin is used in the treatment of __________.
A. Tuberculosis, Leprosy, Brucellosis
B. Tuberculosis, Typhoid, Cholera
C. Leprosy, Tonsillitis, Pneumonia
D. Tuberculosis, UTIs, RTIs.

31. In Mycobacterium Avium Complex (MVA) infection __________ is given.
A. Isoniazid B. Rifampicin
C. Delamanid D. Ethambutol

32. Example of a DNA virus is __________.
A. Smallpox virus
B. Chickenpox virus
C. Herpes virus
D. All of the above

33. Example of an RNA virus is ___________.
A. Yellow fever
B. German measles
C. Rabies
D. All of the above

34. _____________ is the oldest, cheapest and most widely used drug for the treatment of leprosy.
A. Rifampicin B. INH
C. Dapsone D. Ethambutol

35. Penicillin V drug is an example of ___________.
A. Amino penicillins
B. Penicillinase resistant
C. Carboxypenicillins
D. Natural penicillins

36. In 1945 who elucidated the chemical structure of penicillin?

A. D. Hodgkin
B. Alexander Fleming
C. Sheehan and Ferris
D. Florey and co-workers

37. Oxytetracycline is obtained from ________.

A. *Streptomyces rimoss*
B. *Streptomyces aureofaciens*
C. *Streptomyces kanamycleticus*
D. *Streptomyces tenebrarius*

38. Select the class of antibiotics which act by interfering with bacterial protein synthesis, but are bactericidal ________.

A. Tetracyclines
B. Aminoglycosides
C. Cephalosporins
D. Lincosamides

39. Which of the following antibiotics are derived from *Saccharopolyspora erythraea*.

A. Aminoglycoside antibiotics
B. Tetracycline antibiotics
C. Lincosamide antibiotics
D. Macrolide antibiotics

40. β-lactam antibiotics are the antibiotics that contain a ________ ring in their chemical structure.

A. Beta-lactam
B. Delta-lactam
C. Alpha-lactom
D. Gamma-lactam

Answer Key

1 C	2 B	3 C	4 C	5 A	6 D	7 C	8 C	9 B	10 D
11 D	12 C	13 B	14 D	15 B	16 B	17 A	18 A	19 A	20 C
21 D	22 B	23 D	24 B	25 C	26 A	27 D	28 C	29 A	30 B
31 D	32 D	33 D	34 C	35 D	36 A	37 A	38 B	39 D	40 A

CHAPTER 13

Anti-neoplastic Agents

1. **Which of the following is folate antagonist used as antineoplastic agent?**
   A. Busulphan B. 6-mercaptopurine
   C. Methotrexate D. Chlorambucil

2. **Vinblastin and vincristin are alkaloid drugs used in the treatment of ____________.**
   A. Cough B. Cancer
   C. Constipation D. Plague

3. **_____________ is a platinum containing drug with alkylating properties used as antineoplastic agents.**
   A. Radiogold B. Fluorouracil
   C. Cisplatin D. Actinomycin

4. **If cancer cells originate from the skin epithelial cells what type of cancer is it?**
   A. Myeloma B. Lymphoma
   C. Carcinoma D. Sarcoma

5. **In which phase of the cell cycle, the cells prepare to divide?**
   A. G2 phase B. S phase
   C. M phase D. G1 phase

6. **Cisplatin is classified under __________.**
   A. Antimetabolites
   B. Hormonal agents
   C. Radioisotopes
   D. Alkylating agents

7. **Which drug is an antimetabolite and antifolate agent with antineoplastic and immunosuppressant activities?**
   A. Dactinomycin
   B. Methotrexate
   C. Doxorubicin hydrochloride
   D. Vinblastine sulphate

8. **What are the major targets of alkylating agents on DNA?**
   A. 7-position of guanine
   B. 6-position of guanine
   C. Doxorubicin hydrochloride
   D. 5-position of guanine

9. **Metastasis is a process by which the cancer cells spread through ___________.**
   A. Blood B. Lymph
   C. Both A and B D. Cancer in spinal cord

10. **Which of the following are alkylating agents?**
    A. Cyclophosphamide B. Busulfan
    C. Both A and B D. None of the above

11. **Which of the following is alkyl sulphonate derivative?**
    A. Methotrexate B. Doxorubicin
    C. Fluorouracil D. Busulfan

12. **Chemically, mercaptopurine is __________.**
    A. 3,7-dihydropurine-6-thione
    B. 3,7-dihydropurine-4-thione
    C. 3,6-dihydropurine-6-thione
    D. None of the above

13. **Which of the following is Vinca alkaloid?**
    A. Mercaptopurine B. Methotrexate
    C. Vinblastine D. Doxorubicin

14. **Cyclophosphamide is used in the treatment of ________.**
    A. Leukaemia B. Ovarian cancer
    C. Hodgkin's disease D. All of the above

15. **Which of the following is a synthetic androgenic anabolic steroid?**
    A. Dromostanolone B. Mercaptopurine
    C. Methotrexate D. None of the above

16. Which of the following is folate antagonist?

A. Methotrexate
B. Busulfan
C. Trimetrexate
D. Both A and C

17. Which of the following antibiotics is used for treatment of cancer?

A. Doxorubicin
B. Doxycycline
C. Daunorubicin
D. Both A and C

18. Anti-microbial agent which kills microorganism is known as ___________.

A. Bactericidal
B. Bacteriostatic
C. Antibiotic
D. All of the above

19. Broad-spectrum antibiotics act against _________ microorganisms.

A. Gram-positive
B. Gram-negative
C. Both gram-positive and gram-negative
D. None of the above

20. _________ inhibit cell wall synthesis.

A. Penicillin
B. Tetracyclines
C. DNA gyrase
D. Ciprofloxacin

21. Aminoglycoside antibiotic is _________.

A. Streptomycin
B. Gentamicin
C. Amikacin
D. All of the above

22. ___________ is penicillinase-resistant penicillin.

A. Penicillin G
B. Amoxicillin
C. Cloxacillin
D. All of the above

23. Streptomycin is used in treatment of ___________.

A. TB
B. Plague
C. Subacute bacterial endocarditis
D. All of the above

24. ____________ is the drug of first choice for rickettsial infections.

A. Chloramphenicol
B. Doxycycline
C. Erythromycin
D. None of the above

25. Fluorouracil is ___________.

A. Purine analogue
B. Pyrimidine analogue
C. Folic acid analogue
D. All of the above

26. Chlorambucil is an example of ___________.

A. Alkylating agent
B. Antimetabolite
C. Vinca alkaloid
D. Hormone

27. Which of the following drug is used to treat Hodgkin's disease?

A. Chlorambucil
B. Methotrexate
C. Progestin
D. Vinblastin

28. Cyclophosphamide is particularly used to treat _____.

A. Malignant lymphomas
B. Leukemia
C. Ovarian cancer
D. Myelosclerosis

29. Sacroma is the cancer of ____________.

A. Epithelial tissue
B. Leukemia
C. Lymphomas
D. Mesodermal cell

30. Wilms' tumor treated by

A. Doxorubicin
B. Cyclophosphamide
C. Mitomycin
D. Cisplastin

Answer Key

1 C	2 B	3 C	4 C	5 C	6 D	7 B	8 A	9 C	10 C
11 D	12 A	13 C	14 D	15 A	16 D	17 C	18 A	19 B	20 A
21 A	22 C	23 A	24 A	25 B	26 A	27 D	28 A	29 D	30 A

Section III

Pharmacognosy

1. History of Pharmacognosy
2. Classification of Crude Drugs
3. Quality Control of Drugs
4. Chemical Nature of Crude Drugs
5. Pharmacological Grouping of Crude Drugs
6. Plant Fibres used as Surgical Dressings
7. Basic Principles Involved in the Alternative System of Medicine
8. Role of Medicinal and Aromatic Plants
9. Herbs as Health Food
10. Herbal Cosmetics
11. Phytochemical Investigation of Drugs

Syllabus (As per ER 2020) Pharmacognosy

<table>
<tr><th>Chapter</th><th colspan="2">Topics</th></tr>
<tr><td>1</td><td colspan="2">Definition, History, Present Status and Scope of Pharmacognosy</td></tr>
<tr><td>2</td><td colspan="2">Classification of Drugs
■ Alphabetical
■ Taxonomical
■ Morphological
■ Pharmacological
■ Chemical
■ Chemo-taxonomical</td></tr>
<tr><td>3</td><td colspan="2">Quality Control of Crude Drugs
■ Different methods of adulteration of crude drugs
■ Evaluation of crude drugs</td></tr>
<tr><td>4</td><td colspan="2">Brief outline of occurrence, distribution, isolation, identification tests, therapeutic activity and pharmaceutical applications of alkaloids, terpenoids, glycosides, volatile oils, tannins and resins.</td></tr>
<tr><td>5</td><td colspan="2">Biological source, chemical constituents and therapeutic efficacy of the following categories of crude drugs.</td></tr>
<tr><td></td><td>Laxatives</td><td>Aloe, Castor oil, Ispaghula, Senna</td></tr>
<tr><td></td><td>Cardiotonic</td><td>Digitalis, Arjuna</td></tr>
<tr><td></td><td>Carminatives and GI regulators</td><td>Coriander, Fennel, Cardamom, Ginger, Clove, Black Pepper, Asafoetida, Nutmeg, Cinnamon</td></tr>
<tr><td></td><td>Astringents</td><td>Myrobalan, Black Catechu, Pale Catechu</td></tr>
<tr><td></td><td>Drugs acting on nervous system</td><td>Hyoscyamus, Belladonna, Ephedra, Opium, Tea leaves, Coffee seeds, Coca</td></tr>
<tr><td></td><td>Anti-hypertensive</td><td>Rauwolfia</td></tr>
<tr><td></td><td>Anti-tussive</td><td>Vasaka, Tolu Balsam</td></tr>
<tr><td></td><td>Anti-rheumatics</td><td>Colchicum seed</td></tr>
<tr><td></td><td>Anti-tumour</td><td>Vinca, Podophyllum</td></tr>
<tr><td></td><td>Antidiabetics</td><td>Pterocarpus, Gymnema</td></tr>
<tr><td></td><td>Diuretics</td><td>Gokhru, Punarnava</td></tr>
<tr><td></td><td>Anti-dysenteric</td><td>Ipecacuanha</td></tr>
<tr><td></td><td>Antiseptics and disinfectants</td><td>Benzoin, Myrrh, Neem, Turmeric</td></tr>
<tr><td></td><td>Antimalarials</td><td>Cinchona, Artemisia</td></tr>
<tr><td></td><td>Oxytocic</td><td>Ergot</td></tr>
<tr><td></td><td>Vitamins</td><td>Cod liver oil, Shark liver oil</td></tr>
<tr><td></td><td>Enzymes</td><td>Papaya, Diastase, Pancreatin, Yeast</td></tr>
<tr><td></td><td>Pharmaceutical aids</td><td>Kaolin, Lanolin, Beeswax, Acacia, Tragacanth, Sodium alginate, Agar, Guar gum, Gelatine</td></tr>
<tr><td></td><td>Miscellaneous</td><td>Squill, Galls, Ashwagandha, Tulsi, Guggul</td></tr>
<tr><td>6</td><td colspan="2">Plant fibres used as surgical dressings: Cotton, Silk, Wooland regenerated fibres sutures: Surgical Catgut and Ligatures</td></tr>
</table>

Contd...

7	■ **Basic principles involved in the traditional systems of medicine like:** Ayurveda, Siddha, Unani and Homeopathy ■ **Method of preparation of Ayurvedic formulations like:** Arista, Asava, Gutika, Taila, Churna, Lehya and Bhasma
8	**Role of medicinal and aromatic plants in national economy and their export potential**
9	**Herbs as Health Food** Brief introduction and therapeutic applications of—Nutraceuticals, Antioxidants, Pro-biotics, Pre-biotics, Dietary fibres, Omega-3-fatty acids, Spirulina, Carotenoids, Soya and Garlic
10	**Introduction to Herbal Formulations**
11	**Herbal Cosmetics** Sources, chemical constituents, commercial preparations, therapeutic and cosmetic uses of—Aloe vera gel, Almond oil, Lavender oil, Olive oil, Rosemary oil, Sandalwood oil
12	**Phytochemical Investigation of Drugs**

CHAPTER 1.

History of Pharmacognosy

1. **The word "Pharmacognosy" is derived from two Greek words __________.**
   A. Pharmaco and Analycta
   B. Pharmacon and Gignosco
   C. Drug and Medicine
   D. Analycta and Gignosco

2. **The oldest written documents based on Ayurveda is __________.**
   A. De materia medica
   B. Shushruta samhita
   C. Charaka samhita
   D. Papyrus Ebers

3. **Who is known as the Father of Medicine?**
   A. Aristotle B. Seydler
   C. Hippocrates D. Galen

4. **Crude drugs of natural origin that is obtained from plants, animals, and mineral sources and their active chemical constituents are used in __________.**
   A. Cosmetic B. Textile
   C. Food industry D. All of the above

5. **Galen was a __________ scientist.**
   A. German B. Indian
   C. Greek D. France

6. **Who coined the term pharmacognosy?**
   A. Aristotle B. Seydler
   C. Hippocrates D. Galen

7. **The scientist __________ suggested the principle of classification of animal/study of animal kingdom.**
   A. Galen B. Aristotle
   C. Seydler D. Hippocrates

8. **"De materia medica" was written by __________.**
   A. Aristotle B. Dioscorides
   C. Hippocrates D. Galen

9. **__________ published his thesis o sarsaparilla when he was student.**
   A. Charaka B. Sushruta
   C. Galen D. Seydler

10. **Who is the Father of Surgery?**
    A. Seydler B. Hippocrates
    C. Charaka D. Sushruta

11. **Who developed Galenical Pharmacy?**
    A. Aristotle B. Seydler
    C. Hippocrates D. Galen

12. **The Pharmacognosy is explained in the book _______.**
    A. Medicine
    B. Analecta pharmacognostica
    C. Materia medica
    D. None of the above

13. **The word Ayurveda means _______.**
    A. Science of medicine
    B. Science of life
    C. History of people
    D. Knowledge of crude drug

14. **The branch of pharmacy which deals with extraction of chemical constituents from the plants and animals is called _________.**
    A. Galenical pharmacy
    B. Pharmacognosy
    C. Taxonomy
    D. Chemotaxonomy

15. Who is known as the Father of Ayurveda?

A. Hippocrates
B. Galen
C. Charaka
D. Serturner

16. Who has found the methods of extraction?

A. Aristotle
B. Seydler
C. Hippocrates
D. Galen

17. Who wrote the book Analecta Pharmacognostica?

A. Aristotle
B. Seydler
C. Hippocrates
D. Galen

18. Pharmacognosy includes study of drugs obtained from __________.

A. Synthetic source
B. Natural source
C. Only plants
D. Minerals

19. Papyrus Ebers which contains 700 medicinal herbs and more than 570 formulae is an __________.

A. Indian document
B. Egyptian document
C. American document
D. Pakistani document

20. Who discovered Ayurveda system of medicine?

A. Samuel Hahnemann
B. Galen
C. William Withering
D. Charaka

21. Branches of pharmacognosy are _________.

A. Ethanopharmacology
B. Ethnobotany
C. Phytochemistry
D. All of the above

22. Homoeopathic system is developed in _________.

A. 16th Century
B. 17th Century
C. 18th Century
D. None of the above

23. The plant having multiple stems and shorter height is known as _________.

A. Herb
B. Tree
C. Shrub
D. Creeper

24. Pharmakon means _________.

A. Study
B. Drug
C. Knowledge
D. Chemical

25. Gnosis means__________.

A. Knowledge
B. Science
C. Herbal
D. Drug

26. The name Pharmacognosy is coined in the year _____.

A. 1811
B. 1815
C. 1851
D. 1814

27. Growth of the plant is affected by ________.

A. Altitude
B. Fertilizer
C. Rainfall
D. All of the above

28. Chemical substance present in the plant can be identified by _________.

A. Chemical test
B. Chromatography
C. Both A and B
D. None of the above

29. Who is regarded as a First Pharmacist of the world?

A. Galen
B. Aristotle
C. Hippocrates
D. William Withering

30. Which drug is not under the class of organized drug?

A. Flowers
B. Leaves
C. Gums
D. Fruits

Answer Key

1 B	2 C	3 C	4 D	5 C	6 B	7 B	8 B	9 D	10 D
11 D	12 B	13 B	14 A	15 C	16 D	17 B	18 B	19 B	20 D
21 D	22 C	23 C	24 B	25 A	26 B	27 D	28 C	29 A	30 C

CHAPTER 2.

Classification of Crude Drugs

1. **The reason behind classification of drugs is _________.**
   A. Systematic and scientific study
   B. Easy and convenient method
   C. Helps in practical work
   D. All of the above

2. **_________ is a method of classification of crude drugs used in preparing universal, official references books.**
   A. Morphological **B.** Chemical
   C. Alphabetical **D.** Pharmacological

3. **Dried latex of the following drugs is used, *except* __________.**
   A. Opium **B.** Honey
   C. Papain **D.** Balsam

4. **Which of the following is not a method of classification of crude drugs?**
   A. Alphabetical **B.** Geographical
   C. Pharmacological **D.** Chemical

5. **The roots of following drugs are effective, *except* _______.**
   A. Rauwolfia **B.** Ipecacuanha
   C. Turmeric **D.** Aconite

6. **Which of the following drugs is not under the seed class?**
   A. Nux vomica **B.** Digitalis
   C. Cardamom **D.** Isapgula

7. **Taxonomical method of classification of crude is also known as __________.**
   A. Botanical method **B.** Biological method
   C. Chemical method **D.** Zoological method

8. **Drug which does not belong to leaves class is ________.**
   A. Senna **B.** Digitalis
   C. Eucalyptus **D.** Turmeric

9. **Entire parts of the following drugs are effective, *except* __________.**
   A. Ergot **B.** Belladonna
   C. Ephedra **D.** Clove

10. **Classification of drug based on the chemical similarity of taxon is ___________.**
    A. Chemical classification
    B. Sero-taxonomical classification
    C. Chemo-taxonomical classification
    D. Taxonomical classification

11. **Which one of the following drugs is not come under an organized drug?**
    A. Tulsi **B.** Senna
    C. Clove **D.** Acacia

12. **Taxonomical classification is classified according to ___________ of drug.**
    A. Origin **B.** Nature
    C. Content **D.** All of the above

13. **Chemical classifications of drugs are classified according to__________ of the drug.**
    A. Structure
    B. Active chemical constituent
    C. Therapeutic activity
    D. All of the above

14. **Which of the following drug does not come under the unorganized drug?**
    A. Dried latex
    B. Gums
    C. Resins
    D. Rhizomes

15. Which of the following are the methods of classification of crude drug __________.

A. Morphological classification
B. Pharmacological classification
C. Chemical classification
D. All of the above

16. The crude drugs are divided into the parts of plants like leaves, fruits, flowers, woods, barks, dried lattices, extracts, gums, etc. is ___________.

A. Chemical classification
B. Taxonomical classification
C. Morphological classification
D. Alphabetical classification

17. ___________ is a process of removal of soil, dirt and foreign organic parts from the crude drugs.

A. Garbling B. Drying
C. Collection D. Harvesting

18. Which type of classification indicates whether drug is organized or unorganized?

A. Chemical classification
B. Taxonomical classification
C. Morphological classification
D. Alphabetical classification

19. Which part of Fennel is studied in pharmacognosy as a crude drug?

A. Leaves B. Flowers
C. Fruits D. Steam

20. The crude drugs are obtained from __________

A. Plant
B. Animals
C. Minerals
D. All of the above

21. Volatile oils containing crude drugs are ___________.

A. Coriander
B. Cinnamon
C. Clove
D. All of the above

22. Which classification, drug is arranged in according to their kingdom, phylum, order, family, genus, and species is known as ___________.

A. Chemical classification
B. Morphological classification
C. Taxonomical classification
D. Alphabetical classification

23. Drug not under the class of organized drug is _______.

A. Leaves B. Fruits
C. Flowers D. Gums

24. Drug not under the seed class is __________.

A. Nux vomica B. Isapgula
C. Cardamom D. Senna

25. Cellular drugs are also known as __________.

A. Unorganized drugs B. Organized drugs
C. Both A and B D. None of the above

26. Drug which does not belong to leaves class is ________.

A. Senna B. Digitalis
C. Turmeric D. Eucalyptus

27. The crude drugs are classified according to plants or animals from which they are obtained comes under ___________.

A. Morphological classification
B. Taxonomical classification
C. Pharmacological classification
D. Alphabetical classification

28. Drug which does not belong to fruit class is ________.

A. Artemisia B. Fennel
C. Coriander D. Colocynth

29. Unorganized drugs mean __________.

A. Having thorns B. Having acellular parts
C. Having fibrous parts D. None of the above

30. Leaves of the following drugs are effective, *except* __________.

A. Senna B. Digitalis
C. Vasaka D. Clove

Answer Key

1 D	2 C	3 B	4 B	5 D	6 B	7 A	8 D	9 D	10 C
11 D	12 A	13 B	14 D	15 D	16 C	17 A	18 C	19 C	20 D
21 D	22 C	23 D	24 D	25 B	26 C	27 B	28 A	29 B	30 D

CHAPTER 3

Quality Control of Drugs

1. **Confirmation of identity and determination of quality and purity of crude drug is known as ___________.**
   A. Extraction
   B. Perforation
   C. Chromatography
   D. Evaluation

2. **_______________ means worthless admixture of any material in the genuine drug.**
   A. Evaluation B. Adulteration
   C. Combination D. Cultivation

3. **Stomatal Index in Indian senna is in the range of ____________.**
   A. 17 to 20 B. 20 to 23
   C. 23 to 26 D. 26 to 29

4. **Which of the following is not a method of drug evaluation?**
   A. Biological B. Chemical
   C. Taxonomical D. Microscopical

5. **Vein-islet no. of Indian senna is in the range of _________.**
   A. 10.5 to 12.5 B. 13.5 to 16.5
   C. 16.5 to 18.0 D. 19.5 to 22.5

6. **Morphological method of evaluation is also known as ___________ method.**
   A. Physical B. Organoleptic
   C. Chemical D. Biological

7. **The intentional or deliberate type of adulteration is known as __________.**
   A. Deterioration
   B. Sophistication
   C. Substitution
   D. Spoilage

8. **The detail histological examination of organised crude drug is done by ___________.**
   A. Morphological study
   B. Microscopical study
   C. Physical study
   D. Chemical study

9. **Chemical method of classification of drugs includes determination of ___________.**
   A. Percentage of active chemical constituent
   B. Stomatal index
   C. Taste of crude drug
   D. Viscosity of crude drug

10. **The minute openings on epidermal layer of plant are called ___________.**
    A. Stomata B. Trichomes
    C. Both A and B D. Palisade cells

11. **Ash value and extractive value are the parameters used in ___________ evaluation of crude drug.**
    A. Chemical B. Physical
    C. Morphological D. Microscopical

12. **Cocoa butter is adulterated with ___________.**
    A. Paraffin B. Lard
    C. Limestone D. Kokum butter

13. **Karl Fischer reagent is used to determine ___________.**
    A. Viscosity
    B. Moisture content
    C. Extractive value
    D. Ash value

14. **Almond oil is adulterated with ___________.**
    A. Coconut oil B. Linseed oil
    C. Palm oil D. Cotton seed oil

15. **The average number of stomata present per square mm of the epidermis is called ________.**
    A. Stomatal index B. Palisade ratio
    C. Vein islet number D. Stomatal number

16. **Generally, clove is adulterated with ________.**
    A. Mother clove B. Father clove
    C. Clove stalks D. Both A and C

17. **The mixing of original crude drug partially with other similar looking substances is known as ________.**
    A. Adulteration B. Adulterant
    C. Indirect adulteration D. Direct adulteration

18. **________ is the percentage which the number of stomata forms to the number of epidermal cells.**
    A. Stomatal number
    B. Stomatal index
    C. Palisade ratio
    D. Vein islet number

19. **Reason for doing adulteration is the following *except* one ________.**
    A. Enhancement of profit
    B. Increase its purity
    C. For costly drugs
    D. Scarcity of crude drug

20. **When totally different substance is added in place of original drug is called ________.**
    A. Spoilage B. Sophistication
    C. Admixture D. Substitution

21. **________ is the number of vein islets per sq.mm of leaf surface.**
    A. Stomatal number B. Vein islet number
    C. Palisade number D. Vein number

22. **In substitution with inferior drug type of adulteration, adulterant has similar ________ characters as the original drug.**
    A. Biological B. Chemical
    C. Therapeutic D. Morphological

23. **Substitution with artificially manufactured commodities, this type of adulteration is used for ________.**
    A. Toxic drugs B. Costly drugs
    C. Amorphous drugs D. All of the above

24. **Substitution with exhausted drug this type of adulteration is used mainly for drug containing ________.**
    A. Glycosides B. Alkaloids
    C. Volatile oils D. Resins

25. **Lignified trichomes are the characteristics of ______.**
    A. Senna B. Digitalis
    C. Nux vomica D. Vasaka

26. **The quantitative values determined for the identification of leaf drugs remain constant throughout the age of the plant *except* ________.**
    A. Stomatal number
    B. Vein islet number
    C. Stomatal index
    D. Vein islet termination number

27. **Following chemical tests are used for the identification of alkaloids *except* ________.**
    A. Borntrager's test B. Wagner test
    C. Hager test D. Mayer test

28. **When totally different substance is used in place of the original crude drug is called ________.**
    A. Substitution B. Combination
    C. Cultivation D. Collection

29. **Adulteration in simple word is called ________.**
    A. Sophistication
    B. Substitution
    C. Admixture
    D. Debasement of an article

30. **Asafoetida is adulterated with ________.**
    A. Pieces of amber coloured glass
    B. Limestone
    C. Whitestone
    D. Rodent waste matter

Answer Key

1 D	2 B	3 A	4 C	5 D	6 B	7 B	8 B	9 A	10 A
11 B	12 A	13 B	14 D	15 D	16 D	17 A	18 B	19 B	20 D
21 B	22 D	23 B	24 C	25 C	26 C	27 A	28 A	29 D	30 B

CHAPTER 4

Chemical Nature of Crude Drugs

1. Alkaloids are __________ type of substances.

A. Acid
B. Neutral
C. Chemical
D. Basic nitrogenous

2. __________ contains isoprene units.

A. Alkaloids
B. Glycosides
C. Terpenoids
D. Tannins

3. Glycosides are condensation products of __________.

A. Sugar + aglycone
B. Sugar + Protein
C. Protein + aglycone
D. Fats + aglycone

4. Protoalkaloids are also called __________.

A. Amino alkaloid
B. Pseudoalkaloid
C. True alkaloid
D. Extra alkaloid

5. Phlobatannin is an example of __________.

A. Hydrolysable tannins
B. Condensed tannins
C. Both A and B
D. None of the above

6. Stas-otto process is used for extraction of __________.

A. Glycosides
B. Alkaloids
C. Terpenoids
D. Resins

7. Catechin/matchstick test is a chemical test for __________.

A. Alkaloids
B. Glycosides
C. Resins
D. Tannins

8. Resins are classified into following subclasses *except* __________.

A. Acid
B. Ester
C. Resin alcohol
D. Resin ether

9. __________ are either metabolic or pathological products.

A. Resins
B. Tannins
C. Alkaloids
D. Glycosides

10. Oleo gum resins are mixture of __________.

A. Volatile oil + Gum + Resins
B. Fixed oil + Gum + Resin
C. Fats + Gum + Resin
D. Gum + resins

11. Bontrager's test is an identification test for __________.

A. Tannins
B. Resins
C. Alkaloids
D. Glycoside

12. Asafoetida is an example of __________.

A. Acid resin
B. Ester resin
C. Oleo gum resin
D. Resin alcohol

13. Which of the following identification tests positive for volatile oil?

A. Hydro-distillation method
B. Enfleurage
C. Eucelle method
D. All of the above

14. Which of the following identification tests positive for cardiac glycoside?

A. Borntrager's test
B. Killer-Kiliani test
C. Saponin test
D. All of the above

15. What is the taste of tannins?

A. Pungent
B. Astringent
C. Bitter
D. Sweet

16. Which of the following identification tests positive for tannins?

A. Gold beater skin test
B. Phenazone test
C. Matchstick test
D. All of the above

17. __________ drug is an example of amino alkaloid.

A. Ephedrine
B. Aconine
C. Caffeine
D. Theophylline

18. True alkaloids are always present in plants as ______.

A. Salts of inorganic acid

B. Salts of organic acid

B. Salts of meconic acid

C. Salts of benzoic acid

19. Goldbeater skin test is used for identification of_____.

A. Tannins B. Alkaloids

C. Glycosides D. Resins

20. Resins containing benzoic acid or cinnamic acids are called _________.

A. Oleoresins B. Glycoresins

C. Oleogums D. Balsams

21. Terpenes are made up of _________ units.

A. Calcierene B. Pseudopriene

C. Isoprene D. Neoprene

22. Mayer's test gives which colour?

A. Pale yellow precipitate

B. Dark yellow precipitate

C. Dark red precipitate

D. Yellow precipitate

23. Volatile oils have the following characteristics_______.

A. Evaporate at room temperature

B. Saponify with alkali

C. Used as edible oils

D. None of these

24. Glycosides upon hydrolysis gives __________.

A. Double bonds

B. Sugar and non-sugar molecule

C. Covalent bonds

D. None of the above

25. Datura belongs to the class __________.

A. Isoquinoline B. Tropane

C. Steroidal D. Pyridine

26. Indole alkaloid is biosynthesized from __________.

A. Tyrosine

B. Phenyl alanine

C. Tryptophan

D. Anthranilic acid

27. Which of the following is an example of pseudoalkaloid?

A. Reserpine B. Pilocarpine

C. Ephedrine D. Colchicine

28. Potassium mercuric iodide is _________.

A. Wagner reagent

B. Dragendroff reagent

C. Mayer reagent

D. Hager reagent

29. Tropane alkaloids are derived from ______________ amino acid.

A. Ornithine B. Phenyl alanine

C. Tryptophan D. Lysine

30. Choose the right test for identification of anthraquinones.

A. Marquis test

B. Froehde test

C. Liebermann-Burchard test

D. Borntrager test

31. Which is the right test for the cardioactive glycosides of Foxglove leaf?

A. Murexide

B. Liebermann-Burchard

C. Keller-Kiliani

D. Foam test

32. Which one of the following is S-glycoside?

A. Digoxin B. Sennoside A

C. Aloin D. Sinigrin

33. Psoralen is __________.

A. Coumarin

B. Furanocoumarin

C. Sorbic acid derivative

D. Derivative of barbaloin

34. Sesquiterpene contain which of the following number of isoprene units?

A. One B. Two

C. Three D. Four

35. Guggul is an example of __________.

A. Oleo gum resin B. Glycoresins

C. Balsam D. Oleoresin

36. Flower bud of drug showing medicinal importance is _________.

A. Caraway B. Clove

C. Dill D. Saffron

37. Example of pseudo-alkaloid is __________.

A. Arecoline B. Lobeline

C. Caffeine D. Hygrine

38. Alkaloids _________.

A. Contain nitrogen

B. Have a bitter taste

C. Optically inactive

D. Both A and B

39. Ergot is the __________ of the fungus *Claviceps purpurea*.

A. Vegetative form B. Dried sclerotium
C. Ascospore D. Conidiospore

40. Cocaine is used as __________ in the official medicine.

A. Narcotic
B. Emetic
C. Local anaesthetic
D. Cough suppressant

41. __________ is a latex exudates of the unripe incised capsule after air drying.

A. Ergot B. Opium
C. Guggul D. Cannabis

42. Opium is used in the medicine as __________.

A. Tranquillizer
B. Starting material for morphine production
C. Pain killer
D. Laxative

43. Volatile oils are the complex mixture of __________.

A. Mono and sesquiterpenes as well as phenyl-propane derivatives
B. Mono and Diterpene alcohols and ethers
C. Sesquiterpene and other aromatic compounds
D. Monoterpene acids and lactones

44. Saponin containing drug is used as __________.

A. Laxative B. Bitter tonic
C. Expectorant D. Emetic

45. Which of the following compound can be detected by Mayer's reagent?

A. Starches B. Alkaloids
C. Glycosides D. Resins

46. Which one is the right reagent used for the detection of cardioactive glycoside?

A. Hirschson reagent
B. Baljet reagent
C. Kedde reagent
D. Van-urk reagent

47. __________ can be detected by Keller-Kiliani test.

A. The aglycon of digitalis glycoside
B. The digitoxose of digitalis glycoside
C. Digitoxigenin
D. Strophantidine

48. __________ are the derivatives of polyhydroxy benzoic acid which are capable of precipitation of proteins.

A. Alkaloids B. Glycosides
C. Resins D. Tannins

49. Who has first coined the name alkaloid?

A. SW Pelletier
B. Fredrich Serturner
C. Carl FW Meissner
D. Joseph Caventou

50. Gambeir fluorescein test is used for drug __________

A. Arjuna B. Ashoka
C. Pale catechu D. Black catechu

Answer Key

1 D	2 C	3 A	4 A	5 B	6 A	7 D	8 D	9 A	10 A
11 D	12 C	13 D	14 B	15 B	16 D	17 B	18 B	19 A	20 D
21 C	22 A	23 A	24 B	25 B	26 C	27 C	28 C	29 A	30 C
31 C	32 D	33 B	34 C	35 A	36 B	37 C	38 D	39 B	40 C
41 B	42 C	43 A	44 C	45 B	46 B	47 B	48 D	49 B	50 C

CHAPTER

5

Pharmacological Grouping of Crude Drugs

Laxatives, Cardiotonics, Drugs Acting on CNS, Antihypertensives, Antitussives, Antirheumatics, Antitumour, Antileprotic, Antidysentric, Diuretics, Antimalarials, Oxytocics, Vitamins, Enzymes

1. **Senna belongs to which plant family?**
   A. Rubiaceae B. Liliaceae
   C. Leguminosae D. Solaniaceae

2. **Senna is used to treat __________.**
   A. Diabetes B. Cancer
   C. Constipation D. All of the above

3. **Senna leaf comes under the class of glycoside?**
   A. Cardiac
   B. Cyanogenic
   C. Anthracene
   D. Saponin

4. **Senna mainly contains __________.**
   A. O-glycosides B. N-glycosides
   C. C-glycosides D. S-glycosides

5. **Senna is used to treat which syndrome?**
   A. Acquired immune deficiency syndrome
   B. Irritable bowel syndrome
   C. Ackerman syndrome
   D. Cohen syndrome

6. **Borntrager's test is a chemical test for __________.**
   A. Datura B. Opium
   C. Senna D. Digitalis

7. **Myrrh contains important acid __________.**
   A. Camphoric acid
   B. Abietic acid
   C. Benzoic acid
   D. Acetic acid

8. **Mussabar and Korphad are synonyms of __________.**
   A. Castor oil B. Aloe
   C. Senna D. Liquorice

9. **Ginger contains volatile oil in the percentage range of __________.**
   A. 1–4% B. 5–10%
   C. 10–15% D. 15–20%

10. **Swelling factor test is for __________ drug.**
    A. Digitalis B. Rhubarb
    C. Arjuna D. Isphagula

11. **Modified Borntrager's test is positive for drug _______.**
    A. Aloe B. Senna
    C. Digitalis D. Senna pod

12. **Devil's dung is a synonym of ___________.**
    A. Fennel B. Colchicine
    C. Ephedra D. Asafoetida

13. **Keller-Kiliani test is positive for ___________.**
    A. Digitoxose B. Gitoxose
    C. Digitoxigenin D. Ditoxigenin

14. **Banda soap is synonym of drug __________.**
    A. Asafoetida B. Nutmeg
    C. Liquorice D. Coriander

15. **__________ is not the synonym of Liquorice.**
    A. Glycyrrhiza
    B. Liquorice root
    C. Yam
    D. Mulethi

16. **Swelling factor of Ispaghula is __________.**
    A. 1 to 5 B. 5 to 10
    C. 10 to 14 D. 15 to 20

17. **Which oil is showing laxative property?**
    A. Arachis oil B. Sesame oil
    C. Castor oil D. Corn oil

18. What is the shape of leaves of senna?

A. Needle shape B. Lanceolate shape
C. Obovate shape D. Cordate shape

19. Quercetin is chemical constituent of ___________.

A. Benzoin B. Colophony
C. Black catechu D. Myrrh

20. What is the common adulterant of senna?

A. Indigo dye B. Malic acid
C. Dog senna D. All of the above

21. What is the chief chemical constituent of aloe?

A. Vincristine B. Strychnine
C. Protopine D. Emodin

22. Which of the following is an adulterant of aloe?

A. Malic acid B. Glucose
C. Indigo dye D. Both A and B

23. _______ is used as an ingredient of "triphala churna".

A. Ephedra B. Digitalis
C. Myrobalan D. Vinca

24. Leaves of aloe are __________.

A. Rosette shape B. Thick
C. Fleshy D. All of the above

25. Aloe belongs to family __________.

A. Apocynaceae B. Liliaceae
C. Rubiaceae D. Solaneacae

26. Deadly Nightshade leaf is synonym of drug________.

A. Senna B. Digitalis
C. Vasaka D. Belladona

27. Aloe is used to treat ___________.

A. Vaginal infection B. Allergic reaction
C. Herpes D. All of the above

28. Drug not belonging to volatile oil class is __________.

A. Peppermint B. Clove
C. Castor oil D. Garlic

29. Crow-fig is synonym of __________.

A. Nux vomica B. Ephedrine
C. Nutmeg D. Cardamom

30. Castor oil belongs to which family?

A. Leguminosae B. Euphorbiaceae
C. Liliaceae D. Polygonaceae

31. Ma-hung is synonym of __________.

A. Arjuna B. Ashoka
C. Ephedra D. Tulsi

32. What is the botanical name of Castor oil?

A. *Rudbeckia hirta*
B. *Physalis franchetti*
C. *Ricinus communis*
D. *Ricinus vulgaris*

33. Which of the following is chemical constituent of Tulsi?

A. Carvacrol B. Senna
C. Aloe D. Digitalis

34. Castor oil is used as __________.

A. Cathartics B. Carminative
C. Antihypertensive D. None of the above

35. ___________ contains hydnocarpic acid.

A. Linseed oil B. Arachis oil
C. Chaulmoogra oil D. Lemon grass oil

36. Ispaghula belongs to which family?

A. Leguminosae B. Euphorbiceae
C. Liliaceae D. Plantaginaceae

37. Kino red is a chemical constituent of __________.

A. Pterocarpus B. Gymnema
C. Myrrh D. Fennel

38. What is the botanical name of Ispaghula?

A. *Physalis franchetti*
B. *Ricinus communis*
C. *Plantago ovata*
D. None of the above

39. The drug which increases the force of contraction of cardiac muscle and stimulate heart is called ___________.

A. Cardiotonic B. Antihypertensive
C. Antianginal D. Antiarrhythmic

40. Identify the drug showing cardiotonic activity.

A. Cochineal B. Digitalis
C. Aloe D. Rhubarb

41. What is the botanical name of digitalis?

A. *Digitalis purpurea*
B. *Digitalis cascara*
C. *Digitalis vulgaris*
D. All of the above

42. Synonym of turmeric is __________.

A. Indian gentian B. Indian gooseberry
C. Indian saffron D. Indian kino

43. Digitalis belongs to which plant family?

A. Rubiaceae B. Liliaceae
C. Solaniaceae D. Scrophulariaceae

44. Arjuna is used as __________.

A. Cardiotonic B. Antirheumatic
C. Astringent D. Antileprotic

45. __________ drug is used as an oxytocic.

A. Ephedra B. Ergot
C. Vinca D. Gymnema

46. Digitalis contains which glycoside?

A. Cardiac glycoside
B. Anthraquinone glycoside
C. Saponin glycoside
D. Phenol glycoside

47. Arjuna belongs to which plant family?

A. Rubiaceae B. Combretaceae
C. Solamiaceae D. Scrophulariaceae

48. Amylum is synonym of ________.

A. Senna B. Cinnamon
C. Cardamom D. Starch

49. Digitalis is an example of ________.

A. Cardiotonic B. Antidysenteric
C. Antimalarial D. Antileprotic

50. __________ is chemical constituent of Tragacanth.

A. Quercetin B. Catechin
C. Hyoscine D. Bassorin

51. Synonym of Digitalis is ________.

A. Fox glove leaves B. Arjuna bark
C. Fox new leaves D. Fox grow leaves

52. The drugs which expel the flatulence and gas from the GIT are called _________.

A. Carminative B. Laxative
C. Hypertensive D. Cardiotonic

53. What is the botanical name of coriander?

A. *Foeniculum vulgare*
B. *Coriandrum sativum*
C. *Eugenia caryophyllus*
D. *Zingiber officinale*

54. Japanese Isinglass is a synonym of __________.

A. Acacia B. Agar
C. Aconite D. Aloe

55. What is the botanical name of ginger?

A. *Foeniculum vulgare*
B. *Coriandrum sativum*
C. *Eugenia caryophyllus*
D. *Zingiber officinale*

56. What is the botanical name of fennel?

A. *Foeniculum vulgare*
B. *Coriandrum sativum*
C. *Eugenia caryophyllus*
D. *Zingiber officinale*

57. What is the botanical name of clove?

A. *Foeniculum vulgare*
B. *Coriandrum sativum*
C. *Eugenia caryophyllus*
D. *Zingiber officinale*

58. Synonym of Dioscorea is ________.

A. Yam B. Mel
C. Kutki D. Shatmuli

59. What is the botanical name of Ajowan?

A. *Piper nigrum*
B. *Coriandrum sativum*
C. *Trachyspermum ammi*
D. *Zingiber officinal*

60. Allicin is a chemical constituent of ________.

A. Garlic B. Gelatin
C. Guar gum D. Gokharu

61. What is the botanical name of Nutmeg?

A. *Piper nigrum*
B. *Coriandrum sativum*
C. *Myristica fragrans*
D. *Ferula foetida*

62. Which of the following drugs is used as dental analgesic?

A. Fennel B. Cardamom
C. Ginger D. Clove

63. Jasmoline is chemical constituent of _________.

A. Pterocarpus B. Pyrethrum
C. Punarnava D. Papaya

64. Fennel belongs to which plant family?

A. Rubiaceae B. Umbelliferae
C. Zingiberaceae D. Myrtaceae

65. Clove belongs to which plant family?

A. Rubiaceae B. Umbelliferae
C. Zingiberaceae D. Myrtaceae

66. Vitamin C (ascorbic acid) is chemical constituent of __________.

A. Amla B. Arjuna
C. Ashoka D. Aconite

67. Coriander belongs to which plant family?
A. Rubiaceae B. Umbelliferae
C. Zingiberaceae D. Myrtaceae

68. Asafoetida belongs to which plant family?
A. Rubiaceae B. Umbelliferae
C. Zingiberaceae D. Myrtaceae

69. Galls are used as __________.
A. Carminative B. Cardiotonic
C. Astringent D. Antihypertensive

70. Ginger belongs to which plant family?
A. Rubiaceae B. Umbelliferae
C. Zingiberaceae D. Myrtaceae

71. Nutmeg belongs to which plant family?
A. Rubiaceae B. Umbelliferae
C. Zingiberaceae D. Myristicaceae

72. Nicotine is chemical constituent of _________.
A. Pyrethrum B. Neem
C. Tobacco D. Turmeric

73. Ajowan belongs to which plant family?
A. Rubiaceae B. Umbelliferae
C. Zingiberaceae D. Myristicaceae

74. Shatavari is used as __________.
A. Hydrogogue B. Sialogogue
C. Galactogogue D. Hemagogue

75. Cinnamon belongs to which plant family?
A. Lauraceae B. Umbelliferae
C. Zingiberaceae D. Myristicaceae

76. The drug which causes precipitation of protein is known __________.
A. Astringent B. Antihypertensive
C. Antianginal D. Antiarrhythmic

77. Identify the drug showing cardiotonic activity ______.
A. Cochineal B. Digitalis
C. Aloe D. Rhubarb

78. Synonym of linseed oil is ___________.
A. Flax seed B. Cotton seed
C. Nux vomica seed D. Cardamom seed

79. What is the botanical name of Myrobalan?
A. *Terminalia chebula*
B. *Terminalia officinalis*
C. *Terminalia cascara*
D. *Terminalia ledergina*

80. What is the botanical name of Black Catechu?
A. *Terminalia arjuna*
B. *Terminalia chebula*
C. *Terminalia officinalis*
D. *Uncaria gambier*

81. Family of Black Catechu is __________.
A. Combretaceae B. Liliaceae
C. Leguminosae D. Scrophulariaceae

82. Pale Catechu belongs to which plant family?
A. Combretaceae B. Rubiaceae
C. Leguminosae D. Scrophulariaceae

83. Shark liver oil contains __________.
A. Vit. K B. Vit. D
C. Vit. C D. Vit. B_1

84. Botanical name of Opium is __________.
A. *Papaver somniferum*
B. *Terminalia chebula*
C. *Atropa acuminate*
D. *Hyoscymus niger*

85. What is the botanical name of tea leaves?
A. *Coffea arabica*
B. *Terminatia officinalis*
C. *Theobroma cocoa*
D. *Thea sinesis*

86. Hyoscyamus belongs to which plant family?
A. Combretaceae B. Liliaceae
C. Solaniaceae D. Scrophulariaceae

87. Which one of the following is not a stage of life cycle of Ergot?
A. Over wintering stage
B. Stage of flowering
C. Stage of sexual reproduction
D. Stage of asexual reproduction

88. Belladonna belongs to which plant family?
A. Solaniaceae B. Liliaceae
C. Leguminosae D. Scrophulariaceae

89. Opium belongs to which plant family?
A. Combretaceae B. Papaveraceae
C. Leguminosae D. Scrophulariaceae

90. The drugs which have stimulant action on the motility of uterus are called ___________.
A. Astringents B. Oxytocics
C. Carditonics D. Carminative

91. Tea leaves belong to which plant family?
A. Theaceae B. Papaveraceae
C. Leguminosae D. Scrophulariaceae

92. Coca belongs to which plant family?
A. Theaceae B. Papaveraceae
C. Leguminosae D. Sterculiaceae

93. Worm seed is synonym of __________.
A. Arjuna B. Aloe
C. Artemisia D. Aconite

94. Synonym of Hyoscymus is __________.
A. Henbane B. Hencone
C. Hensome D. Hyobromide

95. A synonym of Ephedra is __________.
A. Ma-Haung B. Ephedrine
C. Ma-nung D. Mittha Katha

96. A synonym of tea leaves is __________.
A. Thesa leaves B. Camellia thea
C. Carmoline thea D. Charmolin etheae

97. Curcumin is chemical constituent of __________.
A. Tulsi B. Tolu balsam
C. Turmeric D. Tragacanth

98. The drug containing hyoscyamine is __________.
A. Hyoscyamus B. Belladonna
C. Both A and B D. Coffee

99. Which drug has stimulant action on CNS?
A. Ephedra B. Cocca
C. Coffee D. Belladonna

100. The drug which lowers elevated blood pressure to normal level is called __________.
A. Cardiotonic B. Antihypertensive
C. Antianginal D. Antiarrhythmic

101. Identify the drug showing antihypertensive activity __________.
A. Cochineal B. Digitalis
C. Rauwolfia D. Rhubarb

102. What is the botanical name of Rauwolfia/ sarpagandha?
A. *Rauwolfia sarpagandha*
B. *Rauwolfia sarpentina*
C. *Rauwolfia officinalis*
D. *Rauwolfia vulgaris*

103. Rauwolfia belongs to which plant family?
A. Rubiaceae B. Liliaceae
C. Solaniaceae D. Apocyanaceae

104. Harmin and Harman are chemical constituents of __________.
A. Gokharu B. Guggul
C. Gulvel D. Guar Gum

105. Rauwolfia is used as __________.
A. Cardiotonic B. Antidysenteric
C. Antihypertensive D. Antileprotic

106. Digitalis contain __________.
A. Cardiac glycosides
B. Anthraquinone glycosides
C. Reserpine
D. Phenol

107. What is the botanical name of Vasaka?
A. *Adhatoda vasica*
B. *Myroxy lonbalsamum*
C. *Adhatoda vasaka*
D. None of the above

108. Synonym of Vasaka is __________.
A. Adhatoda B. Adulsa
C. Both A and B D. None of the above

109. Ipecacuanha and Kurchi are used as __________.
A. Antidysenteric B. Antimalarial
C. Antiamoebic D. Antiviral

110. Vasaka belongs to family__________.
A. Acanthaceae B. Leguminosae
C. Combretaceae D. Solaniaceae

111. Tolu balsam belongs to family __________.
A. Acanthaceae B. Leguminosae
C. Combretaceae D. Solaniaceae

112. The drugs which increase rate of urine formation are called __________.
A. Diuretics B. Carminative
C. Cardiotonics D. Galactogogue

113. Vasicine is a chief chemical constituent of__________.
A. Vasaka B. Vinca
C. Arjuna D. Aconite

114. The botanical name of Colchium seed is __________.
A. *Colchicum luteum* B. *Colchicum luenum*
C. *Colchicum lederginum* D. *Colchicum officinalis*

115. Colchium seeds are used in treatment of __________.
A. Rheumatism B. Expectorant
C. Cardiotonic D. Laxative

116. The botanical name of Vinca is _________.

A. *Catharanthus officinalis* B. *Catharanthus roseus*
C. *Catharanthus restoreae* D. *Catharanthus phyllus*

117. What is the botanical name of Podophylum?

A. *Podophyllum hexandrum*
B. *Podophyllum hexanum*
C. *Podophyllum hexonal*
D. *Podophyllum phylaceae*

118. Vinca contain which alkaloid?

A. Indole B. Tropane
C. Phenol D. None of the above

119. Guggul is used as _________.

A. Antimalarial B. Antirheumatic
C. Antigout D. Antitumour

120. What is the synonym of Vinca?

A. Periwinkle B. Sacred basil
C. Chotachand D. Hydocorpus

121. Vinca belongs to which family?

A. Combretaceae B. Liliaceae
C. Podophyllaceae D. Apocyanaceae

122. Holy basil is a synonym of _________.

A. Vasaka B. Turmeric
C. Tulsi D. Vinca

123. The drug which is used in treatment of diabetes is called _________.

A. Astringent B. Antihypertensive
C. Antidiabetics D. Antiarrhythmic

124. Identify the drug showing antidiabetic activity.

A. Gymnema B. Pterocarpus
C. Jambhul D. All of the above

125. Chhotachand is synonym of _________.

A. Rauwolfia B. Belladonna
C. Hyoscymus D. Ashwgandha

126. Family of Gymnema is _________.

A. Asclepiadaceae B. Liliaceae
C. Solaniaceae D. Scrophulariaceae

127. Pterocarpus belongs to which plant family?

A. Combretaceae B. Liliaceae
C. Leguminosae D. Scrophulariaceae

128. Brucine is chemical constituent of _________.

A. Nutmeg B. Nux vomica
C. Neem D. Cinnamon

129. Synonyms of Gymnema is _________.

A. Kattha B. Indian kino tree
C. Fox new leaves D. Madhu nashini

130. A synonym of Pterocarpus is _________.

A. Madhu nashini B. Indian kino tree
C. Fox new leaves D. Mittha Katha

131. The botanical name of Punarnava is _________.

A. *Boerhavia diffusa* B. *Boerhavia ledergina*
C. *Terminalia chebula* D. *Uncaria gambir*

132. What is the botanical name of Gokhru?

A. *Boerhavia diffusa* B. *Tribulus terrestris*
C. *Terminalia chebula* D. *Uncaria gambir*

133. Monkshood is synonym of _________.

A. Acacia B. Aconite
C. Ashoka D. Agar

134. Gokharu belongs to which family?

A. Combretaceae B. Liliaceae
C. Solaniaceae D. Zygophyllaceae

135. Puncture vine is a synonym of _________.

A. Gokharu B. Punarnava
C. Vinca D. Vasaka

136. Which of the following is used as diuretic?

A. Gokharu B. Punarnava
C. Both A and B D. Vasaka

137. Ipecacuanha contains which alkaloid?

A. Quinoline B. Isoquinoline
C. Quinidine D. Phenol

138. The botanical name of benzoin is _________.

A. *Styrax benzoin* B. *Commiphora molmol*
C. *Azadiarachta indica* D. *Curcuma longa*

139. What is the botanical name of myrrh?

A. *Styrax benzoin* B. *Commiphora molmol*
C. *Azadiarachta indica* D. *Curcuma longa*

140. Bishop's weed is synonym of _________.

A. Ajowan B. Lineed oil
C. Cotton seed D. Nux vomica seed

141. The botanical name of neem is _________.

A. *Styrax benzoin* B. *Commiphora molmol*
C. *Azadiarachta indica* D. *Curcuma longa*

142. Marijuana is a synonym of _________.

A. Tobacco B. Neem
C. Pyrethrum D. Cannabis

143. What is the botanical name of turmeric?

A. *Styrax benzoin*
B. *Commiphora molmol*
C. *Azadiarachta indica*
D. *Curcuma longa*

144. Turmeric belongs to which plant family?

A. Styraceae
B. Burseraceae
C. Meliaceae
D. Zingiberaceae

145. Loban is synonym of __________.

A. Benzoin
B. Myrrh
C. Neem
D. Turmeric

146. A synonym of neem is __________.

A. Loban
B. Gum myrrh
C. Margosa
D. Indian saffron

147. Which of the following drug is used as expectorant?

A. Rauwolfia
B. Nux vomica
C. Guggul
D. Vasaka

148. A synonym of turmeric is __________.

A. Loban
B. Gum myrrh
C. Morgosa
D. Indian saffron

149. *Squill* and *Strophanthus* are used as __________.

A. Tranquilizers
B. Cardiotonic
C. Carminatives
D. Antigout

150. Synonym of ashwagandha is __________.

A. Indian Saffron
B. Indian Gentian
C. Indian Ginseng
D. Indian Hemp

Answer Key

1 C	2 C	3 C	4 A	5 B	6 C	7 A	8 B	9 A	10 D
11 A	12 D	13 A	14 B	15 C	16 C	17 C	18 B	19 C	20 C
21 D	22 D	23 C	24 D	25 B	26 D	27 D	28 C	29 A	30 B
31 C	32 C	33 A	34 A	35 C	36 D	37 A	38 C	39 A	40 B
41 A	42 C	43 D	44 A	45 B	46 A	47 B	48 D	49 A	50 D
51 A	52 A	53 B	54 B	55 D	56 A	57 C	58 A	59 C	60 A
61 C	62 D	63 B	64 B	65 D	66 A	67 B	68 B	69 C	70 C
71 D	72 C	73 B	74 C	75 A	76 A	77 B	78 A	79 A	80 D
81 A	82 A	83 B	84 A	85 A	86 C	87 B	88 A	89 B	90 B
91 A	92 D	93 C	94 A	95 A	96 B	97 C	98 C	99 C	100 B
101 C	102 B	103 D	104 A	105 C	106 A	107 A	108 C	109 A	110 A
111 B	112 A	113 A	114 A	115 A	116 B	117 A	118 A	119 B	120 A
121 D	122 C	123 C	124 D	125 A	126 A	127 C	128 B	129 D	130 B
131 A	132 B	133 B	134 D	135 A	136 C	137 B	138 A	139 B	140 A
141 C	142 D	143 D	144 D	145 A	146 C	147 D	148 D	149 B	150 C

CHAPTER 6.

Plant Fibres used as Surgical Dressings

1. **The material used for covering the wound is ________.**
   A. Threads
   B. Ligatures
   C. Sutures
   D. Surgical dressing

2. **Cotton fibres are obtained from __________.**
   A. Cocoons of Antheraea
   B. Epidermal trichomes
   C. Cocoons of Ungulata
   D. Fleece of *Ovies aries*

3. **__________ is a mineral fibre.**
   A. Wool
   B. Silk
   C. Glass
   D. Jute

4. **Cotton consists of __________.**
   A. Protrin-Tobulin
   B. Protein-Keratin
   C. Cellulose
   D. Protein-Myosin

5. **Botanical name of cotton is __________.**
   A. *Cannabis sativa*
   B. *Linium usitatissimum*
   C. *Gossipium herbaceum*
   D. *Ovies aries*

6. **Cotton belongs to family __________.**
   A. Cannabinaceae
   B. Tiliaceae
   C. Bovidae
   D. Malvaceae

7. **Cotton is used as __________.**
   A. Surgical dressing
   B. Filtering media
   C. Insulating material
   D. All of the above

8. **Cotton is soluble in __________.**
   A. NaOH
   B. H_2SO_4
   C. HCl
   D. None of the above

9. **Banana is a __________ fibre.**
   A. Mineral B. Animal
   C. Synthetic D. Plant

10. **Silk fibres are obtained from _________.**
    A. Cocoons of Antheraea
    B. Cocoons of *Bombyx mori*
    C. Cocoons of Ungulata
    D. Fleece of *Ovies aries*

11. **Silk consists of protein __________.**
    A. Tobulin B. Keratin
    C. Fibroin D. Myosin

12. **Silk fibroin on hydrolysis yields amino acids ________.**
    A. Fibroin and keratin
    B. Glycine and alanine
    C. Tyrosine and alanine
    D. None of the above

13. **__________ is a synthetic fibre.**
    A. Terylene B. Glass
    C. Silk D. Wool

14. What is the biological name of silk?

A. *Ovies aries*
B. *Cannabis sativa*
C. *Bombyx mori*
D. *Linium usitatissimum*

15. Silk belongs to family _________.

A. Cannabinaceae B. Bombycidae
C. Tiliaceae D. Bovidae

16. Synonym of jute is _________.

A. Mussabar B. Gunny
C. Gossypol D. Korphad

17. Silk is used as _________.

A. Ligatures B. Sutures
C. Sieves D. All of the above

18. Wool fibers are obtained from _________.

A. Cocoons of *Bombyx mori*
B. Fleece of *Ovies aries*
C. Cocoons of Antheraca
D. Cocoons of Ungulata

19. Wool consists of protein _________.

A. Keratin B. Tobulin
C. Myosin D. Fibroin

20. Which amino acid is present in wool fibre?

A. Alanine
B. Cystine
C. Keratin
D. None of the above

21. Wool belongs to family _________.

A. Canabinaceae B. Bovidae
C. Bombycidae D. Tiliaceae

22. Gossypol is synonym of _________.

A. Rayon B. Terylene
C. Cotton D. Jute

23. Wool is used as _________.

A. Surgical dressing
B. Filtering media
C. Straining media
D. All of the above

24. Cotton is the example of _________.

A. Animal fibre
B. Plant fibre
C. Mineral fibre
D. Synthetic fibre

25. Jute belongs to which family _________.

A. Malvaceae
B. Leguminosae
C. Tiliaceae
D. Rutaceae

26. Epidermal trichomes or hairs of the seeds of Gossypium species are known as _________.

A. Silk B. Jute
C. Wool D. Cotton

27. Silk contains a protein known as _________.

A. Albumin B. Lysin
C. Keratin D. Fibroin

28. Rayon is also known as _________.

A. Regenerated hexose
B. Regenerated pentose
C. Regenerated cellulose
D. Regenerated erythrose

29. Bast fibres are separated from stem by _________.

A. Peeling B. Retting
C. Mulching D. Cutting

30. Example of bast fibre from seed is _________.

A. Flax B. Bamboo
C. Soya D. Palm

31. Example of bast fibre from grass is _________.

A. Coir B. Agave
C. Hemp D. Bamboo

32. Dietary fibres are used for _________.

A. Astringent
B. Laxative
C. Antioxidant
D. Anti-tussive

33. Pulping process is used to remove the _________.

A. Mineral
B. Lignin
C. Cellulose
D. None of the above

34. "Asbestos" is an example of _________.

A. Animal fibre
B. Wool fibre
C. Mineral fibre
D. Synthetic fibre

35. Cotton fibres are separated from seeds by _________.

A. Retting B. Ginning
C. Plucking D. Peeling

36. Hemp contains __________.

A. High cellulose and low protein

B. High lignin and low cellulose

C. High lignin and low protein

D. High cellulose and low lignin

37. Fabric is prepared from_________.

A. Chitin

B. Cellulose

C. Hemicellulose

D. Yarn or thread

38. Jute is obtained from which part of the plant _____.

A. Wood B. Stem

C. Leaves D. Roots

39. _________ gives black precipitate when treated with lead acetate in caustic soda.

A. Rayon B. Silk

C. Wool D. Flax

40. Wool is prepared from __________.

A. Skin B. Bones

C. Scalp D. Fleece

Answer Key

1 D	2 B	3 C	4 C	5 C	6 B	7 D	8 B	9 D	10 B
11 C	12 B	13 A	14 C	15 B	16 B	17 D	18 B	19 B	20 B
21 B	22 C	23 D	24 B	25 C	26 D	27 D	28 C	29 B	30 C
31 D	32 B	33 B	34 C	35 B	36 D	37 D	38 B	39 C	40 D

CHAPTER

7

Basic Principles Involved in the Alternative System of Medicine

Ayurvedic, Siddha, Unani, Homeopathic

1. The word Ayurveda means ________.

A. History of people

B. Science of life

C. Science of medicine

D. Knowledge of crude drugs

2. Panchamahabhuta is related to _________.

A. Siddha B. Ayurveda

C. Unani D. Homeopathy

3. The two basic Vedas of Ayurveda are ________.

A. Vatta and Kapha

B. Pitha and Rigveda

C. Rigveda and Atharvaveda

D. Vipaka and Prabhava

4. Tridosha theory is related to ________.

A. Siddha B. Unani

C. Homeopathic D. Ayurveda

5. Who developed the homeopathic system of medicine?

A. Hippocrates B. Samuel Hahnemann

C. Galen D. CA Seydler

6. The aromatherapy treatment is done by _________.

A. Alkaloids B. Tannins

C. Volatile oils D. Glycosides

7. Which of the following is the fermented infusion?

A. Avaleha B. Ghrita

C. Gutika D. Asava

8. _______ are the natural fermented liquid preparation.

A. Gutika and Churnas

B. Asava and Arista

C. Avaleha and Ghrita

D. All of the above

9. The literature of Sidhha is mostly found in language __________.

A. Marathi B. Hindi

C. English D. Tamil

10. Which of the following is the fermented decoction?

A. Gutika B. Arista

C. Avaleha D. Chrita

11. __________ is the sugar based semi-solid preparations for oral use.

A. Gutika B. Arista

C. Avaleha D. Ghrita

12. Sidhha system is originated in ________.

A. West India

B. South India

C. East India

D. North India

13. _________ are the medicated clarified butters.

A. Arista B. Avaleha

C. Ghrita D. Gutika

14. ___________ is the fine powder of herbal drugs.

A. Churna B. Ghrita

C. Avaleha D. Arista.

15. ___________ is the solid dosage form in the form of pills or tablets.

A. Churna B. Ghrita

C. Paka D. Gutika

16. Lehya is also known as ___________ .

A. Ghrita B. Paka

C. Avleha D. Gutika

17. **In Ayurveda, *Tarkchikitysa* means ___________.**
    A. GIT medicines
    B. Psychological medicine
    C. Orthopaedic medicine
    D. Gynaecological medicine

18. **Which of the following are not the elements of Tridosha theory?**
    A. Vata B. Beta
    C. Pitta D. Kapha

19. **Who is known as the Father of Ayurveda?**
    A. Hippocrates B. Galen
    C. Charaka D. Serturner

20. **According to Ayurveda, Tridosha are __________.**
    A. Vata, Raktta, Pitta
    B. Vata, Rasa, Kapha
    C. Vata, Rakta, Kapha
    D. Vata, Pitta, Kapha

21. **Which is the Perso-Arabic system of medicine?**
    A. Ayurveda B. Unani
    C. Siddha D. Yoga

22. **According to Unani medicine, human body contains _________ elements.**
    A. Three B. Four
    C. Six D. Five

23. **Ayurveda system of medicine was first practiced in which country?**
    A. Greece B. India
    C. Egypt D. China

24. **The Unani System of Medicine includes __________.**
    A. Vatta, Pitta, Kapha B. Madar, Fulfal, Kabab
    C. Like cures like D. Bhakti and Yoga

25. **Aristas and Asavas are preparations in the form of __________.**
    A. Semisolid B. Solid
    C. Alcoholic preparations D. Tablets

26. **Aristas and Asavas are fermented for _________.**
    A. Removal of alcohol
    B. Liberation of alcohol
    C. Removal of water
    D. Liberation of water

27. **Dr Samuel Hahnemann found __________.**
    A. Law of similar B. Law of difference
    C. Law of addition D. Law of substraction

28. **Gutikas are _________.**
    A. Liquid preparations
    B. Solid preparations
    C. Semisolid preparations
    D. Emulsified preparations

29. **Tailas are ________.**
    A. Solid preparations
    B. Semisolid preparations
    C. Emulsified preparations
    D. Liquid preparations

30. **"Veda" stands for __________.**
    A. Life B. Soul
    C. Mind D. Knowledge

31. **"Pitta" is belonging to _________.**
    A. Panchabhuta B. Kapha
    C. Doshas D. Vedas

32. **"Kapha" is composed of _________.**
    A. Fire and water B. Air and water
    C. Water and earth D. Air and earth

33. **The term naturopathy was coined by ___________ in 1895.**
    A. Dr Samuel Hahnemann
    A. Serturner
    B. Hippocrate
    C. Dr John Scheel

34. **Siddha medicine system originated from ________.**
    A. Tamil Nadu
    B. Karnataka
    C. Kerala
    D. Andhra Pradesh

35. **In Ayurveda, *Agadha Tantra* mean. ________.**
    A. Entomology
    B. Toxicology
    C. Psychology
    D. Mycology

36. **"Vaadham" stands for __________.**
    A. Fire B. Earth
    C. Air D. Water

37. **Metals used in Siddha system are ________.**
    A. Mercury and gold
    B. Mercury and sulphur
    C. Sulphur and gold
    D. Gold and copper

38. Which one does not belong to Unani treatment?
A. Naum-o-Yaqzah
B. Hawa
C. Harkat-wo-Mashroob
D. Harkat-o-sakoonnafsaniah

39. "Dau-S-Sadaf" is known as _______.
A. Psoriasis B. Vatiligo
C. Hepatitis D. Fever

40. As per Homeopathy system, potency indicates with the symbol _______.
A. C B. P
C. X D. M

41. "Like cures Like" is the principle of _______.
A. Homeopathy B. Ayurveda
C. Unani D. Siddha

42. Among three *Doshas* in Ayurveda, which *Dosha* is a combination of water and earth?
A. Vata B. Kapha
C. Pitta D. Both A and B

43. In Ayurveda, each *Dosha* is comprised of basic _____ elements.
A. Four B. Five
C. Two D. Eight

44. The main locations of Pitta in the body are the following *except:*
A. Small intestine
B. Spleen
C. Pancreas
D. All of the above

45. Ayurveda is sub-divided into _______ disciplines.
A. Four B. Five
C. Two D. Eight

46. Medicines prepared in the form of tablets or pills are known as _______.
A. Taila B. Lehya
C. Churna D. Gutika

47. Leha and Paka are the synonyms of which preparation?
A. Asava B. Gutika
C. Avaleha D. Artistha

48. Homeopathy was developed in the late 18th century by _______.
A. Aesculapius
B. Samuel Hahnemann
C. Hippocrates
D. Galen

49. Which system of medicines was originated from Dravidian?
A. Unani B. Ayurveda
C. Homeopathy D. Siddha

50. Which system of medicines believed in "like cures like"?
A. Unani
B. Homeopathy
C. Ayurveda
D. Siddha

Answer Key

1 B	2 B	3 C	4 D	5 B	6 C	7 D	8 B	9 D	10 B
11 C	12 B	13 C	14 A	15 D	16 C	17 B	18 B	19 A	20 D
21 B	22 D	23 B	24 B	25 C	26 B	27 A	28 B	29 D	30 D
31 C	32 C	33 C	34 A	35 B	36 C	37 B	38 C	39 A	40 C
41 A	42 B	43 B	44 D	45 D	46 D	47 C	48 B	49 D	50 B

CHAPTER 8

Role of Medicinal and Aromatic Plants

1. MAPs stand for ________.

A. Medicinal and phytochemicals
B. Medicinal and aromatic plants
C. Medicinally active plants
D. None of the above

2. Aromatic plants are defined as those plants which possess ________ in them.

A. Alkaloids B. Glycosides
C. Essential oil D. Flavonoids

3. Which of the following system of medicine is originated in India?

A. Unani B. Chinese
C. Homeopathy D. Ayurveda

4. Which of the following plants contains essential oils?

A. Cinchona B. Sandalwood
C. Rauwolfia D. Senna

5. Which of the following plants contains drug at its bark for curing heart disease?

A. Mango B. Cinchona
C. Arjuna D. Tobacco

6. Ephedrine is used to treat _________.

A. Asthma and hay fever
B. Skin disease
C. Malaria
D. Dengue

7. Which of the following diseases can be cured by using the extract of Vasaka leaf?

A. Cholera B. Tetanus
C. Cold and cough D. Malaria

8. Taxol is used as ________.

A. Antiseptic B. Anticancer
C. Anti-inflammatory D. Astringent

9. The World Health Organization (WHO) estimated that __________ of the population of developing countries relies on traditional medicines.

A. 10% B. 20%
C. 80% D. 40%

10. Which of the following plants is used as purgative?

A. Aloe vera B. Cassia fistula
C. Digitalis purpura D. Plantago ovata

11. The herbal drug market itself is growing at a rate of between ___________ annually.

A. 40% and 60%
B. 60% and 80%
C. 20% and 30%
D. 80% and 100%

12. Cinchona is a native of _______.

A. India B. China
C. Indonesia D. South America

13. Currently, according to industry estimate, total pharmaceutical market is around ________.

A. ₹ 10,000 crore
B. ₹ 5,000 crore
C. ₹ 20,000 crore
D. ₹ 40,000 crore

14. Which of the following leaves is used as mosquito repellent?

A. Eucalyptus B. Digitalis
C. Senna D. Cassia

15. Essential oils are used in making __________ in cooking, in the food, pharmaceutical, cosmetics liquor industries.

A. Cardiotonic **B.** Perfumes
C. Laxative **D.** Analgesic

16. Codeine is an alkaloid obtained from _______.

A. *Papaver somniferum*
B. *Emblica officinalis*
C. *Carum copticum*
D. *Piper nigram*

17. Which constituent in the mint is responsible for bitter cooling taste and harsh odour?

A. Cinthol **B.** Fenchone
C. Terpene **D.** Menthol

18. Which of the following leaves are used in diabetes?

A. Digitalis **B.** Senna
C. *Gymnema sylvestre* **D.** Vasaka

19. *Rauvolfia serpentina* is termed a snake root plant because ________.

A. It possesses venomous poison
B. It smells like snakes
C. It is used in snakebite
D. Its roots appear snake-like

20. The richest source of vitamin C is _______.

A. *Capsicum fruitescence*
B. *Emblica officinalis*
C. Orange
D. Lemon

Answer Key

1 B	2 C	3 D	4 B	5 C	6 A	7 C	8 B	9 C	10 D
11 C	12 D	13 B	14 A	15 B	16 A	17 D	18 C	19 C	20 B

CHAPTER 9

Herbs as Health Food

1. **Herbs are defined as plant with _________.**
   - **A.** Aromatic properties
   - **B.** Flavouring properties
   - **C.** Medicinal property
   - **D.** All of the above

2. **Nutraceuticals are used to _________.**
   - **A.** Treat diseases
   - **B.** Prevent the occurrence of diseases
   - **C.** Cure the diseases
   - **D.** None of the above

3. **Spirulina belongs to which family _________.**
   - **A.** Leguminosae
   - **B.** Liliaceae
   - **C.** Oscillatoriceae
   - **D.** Zygophylaceae

4. **Herbal medicines usually contain __________.**
   - **A.** Specific pharmacological compound
   - **B.** A range of pharmacologically active compounds
   - **C.** Pharmacologically inactive compound
   - **D.** Toxic compound

5. **Soya belongs to which family __________.**
   - **A.** Oscillatoriceae
   - **B.** Liliaceae
   - **C.** Zygophylaceae
   - **D.** Leguminosae

6. **Garlic belongs to which family __________.**
   - **A.** Leguminosae
   - **B.** Oscillatoriceae
   - **C.** Liliaceae
   - **D.** Zygophylaceae

7. **Carotenoids are C40 compounds of which groups?**
   - **A.** Allide **B.** Amide
   - **C.** Glycoside **D.** Terpenoids

8. **Which substances increase the activity of probiotics?**
   - **A.** Prebiotics **B.** Antioxidant
   - **C.** Nutraceuticals **D.** Vitamins

9. **Botanical name of garlic is ___________.**
   - **A.** *Spirulina plantensis*
   - **B.** *Alium sativum*
   - **C.** *Glycine soya*
   - **D.** *Digitalis purpurea*

10. **Probiotics are ___________.**
    - **A.** Chemical substances
    - **B.** Pathogenic bacteria
    - **C.** Helpful bacteria
    - **D.** Nutrients

11. **Polyunsaturated fatty acids (PUFAs) helps in _______.**
    - **A.** Controlling diabetes
    - **B.** Reduce bad cholesterol levels
    - **C.** Fight cancer
    - **D.** Prevent infections

12. **Dietary fibre intake is essential because ___________.**
    - **A.** It prevents infection
    - **B.** Corrects constipation
    - **C.** Helps in digestion
    - **D.** None of the above

13. **Spirulina is obtained from ___________.**
    - **A.** Higher plants **B.** Blue green algae
    - **C.** Animals **D.** Insects

14. **Which of the pharmacological agent is present in periwinkle?**
    A. Vinblastine
    B. Vincristine
    C. Both A and B
    D. None of the above

15. **Which of the following nutraceuticals play a role in immune system?**
    A. Soyabean
    B. Wheat
    C. Carotenoids
    D. Alpha-lipoic acid

16. **Lactobacillus acidophilus is a ___________.**
    A. Vitamin B. Enzyme
    C. Probiotic D. Prebiotics

17. **DHA stands for __________.**
    A. Docosahexaenoic acid
    B. Docosahydranoic acid
    C. Docosaheptanoic acid
    D. None of the above

18. **Beta-carotene is present in the following food sources *except* __________.**
    A. Red peppers B. Mango
    C. Carrot D. Broccoli

19. **Inulin is __________.**
    A. Probiotic B. Vitamin
    C. Prebiotics D. Enzyme

20. **__________ has immunostimulant action.**
    A. Coriander B. Spirulina
    C. Fennel D. Senna

Answer Key

1 C	2 B	3 C	4 B	5 D	6 C	7 D	8 A	9 B	10 C
11 B	12 B	13 B	14 C	15 C	16 C	17 A	18 A	19 C	20 B

CHAPTER 10

Herbal Cosmetics

1. Study of use of medicinal plants are known as ________.

A. Herbarium B. Pharmacognosy
C. Herbalism D. None of the above

2. Herbal drugs are preparations prepared by ________.

A. Decoction B. Infusion
C. Maceration D. All of the above

3. Triphala churna is an example of the following herbal formulations __________.

A. Bhasma B. Churna
C. Tailas D. Gutika

4. _____________ is used as a perfume in cosmetics and incense sticks.

A. Sandalwood oil B. Olive oil
C. Rosemary oil D. Arachis oil

5. Vatika and Gutika available in the following dosage __________

A. Tablets and pills
B. Tablets and capsule
C. Tablets and powder
D. Tablets and paste

6. Herbs are defined as plants with __________.

A. Aromatic property B. Medicinal property
C. Flavouring property D. All of the above

7. Dravaka's are prepared by which of the following processes?

A. Extraction B. Distillation
C. Evaporation D. Drying

8. "King of Nuts" is a synonym of __________.

A. Sandalwood oil B. Olive oil
C. Almond oil D. Aloe

9. Leha and Paka is following type of preparations of drugs _________.

A. Solid B. Liquid
C. Semisolid D. Gaseous

10. How to apply Lepa?

A. External application on the body
B. Internal application
C. Both A and B
D. None of the above

11. ___________ is one of the most well-known essential oil used in aromatherapy.

A. Almond oil B. Olive oil
C. Lavender oil D. Rosemary oil

12. Which type of medicine, whose formulations are reported in books?

A. Classical Ayurvedic medicine
B. Proprietary medicine
C. Siddha medicine
D. Unani medicine

13. Which of the following are the factors affecting herbal formulation?

A. Drug adulteration
B. Faulty drug collection
C. Incorrect storage
D. All of the above

14. Which of the following come under novel drug delivery dosage forms ___________.

A. Herbal syrups B. Herbal ointments
C. Phytosomes D. Herbal mixtures

15. Phytosomes contain active herbal ingredients surrounded and bonded by __________.

A. Phospholipids
B. Nanoparticles
C. Solutions
D. None of the above

16. Traditional herbal formulations include _________.

A. Tablets
B. Syrups
C. Mixtures
D. All of the above

17. __________ is rich in vitamins A and E.

A. Aloe vera
B. Almond oil
C. Lavender oil
D. Olive oil

18. Herbal mixtures are the preparations containing __________.

A. Single herb
B. Combination of one or more herbs
C. Novel dosage forms
D. None of the above

19. Herbal tablets are prepared by ___________.

A. Melting the ingredients
B. Sieving and filtering
C. Sterilising
D. Moulding and compression

20. Amygdaline glycoside is a constituent of which oil?

A. Lavender oil
B. Sandalwood oil
C. Rosemary oil
D. Almond oil

21. Sandalwood oil is also known as __________.

A. Rosemary oil B. Olive oil
C. Chandan oil D. Almond oil

22. Herbal cosmetic product having ___________.

A. Skin healing properties
B. Skin smoothening properties
C. Conditioning properties
D. All of the above

23. Prunus amygdalus var is the biological source of____.

A. Aloe vera gel
B. Almond oil
C. Lavender oil
D. Olive oil

24. Softening skin and soothing effect is obtained by ___________.

A. Aloe vera gel B. Almond oil
C. Lavender oil D. Olive oil

25. Aloe vera gel is prepared from the plant ___________.

A. Ginger
B. Korphad
C. Almond oil
D. Olive oil

26. Linalyl acetate and linalool are chemical constituents of ___________.

A. Aloe vera gel B. Almond oil
C. Lavender oil D. Olive oil

27. Which oil is used therapeutically in urinary tract infection?

A. Lavender oil
B. Sandalwood oil
C. Clove oil
D. Almond oil

28. Which oil is used as a vehicle in parenteral doses?

A. Lavender oil B. Almond oil
C. Sandalwood oil D. Clove oil

29. Which of the following is used in the treatment of disturbance of menstrual dysfunction?

A. Lavender oil
B. Sandalwood oil
C. Aloe vera gel
D. Almond oil

30. "Kumari" is a common name for ____________.

A. Aloe B. Rhubarb
C. Senna D. Digitalis

31. Lavender oil belongs to which family ___________.

A. Oleaceae B. Laminaceae
C. Rosaceae D. Liliaceae

32. Almond oil belongs to which family ___________.

A. Oleaceae B. Liliaceae
C. Rosaceae D. Labiatae

33. Olive oil belongs to which family ____________.

A. Rosaceae B. Liliaceae
C. Oleaceae D. Labiatae

34. Which drug contain palmitic acid?

A. Olive oil B. Almond oil
C. Sandalwood oil D. Rosemary oil

35. Formulation development of herbal cosmetics includes __________.

A. Functional ingredients
B. Supportive ingredients
C. Structural ingredients
D. All of the above

36. Sandalwood oil contains __________.

A. Rhein
B. Emodin
C. Santalol
D. Reserpine

37. Which of the following is used as a colorant?

A. Aloe-emodin
B. Anthocyanins
C. Volatile oils
D. None of the above

38. Biological source of olive oil is __________.

A. Olea europoea
B. Santalum album
C. Prunus amygdalus
D. None of the above

39. Almond plant belongs to which family __________.

A. Umbelliferae
B. Rubiaceae
C. Leguminosae
D. Rosaceae

40. Kumariasava is a commercial preparation __________.

A. Almond oil
B. Aloe vera
C. Sandalwood oil
D. Olive oil

Answer Key

1 C	2 D	3 B	4 A	5 A	6 D	7 B	8 C	9 C	10 A
11 C	12 C	13 D	14 C	15 A	16 D	17 B	18 B	19 D	20 D
21 C	22 D	23 B	24 A	25 B	26 C	27 B	28 B	29 C	30 A
31 B	32 C	33 C	34 B	35 D	36 C	37 B	38 A	39 D	40 B

CHAPTER 11

Phytochemical Investigation of Drugs

1. **The technique used for separation of active principle from the crude drug is called __________.**
   A. Evaporation B. Drying
   C. Extraction D. Filtration

2. **____________ investigation refers to the extraction, screening and identification of the medicinally active substances found in the plants.**
   A. Biological B. Phytochemical
   C. Physical D. Taxonomical

3. **Foam test is used for identification of __________.**
   A. Glycosides B. Alkaloids
   C. Tannins D. Saponins

4. **Following is chromatography technique used for __________.**
   A. Isolation crude drug B. Purification crude drug
   C. Both A and B D. None of the above

5. **Klunges test is used for identification of the drug __________.**
   A. Aloe B. Senna
   C. Digitalis D. Cardamom

6. **Hager's test is used to identify __________.**
   A. Alkaloids B. Glycosides
   C. Tannins D. None of the above

7. **Vitali-Morin test is used for the drug ___________.**
   A. Cascara B. Datura
   C. Belladonna D. Opium

8. **Which of the following test is used to identify tannins?**
   A. Wagner's test
   B. Dragendorff's test
   C. Ferric chloride test
   D. None of the above

9. **Fieche's test is used for ___________.**
   A. Agar B. Tragacanth
   C. Honey D. Ginger

10. **Shinoda's test is used to identify ___________.**
    A. Tannins B. Flavonoids
    C. Alkaloids D. None of the above

11. **Keller-Kiliani is the specific test to detect __________.**
    A. Flavonoids B. Deoxy sugars
    C. Glycoside D. Saponins

12. **Which of the test is used for the identification of anthraquinones?**
    A. Borntrager's test
    B. Liebermann-Burchard test
    C. Shinoda test
    D. Foam test

13. **Which test for identification of Carbohydrates ______.**
    A. Keller-Kiliani test
    B. Liebermann-Burchard test
    C. Fehling test
    D. Foam test

14. **Salkowski test is positive for ___________.**
    A. Deoxy sugars B. Saponins
    C. Triterpenoids D. Glycoside

15. **The following tests are used for the detection of carbohydrates *except* __________.**
    A. Molish test B. Fehling test
    C. Benedict test D. Foam test

16. **Which of the following is a test for cotton?**
    A. Vitali-Morin test B. Keller-Kiliani test
    C. Halaphenes test D. Foam test

17. The following tests are used for the detection of cardiac glycosides, *except* __________.

A. Keller-Killiani test
B. Legal's test
C. Millon's test
D. Baljet's test

18. Guignard test is used for __________.

A. Lavender oil
B. Linseed oil
C. Rosemary oil
D. Cotton seed oil

19. Given the following tests are used for the detection of proteins and amino acids, *except* __________.

A. Biuret test
B. Xanthoprotein test
C. Millon's test
D. Spot test

20. Aluminium chloride colorimetric assay is used for the detection of __________.

A. Phenolics
B. Glycoside
C. Alkaloids
D. Flavonoids

Answer Key

1 C	2 B	3 D	4 C	5 A	6 A	7 B	8 C	9 C	10 B
11 C	12 A	13 C	14 C	15 D	16 C	17 C	18 B	19 D	20 B

Section IV

Human Anatomy and Physiology

1. Scope of Anatomy and Physiology
2. Structure of Cell
3. Tissues of the Human Body
4. The Osseous System (The Skeleton)
5. The Haemopoietic System (The Blood)
6. The Lymphatic System
7. The Cardiovascular System (The Blood Circulation)
8. The Respiratory System
9. The Digestive System
10. The Skeletal Muscles
11. The Nervous System
12. The Sense Organs
13. The Urinary System (The Renal System)
14. The Endocrine System (Hormonal Coordination)
15. The Reproductive System

Syllabus (As per ER 2020) Human Anatomy and Physiology

Chapter	Topics
1	Scope of anatomy and physiology and definition of various terminologies
2	**Structure of Cell:** Components and its functions
3	**Tissues of the Human Body:** Epithelial, connective, muscular and nervous tissues—their sub-types and characteristics.
4	**Osseous system:** Structure and functions of bones of axial and appendicular skeleton Classification, types and movements of joints, disorders of joints
5	**Haemopoietic System** ■ Composition and functions of blood ■ Process of Hemopoiesis ■ Characteristics and functions of RBCs, WBCs, and platelets ■ Mechanism of blood clotting ■ Importance of blood groups
6	**Lymphatic System** ■ Lymph and lymphatic system, composition, function and its formation. ■ Structure and functions of spleen and lymph node.
7	**Cardiovascular System** ■ Anatomy and Physiology of heart ■ Blood vessels and circulation (pulmonary, coronary and systemic circulation) ■ Cardiac cycle and heart sounds, basics of ECG ■ Blood pressure and its regulation
8	**Respiratory System** ■ Anatomy of respiratory organs and their functions. ■ Regulation, and mechanism of respiration. ■ Respiratory volumes and capacities—definitions
9	**Digestive System** ■ Anatomy and physiology of the GIT ■ Anatomy and functions of accessory glands ■ Physiology of digestion and absorption
10	**Skeletal Muscles** ■ Histology ■ Physiology of muscle contraction ■ Disorder of skeletal muscles
11	**Nervous System** ■ Classification of nervous system ■ Anatomy and physiology of cerebrum, cerebellum, midbrain ■ Function of hypothalamus, medulla oblongata and basal ganglia ■ Spinal cord—structure and reflexes ■ Names and functions of cranial nerves. ■ Anatomy and physiology of sympathetic and parasympathetic nervous system (ANS)

Contd...

12	**Sense Organs: Anatomy and Physiology of** ■ Eye ■ Ear ■ Skin ■ Tongue ■ Nose
13	**Urinary System** ■ Anatomy and physiology of urinary system ■ Physiology of urine formation ■ Renin-angiotensin system ■ Clearance tests and micturition
14	**Endocrine System (hormones and their functions)** ■ Pituitary gland ■ Adrenal gland ■ Thyroid and parathyroid gland ■ Pancreas and gonads
15	**Reproductive System** ■ Anatomy of male and female reproductive system ■ Physiology of menstruation ■ Spermatogenesis and oogenesis ■ Pregnancy and parturition

CHAPTER 1

Scope of Anatomy and Physiology

1. **The word anatomy is derived from a Greek word _________.**
   A. Analogy B. Annatto
   C. Anatome D. None of the above
2. **Branch of science that studies the structure of the body _________.**
   A. Physiology B. Anatomy
   C. Homeostasis D. Pathophysiology
3. **The study of tissues is called __________.**
   A. Cytology B. Histology
   C. Anatomy D. Physiology
4. **The study of the function of the body __________.**
   A. Anatomy B. Physiology
   C. Cytology D. Histology
5. **__________ means part "towards the middle" of the body.**
   A. Lateral B. Medial
   C. Proximal D. Superior
6. **The ability to maintain a stable internal environment means __________.**
   A. Stimulus B. Hemopoiesis
   C. Homeostasis D. Response
7. **__________ is a hollow cavity within the bone.**
   A. Sinus B. Condyle
   C. Facet D. Suture
8. **The sagittal plane divides the human body into ______.**
   A. Upper and lower portions
   B. Superior and inferior portions
   C. Left and right portions
   D. Ventral and dorsal portions
9. **Lungs are situated in __________ body cavity.**
   A. Cranial B. Abdominal
   C. Pelvic D. Thoracic
10. **The largest hollow space in the human body is _________.**
    A. The abdominal cavity
    B. The cranial cavity
    C. The pelvic cavity
    D. The thoracic cavity
11. **The part of the structure nearest to a given point is called __________.**
    A. Distal B. Medial
    C. Proximal D. Inferior
12. **The digestion of food takes place in __________.**
    A. Liver B. Heart
    C. Stomach D. Colon
13. **______________ means a line across at right angle to the axis.**
    A. Lateral B. Traverse
    C. Ventral D. Longitudinal
14. **__________ provides an outer covering that protects the body from the external environment.**
    A. Skin
    B. Respiratory
    C. Urinary
    D. Cardiovascular
15. **The fluid portion of blood is called __________.**
    A. Interstitial fluid B. Plasma
    C. Tissue fluid D. Platelets
16. **A tube-shaped cavity within the bone is __________.**
    A. Sinus B. Facet
    C. Condyle D. Meatus

17. **The self-correcting process that helps to maintain stability and restore a homeostatic set point is known as __________.**
    A. Stimulus
    B. Negative feedback
    C. Sensor
    D. Positive feedback

18. **The basic smallest, living, structural and functional unit of the body is called __________.**
    A. Tissue B. Neurone
    C. Cell D. Nephron

19. **The hormone which helps to maintain glucose homeostasis by stimulating liver cells to take up and remove additional glucose is __________.**
    A. Glucagon B. Pancreas
    C. Response D. Insulin

20. **Fixed joint between bones of the skull and cranium is called __________.**
    A. Sulcus B. Suture
    C. Sinus D. Septum

21. **Which system of the body functions for the exchange of oxygen and carbon dioxide between air and blood?**
    A. Respiratory
    B. Cardiovascular
    C. Endocrine
    D. Nervous

22. **Which of the following describes the division of the body by a transverse plane?**
    A. Left and a right
    B. A front and a back
    C. A top and a bottom
    D. An inside and an outside

23. **__________ is a small flat articulating surface.**
    A. Condyle B. Facet
    C. Sinus D. Fossa

24. **The word anatomy is derived from two Greek words which means __________.**
    A. Ana up and tempos up
    B. Ana up and tempos cutting
    C. Ana down and tempos superior
    D. Ana up and tempos axial

25. **The branch of anatomy that deals with the study of specific part of the body __________.**
    A. Gross anatomy
    B. Regional anatomy
    C. Macroscopic anatomy
    D. None of the above

26. **Anatomical term used for 'nearer to midline of body' means**
    A. Fossa B. Foramen
    C. Medial D. Lateral

27. **Following are the body cavities *except* __________.**
    A. Cranial B. Abdominal
    C. Pectoral D. Pelvic

28. **The part of the structure away from a given point means __________.**
    A. Proximal end B. Median
    C. Distal end D. Lateral

29. **Various types of organs join to form a __________.**
    A. Cells B. System
    C. Muscles D. Tissue

30. **__________ means a hole in a structure.**
    A. Sinus B. Foramen
    C. Meatus D. Suture

31. **It is a portion separating two cavities called __________.**
    A. Septum B. Sinus
    C. Meatus D. Suture

32. **Name the term used for 'structure away from the head' __________.**
    A. Superior B. Border
    C. Inferior D. Dorsal

33. **Which one of the following requires magnification/ microscopy to study __________.**
    A. Gross anatomy
    B. Regional anatomy
    C. Histology
    D. Surface anatomy

34. **The other name for anterior __________.**
    A. Dorsal B. Caudal
    C. Ventral D. Cranial

35. **Myology is the study of __________.**
    A. Muscles
    B. Bones
    C. Cartilages
    D. All of the above

36. **Study of blood vessels is called __________.**
    A. Cardiology B. Angiology
    C. Haematology D. Serology

37. The urinary bladder is located in __________ region

A. Umbilical
B. Right inguinal
C. Hypogastric
D. Left inguinal

38. __________ means upper end of the body.

A. Superior
B. Inferior
C. Frontal
D. Ventral

39. A double fold of peritoneum which suspend an organ from the back body wall is called _________.

A. Visceral peritoneum
B. Omentum
C. Mesentery
D. Ligament

40. Tissue found in the outer layer of skin, lining of organs, blood and lymph vessels and body cavities ________.

A. Epithelial tissue
B. Connective tissue
C. Muscle tissue
D. Nerve tissue

Answer Key

1 C	2 B	3 B	4 B	5 B	6 C	7 A	8 C	9 D	10 A
11 C	12 C	13 B	14 A	15 B	16 D	17 B	18 C	19 D	20 B
21 A	22 C	23 B	24 B	25 B	26 C	27 C	28 C	29 B	30 B
31 A	32 C	33 C	34 C	35 A	36 B	37 C	38 A	39 C	40 A

CHAPTER 2

Structure of Cell

1. __________ is the basic living structural and functional unit of the body.
   A. Organ B. Tissue
   C. Organism D. Cell

2. Which organelle of the cell is concerned with autolysis?
   A. Ribosomes B. Golgi bodies
   C. Lysosomes D. Oxysomes

3. Which of the following cell organelles is called the store/powerhouse/energy coin of the cell?
   A. Nucleus
   B. Mitochondria
   C. Lysosomes
   D. Chloroplast

4. __________ is a jelly-like substance found floating inside the plasma membrane.
   A. Cell sap B. Karyoplasm
   C. Cytoplasm D. Mitochondria

5. The cell organelles regulate the entry and exit of molecules is __________.
   A. Lysosomes
   B. Golgi bodies
   C. Mitochondria
   D. Cell membrane

6. Mitochondria is the storehouse or powerhouse of __________.
   A. Fats B. Glucose
   C. ATP D. Glycogen

7. Oxidative enzymes occur mostly in __________.
   A. Lysosomes B. Golgi bodies
   C. Ribosomes D. Mitochondria

8. __________ cell organelles is called a suicidal bag.
   A. Golgi bodies B. Lysosomes
   C. Cell membrane D. Mitochondria

9. Which of the following cell organelles is absent in prokaryotic cells?
   A. Nucleus
   B. Lysosome
   C. Endoplasmic reticulum
   D. All of the above

10. The cell organelles involved in the storage of food, and other nutrients, required for a cell to survive is __________.
    A. Lysosome B. Vacuoles
    C. Mitochondria D. Cell membrane

11. Which of the following cell organelles is involved in the breakdown of organic matter?
    A. Cytoplasm B. Golgi bodies
    C. Mitochondria D. Lysosomes

12. __________ is involved in the synthesis of phospholipids.
    A. Smooth endoplasmic reticulum
    B. Mitochondria
    C. Cytoplasm
    D. Endoplasmic reticulum

13. Which of the following cell organelles is present in plant cells and absent in animal cells?
    A. Nucleus B. Chloroplast
    C. Vacuole D. Cytoplasm

14. Mitochondria are related to __________.
    A. Plastids B. Prokaryotes
    C. Plasmids D. Viruses

15. **The following is a site for cellular respiration?**
A. Nucleus B. Ribosomes
C. ER D. Mitochondria

16. **DNA is present in __________.**
A. Carboxysomes
B. Mitochondria and chloroplast
C. Ribosomes
D. Lysosomes

17. **Centre of phosphorylation is __________.**
A. Peroxisomes B. Ribosomes
C. Oxysome D. Mitochondria

18. **Who observed the 'mitochondria' first?**
A. Albert Von Kolliker B. Robert Brown
C. Robert Hook D. Altmann

19. **ATP is formed in _________.**
A. Nucleus B. Nucleolus
C. Mitochondria D. Ribosomes

20. **The most important function of endoplasmic reticulum is __________.**
A. Nourishing the nucleus
B. Secretion of materials
C. Protein synthesis
D. To give shape to the cell

21. **The endoskeleton of a cell is made up of _________.**
A. Endoplasmic reticulum
B. Cell wall
C. Cytoplasm
D. Mitochondria

22. **Golgi body originated from _________.**
A. Lysosomes
B. Mitochondria
C. Cell membrane
D. Endoplasmic reticulum

23. **The major role of Golgi bodies is _________.**
A. Fermentation B. Glycosidation
C. Phosphorylation D. Translocation

24. **_________ is a site for citric acid, beta-oxidation, urea cycle and ETS, etc.**
A. Golgi complex B. Lysosomes
C. Mitochondria D. Microsomes

25. **The 80S ribosomes are present in _________.**
A. Prokaryotic cells
B. Eukaryotic cells
C. Bacterial cells
D. Cyanobacterial cells

26. **The substances passing through semipermeable membrane depends on the following factors *except* _________.**
A. Particle size
B. Concentration
C. Lipid solubility
D. Acidity

27. **In prokaryotic ribosomes RNA protein ratio is ________.**
A. 3:1 B. 2:1
C. 1:1 D. None of the above

28. **Which of the following cell organs is involved in the breakdown of cellular organic matter?**
A. Ribosomes B. Microsomes
C. Lysosomes D. Autosomes

29. **__________ controls all cellular activities.**
A. Nucleolus B. Mitochondria
C. Nucleus D. Ribosomes

30. **Nucleoli are rich in __________.**
A. DNA and RNA
B. DNA
C. DNA, RNA and proteins
D. RNA

31. **The rupture/breakdown of cell membrane or cell wall and inducing death of the cell is known as _________.**
A. Autolysis
B. Phagocytosis
C. Thrombosis
D. Embolism

32. **DNA was first discovered by _________.**
A. Friedrich Miescher
B. Beadle and Tatum
C. Watson and Crick
D. Kornberg

33. **All of the following are stages of cell division *except* _________.**
A. Prophase B. Metaphase
C. Telophase D. Betaphase

34. **The study of human body cells is termed ________.**
A. Mycology
B. Cytology
C. Physiology
D. None of the above

35. **Aerobic respiration is performed by _________.**
A. Mitochondria
B. Peroxisomes
C. Ribosomes
D. None of the above

36. **The term "suicidal bags" is used for ________.**
A. Peroxisomes B. Lysosomes
C. Mitochondria D. None of the above

37. **Ribosomal subunits are synthesized in ________.**
A. Nucleoplasm B. Cytoplasm
C. Nucleolus D. None of the above

38. **The function of protein sorting, lipid sorting and secretion is performed by ________.**
A. Golgi apparatus B. Rough ER
C. Smooth ER D. None of the above

39. **Chromosome duplication occurs in which of the following phases?**
A. G1 phase B. S phase
C. G2 phase D. Prophase

40. **Endoplasmic reticulum is the centre of ________.**
A. Excretion
B. Blood formation
C. Protein synthesis
D. Carbohydrate synthesis

41. **The network of endoplasmic reticulum is present in the ________.**
A. Cytoplasm B. Chromosome
C. Nucleolus D. Nucleus

42. **Nucleus is the centre of ________.**
A. Digestion B. Gene control
C. Protein synthesis D. Excretion

43. **Chromosomes are present in ________.**
A. Nucleolus B. Cytoplasm
C. Lysosomes D. Nucleus

44. **Mitochondria contain ________.**
A. DNA only B. RNA only
C. Ribosomes only D. All of the above

45. **The name "mitochondria" was given by ________.**
A. Vira B. Flemming
C. Carl Benda D. Palade

46. **________ is a matrix or ground substance in which various cellular components are found.**
A. Nucleus B. Cytoplasm
C. Mitochondria D. Lysosomes

47. **The random movements of molecules from area of high concentration to the area of low concentration is called ________.**
A. Facilitated diffusion B. Osmosis
C. Simple diffusion D. Filtration

48. **________ special type of diffusion referring to the passage of water through a selectively permeable membrane from an area of high-water concentration to lower water concentration.**
A. Osmosis
B. Simple diffusion
C. Facilitated diffusion
D. Filtration

49. **F1 particles /oxysomes are present in ________.**
A. Golgi complex B. Mitochondria
C. Nucleus D. Ribosomes

50. **Which of the following is known as "digestive apparatus of the cell"?**
A. Oxysomes B. Ribosomes
C. Lysosomes D. Microsomes

Answer Key

1 D	2 C	3 B	4 C	5 D	6 C	7 D	8 B	9 D	10 B
11 D	12 A	13 B	14 A	15 D	16 B	17 C	18 A	19 C	20 C
21 A	22 D	23 B	24 C	25 B	26 D	27 B	28 C	29 C	30 C
31 A	32 A	33 D	34 B	35 A	36 B	37 C	38 A	39 B	40 C
41 A	42 B	43 D	44 D	45 C	46 B	47 C	48 A	49 B	50 C

CHAPTER 3

Tissues of the Human Body

1. **The group of cells having similar physical characters and performing same specialized function are called __________.**
   - A. Glands
   - B. Tissues
   - C. Systems
   - D. Organs
2. **Epithelial tissue serves as ___________.**
   - A. Protective covering
   - B. Reproductive structure
   - C. Corpuscles
   - D. None of the above
3. **The following are primary tissues of the body *except***
   - A. Muscle tissue
   - B. Nervous tissue
   - C. Bone tissue
   - D. Connective tissue
4. **Epithelial cells that are adapted for absorption or secretion usually have _________ at their free surface.**
   - A. Many mitochondria
   - B. Nuclei
   - C. Microvilli
   - D. Golgi complexes
5. **Schwann cells are present in __________.**
   - A. Nervous tissue
   - B. Muscle tissue
   - C. Connective tissue
   - D. All of the above
6. **The epithelium that is found lining internal body compartments, blood vessels, and lungs is _________.**
   - A. Simple squamous
   - B. Stratified squamous
   - C. Simple cuboidal
   - D. Stratified cuboidal
7. **The type of epithelium found where absorption or secretion takes place and is found in the kidney tubules is ___________.**
   - A. Simple squamous
   - B. Simple cuboidal
   - C. Stratified squamous
   - D. Transitional
8. **Cells that store fat are called ___________.**
   - A. Fibroblasts
   - B. Macrophages
   - C. Adipose cells
   - D. Mast cells
9. **The muscle tissue which shows no striations is ________.**
   - A. Skeletal muscle
   - B. Smooth muscle
   - C. Cardiac muscle
   - D. Voluntary muscle
10. **The muscle that is located in the walls of hollow internal organs is ___________.**
    - A. Skeletal muscle
    - B. Smooth muscle
    - C. Cardiac muscle
    - D. Voluntary muscle
11. **Cells that remove damaged cells or pathogens from connective tissue are ___________.**
    - A. Fibroblasts
    - B. Adipocytes
    - C. Melanocytes
    - D. Macrophages
12. **Covering of lungs is called ___________.**
    - A. Pericardium
    - B. Pleura
    - C. Peritoneum
    - D. Serosa
13. **___________ is a fluid connective tissue.**
    - A. Bone
    - B. Cuboidal
    - C. Blood
    - D. Cartilage
14. **Ciliated epithelium lines the ___________.**
    - A. Tracheal and fallopian tube
    - B. Bile duct and ureter
    - C. Trachea and oesophagus
    - D. Pharyngeal and stomach mucosae
15. **Squamous epithelium coils are found in __________.**
    - A. Lungs
    - B. Stomach
    - C. Uriniferous tubule
    - D. Testis

16. Ciliated epithelium is found in __________.

A. Ovary and trachea
B. Nephron and trachea
C. Lung and trachea
D. Liver and trachea

17. _______ tissues maintain posture/position of the body.

A. Epithelial B. Connective
C. Muscular D. Nervous

18. Ligaments and tendons are __________.

A. Connective tissue
B. Muscular tissue
C. Fibrous connective tissue
D. Skeletal tissue

19. The strongest cartilage is __________.

A. Fibrous cartilage
B. Hyaline cartilage
C. Elastic cartilage
D. None of the above

20. _______ is a process of formation of RBCs in the red bone marrow.

A. Phagocytosis B. Hemopoiesis
C. Autolysis D. Haemolysis

21. Reticular connective tissue is found in __________.

A. Stomach B. Spleen
C. Kidneys D. Skin

22. The tissue present in umbilical cord is __________.

A. Fatty connective tissue
B. Reticular connective tissue
C. Mucous connective tissue (Wharton's Jelly)
D. Pigmented connective tissue

23. Which of the following muscle gets into fatigue very early __________.

A. Skeletal muscle B. Smooth muscle
C. Cardiac muscle D. All of the above

24. Which of the following is a transparent tissue?

A. Tendon B. Ligament
C. Fibrous cartilage D. Hyaline cartilage

25. Mast cells are found in __________.

A. Connective tissue B. Muscular tissue
C. Nervous tissue D. Blood

26. The gap between two neurones is called __________.

A. Facet B. Fossa
C. Synapse D. Impulse

27. Collagen fibres of connective tissues are __________.

A. White B. Yellow
C. Colourless D. Red

28. The white fibrous tissue occurs in __________.

A. Ligaments B. Tendons
C. Cartilage D. Bone

29. __________ is a chemical substance secreted by nerve cells in the synapse.

A. ICF B. ECF
C. Plasma D. Neurotransmitter

30. A connective tissue __________.

A. Has no matrix
B. Covers the skin
C. Has abundant matrix
D. None of the above

31. The branch of science which deals with study of cell is __________.

A. Biotechnology
B. Microbiology
C. Cytology
D. Myology

32. The cells of a tissue are similar in __________.

A. Structure B. Function
C. Origin D. Both A and B

33. Transitional epithelium is found in __________.

A. Lungs B. Liver
C. Urinary bladder D. Stomach

34. Glandular epithelium is found in __________.

A. Mouth B. Oesophagus
C. Lungs D. Liver

35. Sebaceous gland of the skin is a type of __________.

A. Apocrine gland
B. Merocrine gland
C. Holocrine gland
D. All of the above

36. Haversian system is the characteristic feature in the histology of __________.

A. Muscle B. Bone
C. Cartilage D. All of the above

37. Which of the following muscle tissues can be controlled voluntarily __________.

A. Smooth B. Cardiac
C. Skeletal D. All of the above

38. **Which one of the following is not the primary germ layer?**
A. Protoderm B. Ectoderm
C. Endoderm D. Mesoderm

39. **__________ is a flexible connective tissue.**
A. Nervous tissue B. Squamous tissue
C. Bone D. Cartilage

40. **Pavement epithelial cells is the other name for ________.**
A. Pseudostratified epithelium
B. Squamous epithelium
C. Columnar epithelium
D. Hyalinc cartilage

41. **Those glands which work both as endocrine and exocrine glands, are called __________.**
A. Holocrine B. Apocrine
C. Merocrine D. Heterocrine

42. **Schwann cells are present in _________.**
A. Myofibrils B. Fibroblasts
C. Dendrons D. Axon

43. **Which is the basic structural and functional unit of the nervous system?**
A. Neurone B. Nephron
C. Meninges D. CSF

44. **Adipose tissue can be distinguished from other types of tissue by the presence of _________.**
A. Fat globule
B. Circular cells
C. Large intercellular spaces
D. Absence of nuclei

45. **White fibrous tissue is also called __________.**
A. Ligament
B. Reticular tissue
C. Areolar tissue
D. Collagenous tissue

46. **Tissue which produces movement through its ability to contract is __________.**
A. Epithelial tissue
B. Connective tissue
C. Muscle tissue
D. Nerve tissue

47. **Which of the following is a hardest connective tissue?**
A. Blood B. Cartilage
C. Areolar D. Bone

48. **_________ is also known as skeletal muscles.**
A. Cardiac muscle
B. Involuntary muscle
C. Striated muscle
D. None of the above

49. **Which of the following tissue helps in transmission of impulses in the body?**
A. Connective tissue
B. Nervous tissue
C. Epithelial tissue
D. Muscular tissue

50. **_________ tissue provides support with flexibility.**
A. Cardiac muscle
B. Cartilage
C. Blood
D. Adipose tissue

Answer Key

1 B	2 A	3 C	4 C	5 A	6 A	7 B	8 C	9 B	10 B
11 D	12 B	13 C	14 A	15 A	16 B	17 C	18 C	19 A	20 B
21 B	22 C	23 A	24 D	25 A	26 C	27 A	28 B	29 D	30 C
31 C	32 D	33 C	34 D	35 C	36 B	37 C	38 A	39 D	40 B
41 D	42 D	43 A	44 A	45 D	46 C	47 D	48 C	49 B	50 B

CHAPTER

4

The Osseous System

The Skeleton

1. The branch of science which deals with study of bones is called _________.

A. Histology　　B. Osteology
C. Mycology　　D. Oncology

2. Total number of bones present in the human body are _________.

A. 303　　B. 206
C. 195　　D. 180

3. _________ is a bony framework of the body.

A. Tendon　　B. Ligament
C. Skeleton　　D. Vertebrae

4. Which bone protects the brain?

A. Sternum　　B. The cerebrum
C. The cranium　　D. The cerebellum

5. _________ is a joint between two or more bones.

A. Foramen　　B. Articulation
C. Condyle　　D. Fossa

6. The purpose of the rib cage is to _______.

A. Protect the heart and lungs
B. Protect the stomach
C. Protect the spinal cord
D. Provide an object to which the lungs can attach

7. Which mineral makes the bone stronger?

A. Magnesium
B. Calcium and phosphorous
C. Chloride
D. Sodium

8. The only movable bone of the skull is _______.

A. Maxilla　　B. Mandible
C. Zygomatic　　D. Vomer

9. The hollow space in the middle of bones is filled with _____________.

A. Air　　B. Blood
C. Bone marrow　　D. Bone cells

10. Inflammation of joint is known as _________.

A. Gout　　B. Arthritis
C. Fracture　　D. None of the above

11. What is a joint?

A. The place where two bones are joined
B. A hinge
C. A ball and socket
D. The place where tendons are fastened together

12. The movement of the joint away from the midline of the body is termed ___________.

A. Adduction　　B. Abduction
C. Extension　　D. Reduction

13. Thumb joint is also known as __________.

A. Pivot joint　　B. Gliding joint
C. Saddle joint　　D. Ball and socket joint

14. Which of the following bone is known as knee cap?

A. Scapula　　B. Humerus
C. Patella.　　D. Tibia

15. What is the function of a tendon?

A. To link bones to bones
B. To link muscles to ligaments
C. To link muscles to bones
D. To bind the cells in compact bone closer together

16. There are __________ number of cervical vertebrae in the human body.

A. 5　　B. 7
C. 2　　D. 10

17. **The bone which is horseshoe shaped is _________.**
    A. Frontal B. Vomer
    C. Molar D. Hyoid

18. **The lower jaw is made up of ________.**
    A. One bone B. Two bones
    C. Three bones D. Four bones

19. **Number of bones of the face is __________.**
    A. 30 B. 12
    C. 40 D. 14

20. **_________ vertebrae are 5 fused vertebrae.**
    A. Coccyx B. Sacrum
    C. Lumbar D. Cervical

21. **Cranium of man is made up of __________.**
    A. 12 bones B. 10 bones
    C. 8 bones D. 16 bones

22. **Displacement of bone from its original position is called __________.**
    A. Location B. Sprain
    C. Dislocation D. Osteoporosis

23. **Bone of tongue is __________.**
    A. Maxillary B. Dentary
    C. Hyoid bone D. Palatine

24. **Four fused vertebrae of the vertebral column are known as _________.**
    A. Sacrum B. Lumbar
    C. Thoracic D. Coccyx

25. **Mastoid bone is found in _________.**
    A. Ocular region B. Auditory region
    C. Nasal region D. Occipital region

26. **Immovability of joint means _________.**
    A. Spondylitis B. Ankylosis
    C. Osteoporosis D. Gout

27. **Number of ribs present in man _________.**
    A. 10 B. 12
    C. 24 D. 35

28. **The joint between teeth and maxilla is __________.**
    A. Fixed joint
    B. Slightly movable joint
    C. Synovial joint
    D. None of the above

29. **The number of floating ribs in human body is _______.**
    A. 6 pairs B. 3 pairs
    C. 5 pairs D. 2 pairs

30. **Shoulder joint and hip joint are the examples of _____.**
    A. Ball and socket joint B. Hinge joint
    C. Gliding joint D. Pivot joint

31. **The number of pairs of true ribs is _________.**
    A. 6 B. 7
    C. 9 D. 10

32. **The central shaft of a long bone is known as _______.**
    A. Epiphysis B. Diaphysis
    C. Hypapophysis D. Zygapophysis

33. **Elbow joint and knee joint are the examples of ______.**
    A. Ball and socket joint B. Gliding joint
    C. Hinge joint D. Axial joint

34. **The total number of bones in right arm is _________.**
    A. 32 B. 30
    C. 35 D. 40

35. **__________ helps in mechanism of breathing.**
    A. Humerus B. Ribs
    C. Ulna D. Femur

36. **Ball and socket joints can be seen in __________.**
    A. Wrist B. Shoulders
    C. Fingers D. Neck

37. **Hinge joints _________.**
    A. Are synovial joints
    B. Permit movement in one direction
    C. Are found in knee
    D. All of the above

38. **The joint between radius and ulna is _________.**
    A. Gliding joint B. Pivot joint
    C. Hinge joint D. Saddle joint

39. **The protein present in the bones is known as _______.**
    A. Chondrin B. Sclero protein
    C. Globulin D. Ossein

40. **_________ is a bone of hind arm.**
    A. Clavicle B. Femur
    C. Scapula D. Radius.

41. **All are found in spongy bones *except* _________.**
    A. Osteoblast B. Haversian canal
    C. Bone marrow D. Lacunae and canaliculi

42. **Elbow joint is present in the bones __________.**
    A. Femur, tibia, fibula
    B. Humerus, radius, ulna
    C. Scapula, humerus, clavicle
    D. Ribs, sternum, vertebrae

43. In man the axial skeleton is made up of ________.
A. 100 bones B. 80 bones
C. 103 bones D. 106 bones

44. ________ joint occurs between the vertebrae.
A. Gliding B. Pivot
C. Cartilaginous D. Hinge

45. Study of the bone is known as ________.
A. Osteology B. Craniology
C. Chondrology D. All of the above

46. ________ is a bone of forearm.
A. Patella B. Humerus
C. Fibula D. Tibia

47. In man the thoracic basket is composed of ________.
A. Ribs and thoracic vertebrae
B. Ribs and sternum
C. Ribs, sternum, and thoracic vertebrae
D. Ribs, sternum, and vertebrae

48. The only movable bone of the skull is ________.
A. Maxilla B. Mandible
C. Temporal bone D. Frontal bone

49. The part of a long bone that takes part in the growth of the bone is ________.
A. Diaphysis B. Metaphysis
C. Epiphysis D. None of the above

50. Gout is a condition where ________ crystals are deposited in the joints.
A. Stearic acid B. Pyruvic acid
C. Uric acid D. Tannic acid

51. The lower jaw or mandible is made of ________.
A. One bone B. Two bones
C. Three bones D. Cartilage

52. The small cavity between articulating surfaces of the bone is called ________.
A. Abdominal cavity B. Synovial cavity
C. Thoracic cavity D. Pelvic cavity

53. Which of the following is the most superior of the tarsals and articulates with the distal end of the tibia?
A. Calcaneous B. Talus
C. Navicular D. Cuneiform

54. There are ________ pairs of false ribs in the body.
A. 2 B. 3
C. 4 D. 6

55. The greater sciatic notch is located on the ________.
A. Ischium B. Femur
C. Ilium D. Pubis

56. ________ are the strong fibrous joints between the bones of skull.
A. Sulcus B. Septum
C. Sutures D. Pleura

57. Example of long bone is ________.
A. Femur B. Tibia
C. Fibula D. All of the above

58. ______ suture is present between two parietal bones.
A. Coronal B. Sagittal
C. Lamboidal D. None of the above

59. Example of short bone is ________.
A. Femur B. Carpals (wrist)
C. Tibia D. Fibula

60. Which one of the following is an example of irregular bone?
A. Femur B. Humerus
C. Innominate D. Radius

Answer Key

1 B	2 B	3 C	4 C	5 B	6 A	7 B	8 B	9 C	10 B
11 A	12 B	13 C	14 C	15 C	16 B	17 D	18 A	19 B	20 B
21 C	22 C	23 C	24 D	25 B	26 B	27 C	28 A	29 D	30 A
31 B	32 B	33 C	34 B	35 B	36 B	37 D	38 B	39 D	40 B
41 B	42 B	43 B	44 C	45 A	46 B	47 C	48 B	49 B	50 C
51 A	52 B	53 B	54 B	55 C	56 C	57 D	58 B	59 B	60 C

CHAPTER

5.

The Haemopoietic System

The Blood

1. **The blood is a type of which of the following tissue?**
   A. Epithelial tissue
   B. Connective tissue
   C. Muscular tissue
   D. Nervous tissue

2. **What is not considered as a leucocyte?**
   A. Lymphocyte
   B. Monocyte
   C. Thrombocyte
   D. Neutrophil

3. **WBCs which are the most active phagocytic cells are __________.**
   A. Lymphocytes and macrophages
   B. Neutrophil and eosinophil
   C. Neutrophil and monocyte
   D. Eosinophil and lymphocyte

4. **Haemopoiesis means __________.**
   A. The pooling of blood
   B. The prevention of bleeding
   C. The formation of blood cells
   D. The destruction of red blood cells

5. **The chemical events common to intrinsic and extrinsic pathways systems begin with ___________.**
   A. Blood vessel constriction
   B. Activation of fibrinogen
   C. Activation of factor X
   D. Platelet plug formation

6. **Which of the following blood cells play an important role in blood clotting?**
   A. Thrombocyte
   B. Neutrophil
   C. Leucocyte
   D. Erythrocyte

7. **The intrinsic pathway of blood coagulation is activated by __________.**
   A. Injury to the endothelial lining of the vessel wall
   B. Damage to the vascular wall or external tissue
   C. Factor VII
   D. Activation of factor XII

8. **Serum differs from blood as it lacks __________.**
   A. Antibodies
   B. Clotting factors
   C. Albumin
   D. Globulin

9. **The embolus is __________.**
   A. A venous clot
   B. A clot that is bound to a vessel
   C. A clot that has travelled in the blood vessels
   D. An unformed clot

10. **The normal value of WBCs (leucocytes) is __________ per cubic mm of blood.**
    A. 6000 to 10000
    B. 11000 to 15000
    C. 2000 to 5000
    D. 14000 to 16000

11. **WBCs which release heparin and histamine is ______.**
    A. Basophil
    B. Neutrophil
    C. Monocyte
    D. Eosinophil

12. **Intravascular clotting is also known as __________.**
    A. Embolism
    B. Thrombosis
    C. Oedema
    D. Haemolysis

13. **Erythropoietin controls ___________.**
    A. Rate of leukocyte production
    B. Rate of myeloid production
    C. Rate of stem cell production
    D. Rate of erythrocyte production

14. **Haemolysis (Laking of blood) means breakdown of __________.**
    A. Thrombocytes
    B. Leucocytes
    C. Erythrocytes
    D. Platelets

15. What part of blood is responsible for fighting infections?
A. Red blood cells
B. Platelets
C. White blood cells
D. Plasma

16. Decrease in percentage of haemoglobin or RBCs is known as __________.
A. Polycythemia B. Leukaemia
C. Leucopenia D. Anemia

17. Which one the following is responsible for the red colour of the blood?
A. Plasma B. Haemoglobin
C. WBCs D. Hemocyanin

18. What part of blood is responsible for carrying oxygen and carbon dioxide to body cells?
A. White blood cells B. Red blood cells
C. Platelets D. Plasma

19. __________ is a bleeding disease.
A. Haemostasis
B. Haemophilia
C. Hemopoiesis
D. Haematopoiesis

20. What part of blood is responsible for clotting blood?
A. Platelets B. Red blood cells
C. White blood cells D. Plasma

21. Haemopoiesis is from Greek language meaning ______.
A. To destroy the blood
B. To make new blood
C. To store blood
D. None of the above

22. Rh-factor derives its name from which of the following?
A. Ape B. Human
C. Rat D. Monkey

23. During blood donation, the removal of blood component is called __________.
A. Cytopheresis B. Plasmapheresis
C. Aphaeresis D. Leukopheresis

24. What part of blood is responsible for carrying wastes, nutrients, and minerals?
A. Red blood cells B. Plasma
C. White blood cells D. Platelets

25. Each haemoglobin molecule is able to transport _____ molecules of oxygen.
A. 1 B. 2
C. 4 D. 3

26. The normal platelet (thrombocyte) count in adult is __________ lacs per cubic mm of blood.
A. 3 to 4 B. 6 to 7
C. 8 to 9 D. 9 to 10

27. In which part of the body RBCs are formed?
A. Heart B. Red bone marrow
C. Kidney D. Lungs

28. Clotting time has a normal value of ________ minutes.
A. 7 to 8 B. 9 to 10
C. 3 to 4 D. 1 to 2

29. The nucleus in WBC is _________.
A. Round B. Oval
C. Irregular D. Spindle shaped

30. The excess of white corpuscles in the blood is called __________.
A. Anoxia B. Leukaemia
C. Septicaemia D. Anaemia

31. SVC and IVC are the largest veins carries _________.
A. Oxygenated blood
B. Lymph fluid
C. Deoxygenated blood
D. Pure blood

32. Blood coagulation is assisted by _________.
A. Thrombocytes B. Phagocytes
C. Erythrocytes D. Leucocytes

33. Heredity deficiency of coagulation is referred to as _________.
A. Anaemia B. Haemophilia
C. Haemolysis D. Leukaemia

34. Which of the following acts as a defence against infection?
A. RBCs B. WBCs
C. Platelets D. Fibrinogen

35. Life span of neutrophils is _________.
A. 118 days B. 10–12 hours
C. 24–72 hours D. 120 days

36. The blood group known as the ABO system is based on the presence of __________.
A. Antibodies B. Antigen
C. Agglutinins D. Immunoglobulins

37. T-Lymphocytes originate from __________.
A. Thymus B. Bone marrow
C. Liver D. None of the above

38. Which of the following is not required for blood clotting?
A. Vitamin K B. Calcium
C. Plasmin D. Fibrinogen

39. The normal level of haemoglobin per 100 ml of blood in women is ___________.
A. 18 gm B. 14 gm
C. 12 gm D. 20 gm

40. Platelet plug is associated with _________.
A. Haemostasis B. Fibrin formation
C. Homeostasis D. Clot retraction

41. The blood protein involved in blood coagulation is ________.
A. Serum amylase B. Albumin
C. Fibrinogen D. Globulin

42. The main function of erythrocyte is __________.
A. Transport of nutrients
B. Transport of oxygen
C. Defence of the body
D. Aggregate and prevent bleeding

43. The blood group in man was discovered by _______.
A. Mendel B. Karl Landsteiner
C. Francis Nelson D. S. Miller

44. Coagulation will be retarded by ___________.
A. Lowering of RBC count
B. Increasing temperature
C. Lowering thrombocytes count
D. Removing heparin

45. Haemostasis means ___________.
A. The formation of blood cells
B. The pooling of blood
C. The prevention of bleeding
D. The destruction of blood cells

46. The volume of RBC will increase in _________.
A. Hypotonic solution
B. Isotonic solution
C. Hypertonic solution
D. None of the above

47. The matrix of blood is known as ___________.
A. Serum B. Plasma
C. RBCs D. WBCs

48. Which of the following is capable of carrying oxygen?
A. Lymph B. Serum
C. Plasma D. Blood

49. The life span of RBCs is ___________.
A. 100 days B. 120 days
C. 110 days D. 130 days

50. Haemoglobin contains _________.
A. 70% globin + 30% haematin
B. 95% globin + 05% haematin
C. 80% globin + 20% haematin
D. 90% globin + 10% haematin

51. Basophil cells are the storage and release site for _______.
A. Histamine B. Prothrombin
C. Vitamin K D. Epinephrine

52. During blood coagulation the thromboplastin is released by __________.
A. RBCs B. WBCs
C. Platelets D. Damaged tissues

53. The sample of a healthy human blood is _________.
A. Acidic B. Alkaline
C. Neutral D. None of the above

54. The blood circulation was first explained by__________.
A. Jenner B. William Harvey
C. Mendel D. Pasteur

55. pH of human blood varies between __________.
A. 7.3 to 7.45 B. 6.0 to 7.0
C. 7.0 to 8.0 D. 7.5 to 8.0

56. 'Haemolytic jaundice' is caused due to _________.
A. High mortality rate of WBCs
B. High birth rate of RBCs
C. High mortality rate of RBCs
D. High brain rate of WBCs

57. What is the name of iron containing protein that gives red colour to the blood?
A. Hemocyanin B. Pyrite
C. Haemoglobin D. Myoglobin

58. Breakdown of haemoglobin forms __________.
A. Globulin B. Bile pigment
C. Hb-protein D. Urea

59. Universal donor has a blood group _________.
A. AB B. O –ve
C. O +ve D. O –ve or O +ve

60. The formation clot is also known as _________.
A. Coagulation B. Chemotaxis
C. Leucopoiesis D. Erythropoiesis

61. The viscosity of blood is __________.

A. 2.5 to 3.5 B. 4.5 to 5.5

C. 5.5 to 6.5 D. 7.5 to 8.5

62. Which blood group accepts blood of group A and B?

A. A

B. AB

C. B

D. None of the above

63. Haemopoiesis is a process of the production of________.

A. Blood plasma B. Bone marrow

C. Haemoglobin D. Erythrocytes

64. Which of the following is not required for clot formation?

A. Vitamin K B. Sodium

C. Calcium D. Fibrinogen

65. The total amount of blood present in the human body is about ___________.

A. 3 to 4 litres B. 5 to 5.5 litres

C. 6 to 7 litres D. 10 litres

66. __________ is a connective tissue which provides means of communication between the cells of the body and the external environment.

A. Heart B. Blood

C. Both A and B D. None of the above

67. The normal value of RBCs in an adult is _______ millions per cubic mm of blood.

A. 7 B. 8

C. 5 D. 10

68. Blood makes __________ of body weight.

A. 15% B. 7%

C. 12% D. 2%

69. The fluid remaining after formation of clot is ________.

A. CSF B. Aq. humour

C. Blood serum D. Lymph

70. Constituents of plasma is __________.

A. Albumins

B. Globulins

C. Clotting factors

D. All of the above

Answer Key

1 B	2 C	3 C	4 C	5 C	6 A	7 A	8 B	9 C	10 A
11 A	12 C	13 D	14 C	15 C	16 D	17 B	18 B	19 B	20 A
21 B	22 D	23 A	24 B	25 C	26 A	27 B	28 C	29 C	30 B
31 C	32 A	33 B	34 B	35 B	36 B	37 B	38 C	39 B	40 D
41 C	42 B	43 B	44 C	45 C	46 A	47 B	48 D	49 B	50 B
51 A	52 D	53 B	54 B	55 A	56 C	57 C	58 B	59 D	60 A
61 B	62 B	63 D	64 B	65 B	66 B	67 C	68 B	69 C	70 D

CHAPTER 6

The Lymphatic System

1. **The lymphatic system consists of all the following *except* _________.**
   - **A.** Lymph nodes **B.** Blood
   - **C.** Lymphatic vessels **D.** Lymph

2. **The lymphatic fluid is rich in _________.**
   - **A.** Iron **B.** Antibodies
   - **C.** Neutrophils **D.** Basophils

3. **Lymph node produces ____________ which helps in immunological response of the body.**
   - **A.** Alpha-globulin
   - **B.** Beta-globulin
   - **C.** Gamma-globulin
   - **D.** Delta-globulin

4. **The T-lymphocytes and B-lymphocytes are the major cells of the ___________.**
   - **A.** Lymphatic vessels **B.** Adrenal gland
   - **C.** Lymph nodes **D.** Thymus

5. **___________ acts as a first line of defence guarding respective areas through strategic points in the body.**
   - **A.** Kidney **B.** Liver
   - **C.** Lungs **D.** Lymph nodes

6. **Lymph nodes may be located in the human body in the tissues of the _________.**
   - **A.** Stomach and brain
   - **B.** Ventricle and atrium
   - **C.** Thyroid gland and adrenal gland
   - **D.** Groin and neck

7. **Spleen is a dark-purple coloured _________.**
   - **A.** Epithelial tissue **B.** Lymphoid tissue
   - **C.** Connective tissue **D.** None of the above

8. **Which of the following is not likely to be found in the lymph?**
   - **A.** Protein molecules **B.** Red blood cells
   - **C.** Micro-organisms **D.** Macrophages

9. **Which one the following not a lymphatic organ?**
   - **A.** Spleen **B.** Pancreas
   - **C.** Thymus **D.** Tonsils

10. **The lymphokines secreted by cytotoxic T-lymphocytes increase the activity of _________.**
    - **A.** Macrophages **B.** Red blood cells
    - **C.** Brain cells **D.** B-lymphocytes

11. **Where is the thymus gland located?**
    - **A.** Upper part of mediastinum
    - **B.** Lower part of mediastinum
    - **C.** Behind the mediastinum
    - **D.** In front of mediastinum

12. **Spleen is called the "Graveyard" of the ________.**
    - **A.** Leucocytes **B.** Erythrocytes
    - **C.** Thrombocytes **D.** None of the above

13. **The spleen is situated in _________.**
    - **A.** Pelvic cavity
    - **B.** Abdominal cavity
    - **C.** In the neck
    - **D.** None of the above

14. **Lymph (nodes) gland forms __________.**
    - **A.** Hormone **B.** Lymph
    - **C.** Antibodies **D.** Antigens

15. **The lymphocytes protect from _________.**
    - **A.** Lymph **B.** Leucocytes
    - **C.** Toxins **D.** Pathogens

16. Lymphoid tissue is found in ________.
A. Thymus B. Tonsils
C. Lymph nodes D. All of the above

17. Lymph vessels are united to form ________.
A. Lymph heart B. Cisterna chyle
C. Thoracic duct D. Jugular vein

18. Lymph is colourless because ________.
A. Vitamins are absent B. Minerals are present
C. Haemoglobin is present D. RBCs are absent

19. The lymph serves to ________.
A. Transport O_2 to the brain
B. Transport CO_2 to the lung
C. Return the interstitial fluid to the blood
D. Return the WBCs and the RBCs to the lymph nodes

20. The lymphocytes provide the principal defence mechanism by producing ________.
A. Antigens B. Haemoglobin
C. Immunoglobulin D. Myoglobin

21. A yellow substance oozing out from wound has _______.
A. Lymph + RBC + WBC
B. Lymph + RBC + dead bacteria
C. Lymph + WBC + dead bacteria
D. Lymph + dead Leucocytes

22. Humoral antibodies are produced by _______.
A. β-cells B. T cells
C. Globulin D. Plasma cells

23. Which organ serves as storage depot for RBCs?
A. Spleen B. Bone marrow
C. Liver D. Gall bladder

24. Which of the following fluid is colourless?
A. Plasma B. Lymph
C. Cerebrospinal fluid D. All of the above

25. After vaccination, the body build up _______.
A. Toxins B. Antibodies
C. Lymph D. Plasma

26. Antibodies of the plasma are partly manufactured by ________.
A. Monocytes B. Lymphocytes
C. Eosinophils D. Neutrophils

27. The main function of the lymph node in the man is ________.
A. Destruction of old RBC
B. Destruction of old WBC
C. Collection and destruction of pathogens blood
D. Production of WBC

28. Lymph glands and nodes help to ________.
A. Excrete the urea
B. Eliminate the ammonia
C. Prepare blood
D. Destroy the bacteria

29. "Crypts" are present in the tissue of _______.
A. Thymus
B. Tonsils
C. Spleen
D. Reticule-endothelial system

30. The function of spleen is _________.
A. Phagocytosis
B. Storage of blood
C. Immune response
D. All of the above

Answer Key

1	B	2	B	3	C	4	C	5	D	6	D	7	B	8	B	9	B	10	A
11	B	12	B	13	B	14	C	15	D	16	D	17	C	18	D	19	C	20	C
21	C	22	A	23	A	24	D	25	B	26	B	27	C	28	D	29	B	30	D

CHAPTER 7

The Cardiovascular System
The Blood Circulation

1. **The study of blood circulation is called _________.**
   A. Haematology B. Osteology
   C. Angiology D. Myology

2. **Cardiac muscles are exclusively found in ___________ of the heart.**
   A. Pericardium B. Myocardium
   C. Endocardium D. Epicardium

3. **The bundle of His is present in ________.**
   A. Aorta B. Right atrium
   C. Septum D. Left atrium

4. **The first branch of the human aorta is ________.**
   A. Brachiocephalic artery
   B. Coronary artery
   C. Left subclavian artery
   D. Left common carotid artery

5. **The cardiac cycle time is ________.**
   A. 0.2 seconds B. 0.4 seconds
   C. 0.8 seconds D. 0.5 seconds

6. **Hepatic portal system originates from ________.**
   A. Kidney
   B. Different parts of the alimentary canal
   C. Diaphragm
   D. Liver

7. **_________ means contraction of chamber of heart.**
   A. Diastole B. Pulse
   C. Pause D. Systole

8. **Least blood pressure is present in ________.**
   A. Vena cava B. Aorta
   C. Capillary D. Vein

9. **________ is an origin of impulse of contraction in the heart.**
   A. AV node B. SA node
   C. SVC D. IVC

10. **The left border of the heart is formed by ________.**
    A. Right ventricle
    B. Left atrium and left ventricle
    C. Left atrium
    D. Left ventricle

11. **A blood clot inside a blood vessel is known as _______.**
    A. Fibrinolysis B. Thrombosis
    C. Thrombus D. Clot

12. **The thickest layer in the heart is __________.**
    A. Myocardium B. Endocardium
    C. Epicardium D. Pericardium

13. **Pacemaker of the heart is __________.**
    A. AV node B. SA node
    C. AV septum D. IA septum

14. **Bicuspid valve is also called ___________.**
    A. Eustachian valve B. Pulmonary valve
    C. Mitral valve D. Ventricular valve

15. **AV node means _________.**
    A. Axillary ventricular node B. Artery ventricular node
    C. Aorta ventricular node D. Atrioventricular node

16. **Normal diastolic pressure in young man about ______.**
    A. 20 mmHg B. 110 mmHg
    C. 80 mmHg D. 130 mmHg

17. **The blood pressure is high in ________.**
    A. Veins B. Capillaries
    C. Veins of portal system D. Arteries

18. ________ blood circulation helps in purification of blood.

A. Hepatic portal B. Pulmonary
C. Systemic D. Coronary

19. Which of the following is a repolarization wave?

A. P B. T
C. QRS D. R

20. The normal value of stroke volume is __________.

A. 100 ml B. 120 ml
C. 70 ml D. 90 ml

21. ECG records ________.

A. Potential differences
B. Electric current of the body
C. Pulse rate
D. Quantity of blood pumped per minute

22. ________ blood circulation helps in regulating the nutrient material supply to various parts of the body.

A. Systemic B. Pulmonary
C. Hepatic portal D. Coronary

23. An abnormal narrowing of blood vessels means _____.

A. Stenosis B. Thrombosis
C. Ankylosis D. Fibrinolysis

24. The pulse beat is measured by the _________.

A. Capillary B. Vein
C. Artery D. None of the above

25. Long form of ECG is ________.

A. Electron cardiogram B. Epic cardiogram
C. Electrocardiogram D. Endo cardiogram

26. The diastole means _________.

A. Relaxation of chamber of heart
B. Expansion of chamber of heart
C. Contraction of chamber of heart
D. None of the above

27. Heart beat below normal level is called ________.

A. Tachycardia B. Hyperpiesia
C. Bradycardia D. All of the above

28. _________ blood circulation supplies blood to heart muscle (myocardium).

A. Systemic B. Hepatic portal
C. Coronary D. None of the above

29. Heart sounds are described as _________.

A. Zigzag B. Slow–Fast
C. Lup–Dup D. Sharp–Faint

30. The smallest lumen blood vessels in the body are ______.

A. Artery B. Vein
C. Capillary D. Vena-cava

31. The amount of blood ejected from the heart by each contraction of the ventricle is called ________.

A. Cardiac output B. Stroke volume
C. Pulse rate D. Heart rate

32. Which one of the following are largest blood vessels in body?

A. Carotid artery B. Chronic artery
C. Dorsal aorta D. Coronary artery

33. Which of the following chamber of the heart receives oxygenated blood?

A. Right atrium B. Left atrium
C. Right ventricle D. None of the above

34. The normal value of cardiac output is ________.

A. 2000 ml B. 3040 ml
C. 4040 ml D. 5040 ml

35. All arteries carry oxygenated blood *except* ________.

A. Pulmonary artery B. Systemic artery
C. Hepatic artery D. Cardiac artery

36. _______ is an interruption of blood supply to the brain.

A. Sprain B. Stroke
C. Strain D. Blood pressure

37. Which of the following hormone regulate blood pressure?

A. Insulin B. Thyroxine
C. Adrenaline D. Estrogens

38. The main systemic artery which originates from the left ventricle is __________.

A. Carotid B. Aorta
C. Pulmonary D. Jugular

39. SA node is situated in __________.

A. Right atrium B. Left atrium
C. Right ventricle D. Right atrium

40. Oxygen Fick method is used to measure __________.

A. Blood pressure B. Cardiac reserve
C. Cardiac output D. Capillary blood flow

41. What is the normal blood pressure range value for an adult healthy individual?

A. 140/90 mmHg B. 120/80 mmHg
C. 100/60 mmHg D. 145/95 mmHg

42. The difference between systolic and diastolic pressure is called ________.

A. High pressure B. Low pressure
C. Medium pressure D. Pulse pressure

43. **Which part of the body can be called a kind of "Blood Bank".**
   A. Heart B. Liver
   C. Spleen D. Lungs

44. **Heart beat and pulse rate is increased under conditions of __________.**
   A. Psychogenic stress B. Fever
   C. Muscular exercise D. All of the above

45. **The amount of blood ejected from heart in each minute by the contraction of ventricles is called ________.**
   A. Respiratory output
   B. Cardiac output
   C. Urinary output
   D. None of the above

46. **What is the approximate weight of human heart?**
   A. 250 to 300 gm B. 250 to 450 gm
   C. 450 to 500 gm D. 300 to 400 gm

47. **The covering of heart is called _________.**
   A. Peritoneum B. Pericardium
   C. Perineurium D. Periosteum

48. **__________ is a deposition of fat in the walls of artery.**
   A. Arteritis B. Atherosclerosis
   C. Aneurysm D. None of the above

49. **___________ is present at the base of the septum.**
   A. SA node B. Pacemaker
   C. AV node D. SVC

50. **The rate of heart beat is controlled by __________.**
   A. CNS
   B. Autonomic nervous system
   C. Endocrine gland
   D. Renal system

51. **Pains in the chest means ___________ condition.**
   A. Blood pressure B. Angina pectoris
   C. CHD D. Arteriosclerosis

52. **Blood return from lungs to heart through ___________.**
   A. Right auricle B. Left auricle
   C. Right ventricle D. Left ventricle

53. **The blood pressure is measured by an instrument called ___________.**
   A. Stethoscope B. Sphygmomanometer
   C. Sonometer D. Glucometer

54. **The blood circulation in the human body was first discovered by ___________.**
   A. William Harvey B. Waldeyer
   C. Aristotle D. Palade

55. **Tricuspid valve is present __________.**
   A. Between LA and LV B. In the pulmonary arch
   C. Between RA and RV D. In the aortic arch

56. **AV node is located ___________.**
   A. On the tricuspid valve
   B. On the bicuspid valve
   C. Near the bicuspid valve
   D. Near the tricuspid valve

57. **The BP is measured in terms of __________.**
   A. mmHg B. mgHg
   C. mlHg D. Litre of Hg

58. **The heart beat is regulated by ___________.**
   A. Vagas nerve B. Pacemaker
   C. Sympathetic nerve D. All of the above

59. **The wave of contraction is under the control of ______.**
   A. Auditory nerve
   B. Parasympathetic nerve
   C. Phrenic nerve
   D. Auditory nerve

60. **Which of the following method is not a method of measurement of blood pressure?**
   A. Oscillatory method B. Spirometry
   C. Auscultatory D. Palpatory

Answer Key

1 C	2 B	3 C	4 C	5 C	6 B	7 D	8 A	9 B	10 B
11 C	12 A	13 B	14 C	15 D	16 C	17 D	18 B	19 B	20 C
21 A	22 C	23 A	24 C	25 C	26 A	27 C	28 C	29 C	30 C
31 B	32 C	33 B	34 D	35 A	36 B	37 C	38 B	39 A	40 C
41 B	42 D	43 C	44 D	45 B	46 A	47 B	48 B	49 C	50 B
51 B	52 B	53 B	54 A	55 C	56 D	57 A	58 D	59 B	60 B

CHAPTER

8

The Respiratory System

1. **In which part of the respiratory system, gaseous exchange takes place?**

   A. Alveoli B. Pharynx
   C. Larynx D. Trachea

2. **__________ are the principal organs of the respiratory system.**

   A. Alveoli B. Nose
   C. Lungs D. Larynx

3. **Which is the common passage of both the respiratory and digestive system?**

   A. Trachea B. Larynx
   C. Bronchioles D. Pharynx

4. **__________ is located between two pleural sacs and is the central compartment of the thoracic cavity.**

   A. Mediastinum B. Hilum
   C. Pleura D. Thoracic cage

5. **Parietal and visceral pleura are the coverings of_____.**

   A. Heart B. Lungs
   C. Kidney D. Ovary

6. **Which of the following are parts of the human respiratory system?**

   A. Larynx
   B. Diaphragm
   C. The lungs
   D. All of the above

7. **__________ is a wind pipe which is continuous with the larynx.**

   A. Trachea B. Pharynx
   C. Lungs D. Alveoli

8. **Which of the following gas is released out during the process of respiration?**

   A. Carbon dioxide B. Oxygen
   C. Hydrogen D. None of the above

9. **The trachea is made up of 16–20 C-shaped rings of __________.**

   A. White fibrocartilage
   B. Hyaline cartilage
   C. Yellow elastic cartilage
   D. None of the above

10. **The tiny air sacs present in human lungs are called __________.**

    A. Bronchus B. Alveoli
    C. Bronchioles D. All of the above

11. **The normal value of vital capacity is __________.**

    A. 1 to 2 litres B. 5 to 6 litres
    C. 8 to 10 litres D. 3 to 5 litres

12. **__________ functions for filtering and keeping the mucus and dirt away from our lungs?**

    A. Bronchioles B. Cilia
    C. Hairs in the lungs D. All of the above

13. **The total number of alveoli present in the human lungs is around __________.**

    A. 2000 million B. 1 billion
    C. 500 million D. 1500 million

14. **__________ means deficiency of oxygen to the lungs and tissues.**

    A. Anoxia B. Hypocapnia
    C. Dysphonia D. Hypercapnia

15. **The exchange of gases between the external environment and the lungs is called _________.**
A. Respiration
B. Cellular respiration
C. External respiration
D. None of the above

16. **The amount of air remaining in the lungs after the most powerful expiration is known as _________.**
A. Residual volume
B. Tidal volume
C. Vital capacity
D. Inspiratory reserve volume

17. **______________ means the condition of difficulty in breathing.**
A. Anoxia B. Hypocapnia
C. Dysphonia D. Hypercapnia

18. **The maximum volume of air contained in the lung by a full forced inhalation is called __________.**
A. Total lung capacity
B. Tidal volume
C. Vital capacity
D. Ventilation rate

19. **The following is the function of the trachea?**
A. Gaseous exchange
B. Exhales the air from the body
C. Filters the air we breathe
D. All of the above

20. **Which of the following organs functions as an air conditioner?**
A. Larynx B. Nasal chambers
C. Pharynx D. All of the above

21. **__________ is a common passage in swallowing food and breathing.**
A. Larynx B. Gullet
C. Pharynx D. Glottis

22. **Which organ of the respiratory system is known as voice box/sound box?**
A. Larynx B. Bronchus
C. Trachea D. Bronchioles

23. **The function of nasal cavity is_________.**
A. Air is filtered
B. Air is warmed
C. Air is humidified
D. All of the above

24. **The left and right bronchi are _________.**
A. Lobes of lungs
B. Subdivisions of the trachea
C. Fine branches of the tracheoles
D. All of the above

25. **The normal value of tidal volume in human is ______.**
A. 500 ml B. 1000 ml
C. 1500 ml D. 4.5 litres

26. **The greatest quantity of air that can be expired after a maximum inspiration is its _________.**
A. Residual volume
B. Tidal volume
C. Lung volume
D. Vital capacity

27. **Rate of breathing/ respiratory rate in an adult human is __________.**
A. 14–18/min B. 10–12/min
C. 20–25/min D. 25–30/min

28. **Which one has the lowest value?**
A. Vital capacity
B. Inspiratory reserve volume
C. Tidal volume
D. Expiratory reserve volume

29. **During forced expiration, actively contracting muscles include the _________.**
A. Abdominal muscles
B. Diaphragm
C. External intercostals
D. Diaphragm and intercostal muscle

30. **Amount of air exchanged in breathing can be measured with a _________.**
A. Spherometer
B. Barometer
C. Spirometer
D. Sphygmomanometer

31. **In human beings the number of lobes in right and left lungs is _________.**
A. 2 and 3 B. 3 and 2
C. 2 and 2 D. 4 and 2

32. **Lungs have a large number of narrow tubes called _________.**
A. Alveoli B. Bronchi
C. Bronchioles D. Alveolar ducts

33. **Exchange of gases between the blood and the cells is called ________.**
   A. External respiration
   B. Internal respiration
   C. Both A and B
   D. None of the above

34. **During expiration diaphragm becomes________.**
   A. Flattened B. Oblique
   C. Normal D. Dome-shaped

35. **The internal lining of trachea has a membrane of ________.**
   A. Squamous epithelium
   B. Connective tissue cells
   C. Ciliated endothelium
   D. Mucous cells

36. **Lecithin is a substance present in the _______.**
   A. Alveoli
   B. Nasal chambers
   C. Oropharynx
   D. Bronchial tubes

37. **During normal breathing, the amount of air that moves into the lungs and comes out is called _______.**
   A. Inspiratory reserve volume
   B. Residual volume
   C. Expiratory reserve volume
   D. Tidal volume

38. **Smoking is one of the causes of_________.**
   A. Hypoxia B. Narcosis
   C. Emphysema D. Pharyngitis

39. **The various organs of respiration are ________.**
   A. Nasal cavity
   B. Pharynx
   C. Larynx
   D. All of the above

40. **Exchange of gases between the blood and the lungs is called _________.**
   A. Internal respiration
   B. External respiration
   C. Both A and B
   D. None of the above

Answer Key

1 A	2 C	3 D	4 A	5 B	6 D	7 A	8 A	9 B	10 B
11 D	12 B	13 A	14 C	15 C	16 A	17 A	18 A	19 C	20 B
21 C	22 C	23 D	24 B	25 A	26 D	27 A	28 C	29 A	30 C
31 B	32 C	33 B	34 D	35 C	36 A	37 D	38 C	39 D	40 A

CHAPTER 9

The Digestive System

1. **The process of conversion of complex food substances into simple absorbable form is called ________.**
   A. Ingestion B. Digestion
   C. Mastication D. Excretion

2. **The muscular tube that extends from the mouth to the anus is called ________.**
   A. The gullet
   B. The intestine
   C. The colon
   D. The alimentary canal

3. **Deglutition is the main function of ________.**
   A. Oesophagus B. Pharynx
   C. Mouth D. Intestine

4. **Which organ in the list is the largest gland in the human body?**
   A. Parotid B. Liver
   C. Pancreas D. Thyroid

5. **There are ________ of salivary glands in mouth.**
   A. 1 pair B. 2 pairs
   C. 3 pairs D. 4 pairs

6. **Which layer of GI tract forms the innermost lining and continuously secretes mucus?**
   A. Serosa B. Muscularis externa
   C. Muscularis D. Mucosa

7. **Deglutition means the process of ________.**
   A. Digestion B. Mastication
   C. Swallowing D. Ingestion

8. **________ is a salivary enzyme.**
   A. Trypsin B. Chymotrypsin
   C. Ptyalin D. Renin

9. **Food and chyme are pushed through the digestive system by ________.**
   A. Ingestion B. Mastication
   C. Assimilation D. Peristalsis

10. **Stomach is a ________ portion of the alimentary canal.**
    A. T-shaped B. J-shaped
    C. L-shaped D. U-shaped

11. **Which of the following secretions is not produced by gastric glands?**
    A. Hydrochloric acid B. Intrinsic factor
    C. Pepsin D. Sebum

12. **Which of the following digestive enzymes is not found in intestinal juice?**
    A. Sucrase B. Trypsin
    C. Lactase D. Maltase

13. **Which portion of the stomach opens into small intestine?**
    A. Cardiac portion B. Fundic portion
    C. Pyloric portion D. Body portion

14. **Blood from the intestines travels to the liver via the ________.**
    A. Hepatic artery B. Mesenteric artery
    C. Hepatic vein D. Hepatic portal vein

15. **The hard chewing surface of the teeth is ________.**
    A. Tongue B. Enamel
    C. Frenulum D. Papillae

16. **The length of small intestine is about ________.**
    A. 2 meters B. 3 meters
    C. 4 meters D. 5 meters

17. **The end product of digestion of starch which is absorbed into the blood stream is ________.**
    A. Amino acid B. Fatty acid
    C. Glucose D. Sucrose

18. **Duodenum, jejunum, ileum are the parts of________.**
    A. Large intestine B. Anus
    C. Rectum D. Small intestine

19. **Which of the following is a function of bile?**
    A. Acidification of GI contents
    B. Emulsification of GI contents
    C. Digestion of proteins
    D. Speeding up GI transit time

20. **__________ is called both exocrine and endocrine gland.**
    A. Liver B. Gall bladder
    C. Duodenum D. Pancreas

21. **Which of the following glands produces saliva?**
    A. Parotid B. Pancreas
    C. Thyroid D. Pituitary

22. **The primary site for absorption of water by the digestive system is the ________.**
    A. Oesophagus
    B. Colon (large intestine)
    C. Small intestine
    D. Liver

23. **Large intestine has _________ colons.**
    A. 2 B. 3
    C. 5 D. 4

24. **Submucosa is thickest in _________.**
    A. Stomach B. Oesophagus
    C. Intestine D. Rectum

25. **Cirrhosis is a disease that affects which among the following organs?**
    A. Kidney B. Pancreas
    C. Liver D. Duodenum

26. **Appendix is a finger-like projection that protrude from the lower right end of the _________.**
    A. Small intestine B. Duodenum
    C. Rectum D. Large intestine

27. **What are the functions of goblet cells?**
    A. Production of enzyme
    B. Production of mucin
    C. Production of hormone
    D. Production of HCI

28. **What does the pancreatic duct directly joins to ______.**
    A. Jejunum B. Liver
    C. Duodenum D. Ileum

29. **Kupffer cells of liver are __________.**
    A. Loose connective tissue B. Phagocytic cell
    C. Mast cell D. Fat cell

30. **Trypsin and chymotrypsin are the enzymes found in __________.**
    A. Gastric juice B. Intestinal juice
    C. Pancreatic juice D. Saliva

31. **The number of salivary glands in man is __________.**
    A. Two pairs B. Three pairs
    C. Four pairs D. Five pairs

32. **The islets of Langerhans cells are found in the ______.**
    A. Stomach B. Liver
    C. Pancreas D. Intestine

33. **The name of an enzyme produced by the salivary gland is _________.**
    A. Pepsin B. Rennin
    C. Ptyalin D. Pancreatic juice

34. **What is the largest gland in the body?**
    A. Liver B. Gall bladder
    C. Pancreas D. Large intestine

35. **The length of large intestine is about ________.**
    A. 2.5 meters B. 3.5 meters
    C. 1.5 meters D. 4.5 meters

36. **Saliva converts ________.**
    A. Proteins into amino acids
    B. Glycogen into glucose
    C. Starch into maltose
    D. Fats into vitamins

37. **Alpha cells of islets of Langerhans secretes ________.**
    A. Renin B. Glucagon
    C. Insulin D. Melanin

38. **The activator of intestinal juice is _________.**
    A. Succus entericus B. Secretin
    C. Enterocrinin D. Enterozymase

39. **Fat digestion is facilitated by _______.**
    A. Bile juice B. Pancreatic juice
    C. Gastric juice D. None of the above

40. **Beta cells of Islets of Langerhans secrete ________.**
    A. Glucagon B. Renin
    C. Insulin D. Oxytocin

41. **Bilirubin and biliverdin are ________.**
A. Bile salts
B. Bile pigments
C. Hormones
D. Enzymes

42. **Gall bladder is stimulated by ________.**
A. Secretin
B. Cholecystokinin
C. Enterogastrone
D. Enterokinase

43. **The trypsin enzyme is secreted by ________.**
A. Stomach
B. Duodenum
C. Pancreas
D. Liver

44. **Bile is secretion of ________.**
A. Pancreas
B. Intestine
C. Liver
D. Salivary glands

45. **In pancreas, pancreatic juice and hormones are secreted by ________.**
A. Same cells
B. Different cells
C. Same cells at different times
D. None of the above

46. **Which of the following is the end product of digestion of protein?**
A. Glucose
B. Fat
C. Amino acids
D. Bile

47. **pH of the pancreatic juice is about ________.**
A. 6.4
B. 8.4
C. 12.0
D. 7.0

48. **The amount of gastric juice secreted per day from man's stomach is about ________.**
A. 5000 ml to 10000 ml
B. 2000 ml to 3000 ml
C. 100 ml to 500 ml
D. 10 ml to 15 ml

49. **BMR means ________.**
A. Basic modification rate
B. Basic molecular rate
C. Basal metabolic rate
D. Basal morphological rate

50. **Which word best describe the action of bile on fats?**
A. Neutralizes
B. Digests
C. Emulsifies
D. Absorbs

51. **Absence of dil.HCl in gastric juice is called ________.**
A. Hyperchlorhydria
B. Achlorhydria
C. Hypochlorhydria
D. None of the above

52. **The pH of amylase present in saliva is ________.**
A. 6
B. 6.8
C. 7.2
D. 8

53. **Saliva is secreted from ________.**
A. Submaxillary and sublingual glands
B. Gastric gland
C. Pancreas
D. Gall bladder

54. **Tonsils are also named ________.**
A. Adrenal glands
B. Adenoids
C. Adenohypophysis
D. Androgens

55. **The functional unit for the absorption of digested food is ________.**
A. Crypts of Lieberkuhn
B. Peyer's patches
C. Villi
D. Brunner's gland

56. **Which region of the alimentary canal is principal organ for the absorption of nutrients and digested food?**
A. Small intestine
B. Large intestine
C. Stomach
D. Liver

57. **The enzyme pepsin of gastric juice gets activated in ________.**
A. Neutral medium
B. Alkaline medium
C. Acidic medium
D. None of the above

58. **The gas which stimulates respiration is ________.**
A. Nitrogen
B. Oxygen
C. Carbon dioxide
D. None of the above

59. **Digestion of carbohydrates starts in the ________.**
A. Large intestine
B. Small intestine
C. Buccal cavity
D. Stomach

60. **The digestive system comprises of ________.**
A. Mouth
B. Pharynx
C. Oesophagus
D. All of the above

61. **Bile juice is formed in ________.**
A. Kidney
B. Liver
C. Mouth
D. Stomach

62. **The functions of the digestive system are ________.**
A. Ingestion
B. Digestion
C. Absorption of food
D. All of the above

63. **Saliva helps in digestion of ________.**
A. Starch
B. Fat
C. Proteins
D. Oils

64. Which of the following enzyme in the human body starts the digestion of proteins?

A. Trypsin

B. Hydrase

C. Amylase

D. Pepsin

65. C-shaped fixed part of the alimentary canal is ______.

A. Duodenum

B. Jejunum

C. Ileum

D. None of the above

66. Which is the longest organ of digestive system in human body?

A. Large intestine

B. Small intestine

C. Pancreatic duct

D. Bile duct

67. It is the continuation of duodenum and the middle portion of small intestine ________.

A. Ileum B. Jejunum

C. Appendix D. None of the above

68. The part of alimentary canal present in between pharynx and stomach is ________.

A. Duodenum

B. Large intestine

C. Oesophagus

D. Liver

69. Saliva is a ________.

A. Endocrine secretion

B. Exocrine secretion

C. Hormone

D. Chemical

70. Chewing of the bolus in the mouth cavity is ________.

A. Ingestion B. Digestion

C. Mastication D. Excretion

Answer Key

1 B	2 D	3 A	4 B	5 C	6 D	7 C	8 C	9 D	10 B
11 D	12 B	13 B	14 A	15 B	16 D	17 C	18 D	19 B	20 D
21 A	22 B	23 D	24 B	25 C	26 D	27 B	28 C	29 B	30 C
31 B	32 C	33 C	34 A	35 C	36 C	37 B	38 B	39 A	40 C
41 B	42 B	43 C	44 C	45 B	46 C	47 B	48 B	49 C	50 C
51 B	52 B	53 A	54 B	55 C	56 A	57 C	58 C	59 C	60 D
61 B	62 D	63 A	64 D	65 A	66 B	67 B	68 C	69 B	70 C

CHAPTER 10.

The Skeletal Muscles

1. **Striated muscles are found attached to ________.**
   A. Liver B. Skeleton
   C. Heart D. Lungs

2. **_________ in the skeletal muscle is responsible for maintaining posture of the body.**
   A. Muscle tone B. Muscle fatigue
   C. Refractory period D. Conductivity

3. **The contraction of muscle of shortest duration is seen in __________.**
   A. Heart B. Jaws
   C. Eyelids D. Intestine

4. **Which of the following muscle surrounds the eye?**
   A. Oculi B. Orbicularis
   C. Levator D. Buccinator

5. **Triceps muscle joins ulna with ________.**
   A. Radius B. Phalanges
   C. Suprascapular D. Humerus

6. **In muscle contraction, which of the following ion is essential?**
   A. Cl B. Ca
   C. K D. Na

7. **Which muscle moves the forelimb/forearm?**
   A. Latissimus dorsi B. Brachialis
   C. Dorsal scapularis D. Triceps brachii

8. **The superior rectus muscle ________.**
   A. Closes lips
   B. Closes eyes
   C. Rolls eye ball upward
   D. Flexes vertebral column

9. **In the skeletal muscle the functional unit of contractile system is _________.**
   A. Z-band B. Cross-bridge
   C. Sarcomere D. Myofibril

10. **Abductor muscles are antagonist of _________.**
    A. Flexor B. Adductor
    C. Pronator D. Rotator

11. **Completely involuntary unstriated muscles occur in ___________.**
    A. Base of pinna B. Diaphragm
    C. Pylorus D. Eyelids

12. **The two principal proteins in skeletal muscle are __________.**
    A. Actin and troponin
    B. Actin and tropomyosin
    C. Actin and myosin
    D. Myosin and tropomyosin

13. **A muscle bends a part over another. It is _______.**
    A. Extensor B. Abductor
    C. Adductor D. Flexor

14. **What is the basic functional unit of skeletal muscle tissue?**
    A. Sarcomere
    B. Muscle fibre
    C. Myofibril
    D. Sarcoplasmic reticulum

15. **Biceps are attached with _______.**
    A. Radius B. Scapula
    C. Femur D. Both A and B

16. In the structure of skeletal muscle which of the following surrounds the bundle of muscle fibres?

A. Epimysium B. Endomysium
C. Perimysium D. Aureomysium

17. Biceps and triceps surround ________.

A. Radius B. Humerus
C. Ulna D. Femur

18. In the organization of skeletal muscle, myofilament is a part of ________.

A. Tissue B. Organ
C. Organelle D. Sarcomere

19. The strongest muscle of the body is found in _______.

A. Thigh B. Jaw
C. Wrist D. Finger

20. The total number of muscles in the body of man is ________.

A. 409 B. 639
C. 439 D. 539

21. The longest visceral muscle cell is present in _______.

A. Pregnant uterus B. Vas deferens
C. Normal uterus D. Abdomen

22. A muscle consists of packages of muscle cells is known as _______.

A. Fundibulum B. Inverted
C. Invading D. Fascicles

23. Largest smooth muscle present in ________.

A. Leg
B. Uterus of pregnant woman
C. Urethra
D. Thigh

24. A tendon joins __________.

A. Bone with bone
B. Muscle with bone
C. Muscle with muscle
D. Muscle with ligament

25. Which of the following is the contractile protein of muscle?

A. Tubulin B. Myosin
C. Troponin D. None of the above

26. The repeating functional unit of a myofibril is ______.

A. Sarcoplasm
B. Sarcomere
C. Sarcosome
D. Sarnuclease

27. A ligament joins ________.

A. Bone with tendon
B. Muscle with bone
C. Bone with bone
D. Tendon with ligament

28. The muscle which opens the mouth is called _______.

A. Depressor mandibula B. Masseter
C. Supinator D. Dilatator

29. "All-or-none" is a phenomenon related to ________.

A. Muscle relaxation
B. Muscle fatigue
C. Muscle contraction
D. Action potential

30. ___________ is made up of a large number of muscle fibres.

A. Skin B. Skeletal muscles
C. Bone D. Teeth

Answer Key

1 B	2 A	3 C	4 B	5 D	6 B	7 B	8 C	9 C	10 B
11 C	12 C	13 D	14 A	15 D	16 C	17 B	18 D	19 B	20 B
21 A	22 D	23 B	24 B	25 B	26 A	27 C	28 A	29 C	30 B

CHAPTER

11.

The Nervous System

1. What are the functional units of the nervous system?

A. Nephrons B. Neurons

C. Fibres D. Ligaments

2. The neurone that carries information from the peripheral nervous system to central nervous system is __________.

A. Afferent nerve B. Efferent nerve

C. Motor nerve D. None of the above

3. Cerebrospinal fluid is produced by __________.

A. Ependymal cells

B. Choroid plexus

C. Neuroglial cells

D. Neurons

4. __________ are the coverings of the brain and spinal cord.

A. Membranes B. Tissues

C. Meninges D. Cells

5. _________ is the ability of neurone to initiate nerve impulses.

A. Myelination B. Conductivity

C. Neurotransmitter D. Irritability

6. The space between the cranium and dura mater of the brain is called __________.

A. Subarachnoid

B. Subdural

C. Epidural

D. Foramen of magnum

7. Which is the smallest cranial nerve?

A. Olfactory nerve B. Abducent nerve

C. Trochlear nerve D. Accessary nerve

8. Learning is related to which part of the human brain _________.

A. Medulla oblongata B. Hypothalamus

C. Cerebrum D. Cerebellum

9. Which fluid is present in between meninges of the brain and spinal cord?

A. Tear fluid

B. Cerebrospinal fluid

C. Intracellular fluid

D. Extracellular fluid

10. Which part of brain controls emotions like love, anger, and pleasure?

A. Medulla oblongata B. Hypothalamus

C. Cerebrum D. Cerebellum

11. __________ acts as a cushion and shock absorber of the brain.

A. ICF B. ECF

C. CSF D. Lymph

12. What is the structural and functional unit of the nervous system?

A. Brain B. Spinal cord

C. Neurone D. Synapse

13. Nearly 80% of the human brain is made up of________.

A. Cerebellar cortex

B. Cerebral cortex

C. Medulla oblongata

D. Meninges

14. Which of the following separates the lobes of the brain?

A. Sutures B. Septum

C. Sulcus D. None of the above

15. Which of the following is not a part of the CNS?

A. Brain B. Spinal cord
C. PNS D. Retina

16. ________ means inflammation of brain and spinal cord membranes.

A. Arthritis B. Meningitis
C. Spondylitis D. Appendicitis

17. The fluid present between the meninges for protection of the CNS is called ________.

A. Intracellular fluid B. Extracellular fluid
C. Cerebrospinal fluid D. Protoplasmic fluid

18. Weight of the human brain is approximately ________.

A. 2.5 lbs B. 3.5 lbs
C. 4.0 lbs D. 4.5 lbs

19. The nervous system is divided into the ________.

A. Brain and spinal cord
B. SNS and PSNS
C. PNS and CNS
D. Sensory and motor system

20. The length of spinal cord is about ________.

A. 20 cm B. 30 cm
C. 45 cm D. 60 cm

21. Hypothalamus contains regulatory center for ________.

A. Feeding and satiety
B. Thermoregulation and water balance
C. Sex drives (libido)
D. All of the above

22. There are ________ ventricles in the brain.

A. 4 B. 2
C. 5 D. 6

23. The second cranial nerve is ________.

A. Optic B. Trigeminal
C. Olfactory D. Abducens

24. Which of the following structure connects the cerebral hemisphere?

A. Corpus luteum
B. Corpus albicans
C. Corpus callosum
D. Corpora quadrigemina

25. Which of the following is the largest cranial nerve?

A. Facial nerve
B. Trigeminal nerve
C. Vagus nerve
D. Accessary nerve

26. Heart is innervated by ________.

A. Trigeminal B. Vagus
C. Glossopharyngeal D. Facial

27. Subdural space in the brain is present in between ________.

A. Pia mater and dura mater
B. Dura mater and arachnoid mater
C. Arachnoid mater and pia mater
D. Inbetween cerebral hemispheres

28. The spinal cord originates from which part of brain?

A. Cerebellum
B. Medulla oblongata
C. Pons varolii
D. Cerebrum

29. The outer covering of the brain is called ________.

A. Arachnoid mater
B. Pia mater
C. Dura mater
D. Corpus callosum

30. Which part of the brain regulates posture and balance of the body?

A. Forebrain
B. Medulla oblongata
C. Midbrain
D. Hindbrain

31. Which of the following part of the brain controls the body temperature and urge of eating?

A. Thalamus
B. Cerebellum
C. Pons varolii
D. Hypothalamus

32. The second largest part of human brain is ________.

A. Midbrain
B. Cerebellum
C. Cerebrum
D. Medulla

33. One of the following nerves does not go to eyes ________.

A. Oculomotor B. Ophthalmic
C. Abducens D. Facial

34. In a reflex arc, the connector neuron (interneuron) is present in the ________.

A. Spinal cord
B. Effector
C. Receptor
D. White matter of spinal cord

35. A cranial nerve with the highest number of branches is __________.

A. Facial nerve
B. Trigeminal nerve
C. Optic nerve
D. Ocular nerve

36. Central nervous system includes __________.

A. Brain
B. Spinal cord
C. Both A and B
D. None of the above

37. Name the nerve which functions for sense of smell?

A. Olfactory nerve
B. Optic nerve
C. Vagas nerve
D. Ocular nerve

38. Peripheral nervous system includes __________.

A. Cranial nerves
B. Spinal nerves
C. Autonomic nervous system
D. All of the above

39. Which part of the central nervous system controls "reflex actions"?

A. Cerebrum
B. Spinal cord
C. Cerebellum
D. Medulla oblongata

40. Parasympathetic nervous system increases the activity of __________.

A. Gut, iris and urinary bladder
B. Heart, adrenal and sweat gland
C. Heart, pancreas and lacrimal gland
D. Lacrimal and sweat gland

Answer Key

1 B	2 A	3 B	4 C	5 D	6 C	7 C	8 C	9 B	10 B
11 C	12 C	13 B	14 C	15 D	16 B	17 C	18 B	19 C	20 C
21 D	22 A	23 A	24 C	25 B	26 B	27 B	28 B	29 C	30 D
31 B	32 B	33 D	34 A	35 B	36 C	37 A	38 D	39 B	40 A

CHAPTER

12

The Sense Organs

1. **Photoreceptors are located __________.**
   A. On the surface of the tongue
   B. In the eye
   C. In the ear
   D. On the skin

2. **Sweat gland and sebaceous gland are found in the structure of __________.**
   A. Eye   B. Nose
   C. Ear   D. Skin

3. **Cones are more numerous in the part of the retina opposite to the pupil, which is known as ________.**
   A. The macula lutea
   B. Blind spot
   C. Aqueous humour
   D. Optic disc

4. **Which of the following are not papillae of tongue?**
   A. Vallate papillae   B. Filiform papillae
   C. Uniform papillae   D. Fungiform papillae

5. **__________ is a hammer-shaped bone.**
   A. Incus   B. Malleus
   C. Stapes   D. Auricle

6. **The amount of light passing through the pupil of the eye is adjusted by the __________.**
   A. Iris   B. Lens
   C. Optic nerve   D. Retina

7. **Membranous labyrinth is filled with a fluid called _________.**
   A. Ecolymph   B. Perilymph
   C. Endolymph   D. Exolymph

8. **__________ means an abnormal sensitiveness of the eye to the bright light.**
   A. Glaucoma   B. Xerophthalmia
   C. Myopia   D. Photophobia

9. **Eye is also called _________.**
   A. Chemoreceptors   B. Photoreceptors
   C. Neurotransmitter   D. Chemotrasmitters

10. **_________ layer of eye is described as "White of Eye".**
    A. Sclera   B. Retina
    C. Cornea   D. Iris

11. **__________ means short sightedness.**
    A. Presbyopia   B. Myopia
    C. Hypermetropia   D. Cataract

12. **Light is focused on the lens through the action of __________ on suspensory ligaments.**
    A. The optic nerve   B. The iris
    C. The ciliary muscles   D. The retina

13. **"Organ of Corti" is a part of __________.**
    A. External ear   B. Inner ear
    C. Middle ear   D. Nasal chamber

14. **Which of the following conditions means extreme dryness of conjunctiva of the eye?**
    A. Xerophthalmia   B. Cataract
    C. Night blindness   D. Myopia

15. **The distant objects can be seen but not the near objects, this condition is called __________.**
    A. Myopia   B. Presbyopia
    C. Hypermetropia   D. Night blindness

16. Which of the following is anvil-shaped bone of the middle ear?

A. Incus **B.** Malleus
C. Stapes **D.** Vomer

17. A sudden flash of light would __________.

A. Shrink the vitreous humour
B. Cause constriction of the pupil
C. Cause dilation of the pupil
D. Increase the size of the lens

18. ___________ helps in regulation of body temperature.

A. Nose **B.** Tongue
C. Skin **D.** Ear

19. Which of the following anatomical structures would not be found in the ear?

A. Olfactory glomerulus
B. Cochlea
C. Tympanic membrane
D. Incus

20. ___________ is sometimes called Window of Eye.

A. Retina **B.** Cornea
C. Iris **D.** Pupil

21. ___________ secretion prevents drying and cracking of the skin.

A. Cerumen **B.** Sweat
C. Sebum **D.** Lymph

22. The central aperture of the iris is called _________.

A. Pupil B. Iris
C. Retina D. Choroid

23. The Eustachian tube connects __________.

A. The auditory canal with the cochlea
B. The incus with the stapes
C. The pharynx with the middle ear
D. Cerumen and the tympanic membrane

24. __________ layer of eye contains rod and cone cells.

A. Retina
B. Choroid
C. Sclera
D. None of the above

25. Thickening of fibrosis of lens means __________.

A. Cataract
B. Diplopia
C. Myopia
D. Photophobia

26. Sound waves are transmitted from the outer ear to the cochlea because of movement of the __________.

A. Ossicles
B. Oval window
C. Tympanic membrane
D. Semicircular canals

27. Which of the following is an organ of sense of vision/ sight?

A. Eye **B.** Ear
C. Nose **D.** Tongue

28. The structure(s) associated with sensing changes in the position of the head are __________.

A. The ossicles
B. The cochlea
C. The semicircular canals
D. The fovea

29. The eyeballs are situated in the bony socket called __________.

A. Circles
B. Depression
C. Orbits
D. Cavity

30. Which of the following structures is not part of the vestibular apparatus of the inner ear?

A. The pinna
B. The utricle
C. The saccule
D. The ampulla

31. Sensation of heat is picked up by _________.

A. Meissner's capsules
B. Organs of Golgi-Mazzoni
C. Ruffini's corpuscles
D. Pacinian corpuscles

32. Which part of the eye controls the amount of light entering in it?

A. Iris
B. Cornea
C. Ciliary body
D. Suspensory ligaments

33. The cones are located in __________.

A. Iris **B.** Retina
C. Sclerotic **D.** Choroid

34. Vitreous humour is seen in __________.

A. Ear **B.** Brain
C. Bone marrow **D.** Eye

35. Receptors of skin are called _________.
A. Somatic receptors
B. Interceptors
C. Gland receptors
D. Visceral receptors

36. _________ layer of the eye contains rod and cone cells.
A. Sclera B. Choroid
C. Retina D. None of the above

37. Function of ciliary muscles is _________.
A. To contract pupil when one move in sunlight
B. To keep valve in position
C. To change shape of lens
D. To rotate eyeball

38. Our taste organs located on the tongue are examples of _________.
A. Interoceptors B. Photoreceptors
C. Gustatoreceptors D. Tenoreceptors

39. Photosensitive pigment found in the rod cells of retina layer of the eye is called _________.
A. Renin B. Rhodopsin
C. Melanin D. Keratin

40. The sweet and acidic tastes are better detected by _________.
A. Base of the tongue
B. Tip of the tongue
C. Middle of the tongue
D. Lateral sides of the tongue

41. Colour to the eye is imparted by _________.
A. Iris B. Lens
C. Pupil D. Vitreous humour

42. In man's eye, the sclerotic is made up of _________.
A. Bone
B. Fibrous connective tissue
C. Cartilage
D. Muscles and cartilage

43. The site from which the nerve impulse for hearing originates _________.
A. Cochlea B. Ear ossicles
C. Auditory nerve D. Tympanum

44. The lens becomes opaque in _________.
A. Myopia B. Hypermetropia
C. Cataract D. Astigmatism

45. Too short eyeball and flat lens produce _________.
A. Nearsightedness
B. Astigmatism
C. Farsightedness
D. Presbyopia

46. Sound is amplified by the _________.
A. Ear ossicles
B. Pinna
C. Tympanic membrane
D. Round window

47. Cone cells of the eye are responsible for _________.
A. Dim vision
B. Colour vision
C. Bright vision
D. Dark vision

48. The sense of equilibrium is determined by _________.
A. Basilar membrane of cochlea
B. Sensory crista of ampulla
C. Tectorial membrane of cochlea
D. Sensory cells of organ of Corti

49. Night blindness is caused by deficiency of _________.
A. Vitamin K B. Vitamin C
C. Vitamin A D. Vitamin E

50. The first cranial nerve is _________.
A. Oculomotor
B. Olfactory
C. Optic
D. None of the above

51. Thickness of lens is controlled by _________.
A. Pupil B. Choroid
C. Iris D. Ciliary body

52. From outside to inside the arrangement of the bones of middle ear is _________.
A. Malleus-incus-stapes
B. Incus-malleus-stapes
C. Stapes-malleus-incus
D. Incus-stapes-malleus

53. The central aperture of the iris is known as _________.
A. Iris B. Pupil
C. Rods D. Cones

54. "Organ of Corti" is a part of _________.
A. External ear B. Middle ear
C. Nasal chambers D. Inner ear

55. ________ fluid is present in the anterior chamber of the eye.

A. Sebum
B. Aqueous humour
C. Vitreous humour
D. Lymph

56. The corpuscles in the skin, which are sensitive to pressure are called ________.

A. Ruffini corpuscles
B. Pacinian corpuscles
C. Krause corpuscles
D. Meissner's corpuscles

57. Layers of tissue in the walls of the eye are ________.

A. The middle vascular layer
B. The outer fibrous layer
C. The inner nervous tissue layer
D. All of the above

58. ________ are also called auditory ossicles.

A. Ear ossicles
B. Semicircular canals
C. Auricular ossicles
D. Auditory tube

59. The inner nervous tissue layer of the eye includes ________.

A. Retina
B. Choroid
C. Ciliary body
D. Iris

60. Which of the following are present in the external acoustic meatus?

A. Sebaceous glands
B. Lacrimal glands
C. Ceruminous glands
D. Nasal glands

Answer Key

1 B	2 D	3 A	4 C	5 B	6 A	7 C	8 D	9 B	10 A
11 B	12 C	13 B	14 A	15 C	16 A	17 B	18 C	19 A	20 B
21 C	22 A	23 C	24 A	25 A	26 A	27 A	28 C	29 C	30 A
31 C	32 A	33 B	34 D	35 A	36 C	37 C	38 C	39 B	40 B
41 A	42 B	43 A	44 C	45 C	46 A	47 B	48 B	49 C	50 B
51 D	52 A	53 B	54 D	55 B	56 B	57 D	58 A	59 A	60 C

CHAPTER 13

The Urinary System

The Renal System

1. **The basic structural and functional unit of the urinary system/renal system is __________.**
   A. Neurone B. Nephron
   C. Medulla D. Cortex

2. **Nephron is also known as __________.**
   A. Seminiferous tubule
   B. Convoluted tubule
   C. Collecting duct
   D. Uriniferous tubule

3. **Which of the following structures is found within the urinary system?**
   A. Gall bladder B. Sphincter of Oddi
   C. Ureter D. Larynx

4. **The hormone secreted by the hypothalamus to increase fluid reabsorption is __________.**
   A. ACTH B. TSH
   C. Renin D. ADH

5. **Which of the following substances would not normally be expected to appear in urine?**
   A. Water B. Glucose
   C. Urea D. Sodium ions

6. **The blood vessel which carries blood to the glomerulus is the __________.**
   A. Renal artery B. Renal vein
   C. Efferent arteriole D. Afferent arteriole

7. **Which of the following structures is not a part of a nephron?**
   A. Renal pelvis B. Distal tubule
   C. Collecting duct D. Proximal tubule

8. **The urinary bladder stores about __________ urine temporarily.**
   A. 2 litres B. 3 litres
   C. 0.5 litres D. 4 litres

9. **The outermost covering of the kidney is the _______.**
   A. Cortex B. Capsule
   C. Medulla D. Pelvis

10. **Each kidney contains about a million nephrons, each of which begins in a filtration apparatus called ______.**
    A. The glomerular capsule B. The distal tubule
    C. The proximal tubule D. The loop of Henle

11. **The entrance of the kidney is called ________.**
    A. Sinus B. Column
    C. Hilum D. Pyramid

12. **What is the volume of glomerular filtrate per day in an adult?**
    A. 1–5 litres B. 130 litres
    C. 80 litres D. 180 litres

13. **In an adult each kidney weighs about _________.**
    A. 60 gm B. 70 gm
    C. 80 gm D. 140 gm

14. **Which of the following substances does not normally pass through capillaries into the filtrate?**
    A. Sodium ions B. Albumin
    C. Water D. Urea

15. **The act of contraction of urinary bladder to pass the urine is called ________.**
    A. Mastication B. Ingestion
    C. Micturition D. Deglutition

16. **The urine of man suffering from diabetes insipidus is ________.**
A. Tasteless and watery
B. Sweaty and watery
C. Sweaty and thick
D. Tasteless and thick

17. **The __________ cells in the kidney are responsible for maintaining blood pressure.**
A. Epithelial cells
B. Testicular cells
C. Adrenal cells
D. Juxtaglomerular cells

18. **Which structure carries urine from kidneys to urinary bladder?**
A. Urethra B. Nephron
C. Ureter D. Pelvis

19. **Each kidney is composed of about ____________ of nephrons.**
A. 5 millions B. 4 millions
C. 3 millions D. 1 to 1.5 millions

20. **The filtration of blood under pressure is called ________.**
A. Meta filtration
B. Ultrafiltration
C. Uni filtration
D. Semifiltration

21. **A man excretes about urine per day ________.**
A. 1 litre B. 2 litres
C. 2.5 litres D. 1.5 litres

22. **Which of the following is an example of high threshold substances?**
A. Glucose B. Urea
C. Uric acid D. Creatine

23. **Glomerular capsule is also known as ________.**
A. Globular capsule
B. Bowman's capsule
C. Tubular capsule
D. Convoluted capsule

24. **A person feels the sensation of micturition when the quantity of urine in the bladder is about**
A. 300 cc B. 100 cc
C. 200 cc D. None of the above

25. **When bile appears in the urine, the condition is called ________.**
A. Glycosuria B. Ketonuria
C. Jaundice D. Pyuria

26. **GFR means ________.**
A. Globular filtration rate
B. Glomerular filtration rate
C. Both A and B
D. None of the above

27. **Which one of the following is not an abnormal constituent of urine?**
A. Protein B. Blood
C. Pus D. Urea

28. **Glomeruli fail to filter from plasma is _________.**
A. Glucose B. Globin
C. Lipids D. Both B and C

29. **Inflammation of kidney means _________.**
A. Kidney stone B. Arthritis
C. Nephritis D. Oedema

30. **In the kidney, the formation of urine involves the following processes arranged as __________.**
A. Reabsorption, filtration, and secretion
B. Glomerular filtration, reabsorption, and tubular secretion
C. Secretion, absorption, and filtration
D. Filtration, secretion, and reabsorption

31. **An abnormal accumulation of tissue fluid in the intracellular spaces of the body is called _________.**
A. Gout B. Oedema
C. Arthritis D. Glaucoma

32. **Normal odour of human urine is __________.**
A. Like bitter almond
B. Like pineapple
C. Aromatic
D. Like decaying fruit

33. **About _________ of blood is filtered out per minute as a glomerular filtration.**
A. 50 ml B. 70 ml
C. 125 ml D. 90 ml

34. **The action of aldosterone is _______.**
A. Sodium elimination
B. Sodium reabsorption
C. Potassium reabsorption
D. Chloride excretion

35. **The complete suppression of urine means ________.**
A. Oliguria B. Polyuria
C. Anuria D. Dysuria

36. **Secretion of urine is called _______.**
   A. Diuresis B. Parturition
   C. Micturition D. None of the above

37. **The glomerular filtration rate is about ________.**
   A. 1% B. 4%
   C. 8% D. 10%

38. **The tubular reabsorption occurs at the _______.**
   A. Loop of Henle B. DCT
   C. PCT D. Glomerulus

39. **The anterior half of the proximal convoluted tubules is the site of ________.**
   A. Reabsorption of glucose B. Diuresis
   C. Action by ADH D. Action of aldosterone

40. **Loop of Henle is meant for absorption of ________.**
   A. Potassium B. Water
   C. Glucose D. Salt

41. **The presence of pus in the urine is called ________.**
   A. Polyuria B. Pyuria
   C. Pyloritis D. Polymorph

42. **Urea cycle in liver was discovered by __________.**
   A. Hans Krebs and Kurt Henseleit
   B. Bowman and Krebs
   C. Bayliss and Starling
   D. Landsteiner and Weiner

43. **The amount of liquid filtered by glomerulus of kidney in a 24 hours period is ________.**
   A. 100 litres B. 170 litres
   C. 200–250 cc D. 500–1000 cc

44. **Reabsorption of glucose from the glomerular filtrate in the kidney tubule is carried out by _________.**
   A. Osmosis
   B. Brownian movement
   C. Diffusion
   D. Active transport

45. **Proximal and distal convoluted tubules are parts of a ________.**
   A. Oviduct B. Nephron
   C. Vas deferens D. Caecum

46. **All Bowman's capsules of the kidney are found in __________.**
   A. Medulla B. Cortex
   C. Pelvis D. None of the above

47. **An upper expanded end of ureter called _________.**
   A. Nephrons B. Pelvis
   C. Both A and B D. None of the above

48. **_________ canal through which urine passes from bladder to outside which differs in males and females having a sphincter which is common.**
   A. Nephron B. Urethra
   C. Both A and B D. None of the above

49. **Which tests are used to access the rate of glomerular filtration?**
   A. Chemical tests B. Clearance tests
   C. Colour tests D. Odour tests

50. **Which glands are present at the top of each kidney?**
   A. Pituitary gland B. Thyroid glands
   C. Adrenal glands D. Pineal gland

Answer Key

1	B	2	D	3	C	4	D	5	B	6	A	7	A	8	C	9	B	10	A
11	C	12	C	13	D	14	B	15	C	16	A	17	D	18	C	19	D	20	B
21	D	22	A	23	B	24	A	25	C	26	B	27	D	28	D	29	C	30	B
31	B	32	C	33	C	34	B	35	C	36	C	37	D	38	C	39	A	40	B
41	B	42	A	43	B	44	D	45	B	46	B	47	B	48	B	49	B	50	C

CHAPTER

14

The Endocrine System

Hormonal Coordination

1. **Which gland of the body is called master gland of the body?**
   A. Thyroid gland B. Adrenal gland
   C. Pituitary gland D. Pineal gland

2. **The gland that secretes the hormone that determines the basal rate of metabolism and normal growth is located _________.**
   A. In the brain
   B. In front of the trachea
   C. In bones
   D. In the pelvis

3. **The exocrine cells of the pancreas produce _________.**
   A. Adrenaline B. Insulin
   C. Digestive juices D. Cortisol

4. **Which hormone is primarily responsible for uptake of glucose from blood by cells?**
   A. Renin B. Angiotensin
   C. Insulin D. Aldosterone

5. **Endocrine glands are ductless glands which secretes _________.**
   A. Enzymes B. Sebum
   C. Hormones D. None of the above

6. **Which of the following cell types is not found in the pancreas?**
   A. Acinar cells B. Kappa cells
   C. Alpha cells D. Beta cells

7. **All of the following are endocrine glands *except* _____.**
   A. Adrenal gland B. Testes
   C. Thyroid gland D. Gastric glands

8. **Which of the following hormones are produced and secreted by the adrenal medulla?**
   A. T4 (thyroxine) and T3 (triiodothyronine)
   B. Insulin and glucagon
   C. Adrenaline and noradrenaline
   D. Calcitonin and parathyroid hormone (PTH)

9. **TSH stands for _________.**
   A. Thyroid stimulating hormone
   B. Thrombin stimulating hormone
   C. Troponin stimulating hormone
   D. None of the above

10. **Which hormone from the anterior pituitary gland regulates the release of corticosteroid hormones from the adrenal cortex?**
    A. TSH B. FSH
    C. LH D. ACTH

11. **Which of the following hormones does not affect Na, Cl, and water reabsorption and K secretion by the renal tubules?**
    A. Angiotensin II
    B. Thyroid hormone
    C. Aldosterone
    D. Antidiuretic hormone

12. **Name the hormone, which is released by the posterior lobe of pituitary gland.**
    A. Oxytocin B. TSH
    C. ACTH D. Prolactin

13. **Which of the following is not an endocrine gland?**
    A. Pituitary gland B. Adrenal gland
    C. Sweat gland D. Testis

14. **Oxytocin and vasopressin are the hormones secreted by __________ lobe of the pituitary gland.**
A. Adenohypophysis B. Neurohypophysis
C. Middle lobe D. None of the above

15. **ACTH stands for ________.**
A. Adrenocorticotropic hormones
B. Adenocorticotropic hormones
C. Adeninocorticotropic hormones
D. Anticorticptropic hormones

16. **Which of the following hormone is not secreted by thyroid gland?**
A. Thyroxin B. Triiodothyronine
C. Calcitonin D. Oxytocin

17. **ADH stands for ________.**
A. Anti-derived hormone
B. Antidiuretic hormone
C. Adenoid diuretic hormone
D. Albumin developing hormone

18. **Myxoedema is caused by the deficiency of a hormone secreted by __________.**
A. Parathyroid B. Thyroid
C. Hypothalamus D. Pineal body

19. **A gland that disappears in the adult but is active during childhood is __________.**
A. Hypothalamus B. Thymus
C. Parathyroid D. Adrenal cortex

20. **Low secretion of the growth hormone causes which of the following disease?**
A. Acromegaly B. Goitre
C. Dwarfism D. Gigantism

21. **Which hormone stimulates secretion of milk?**
A. Prolactin B. Growth hormone
C. TSH D. Oestrogen

22. **__________ located at the base of the brain in the sphenoid bone.**
A. Pituitary gland B. Thyroid gland
C. Both A and B D. None of the above

23. **Which of the following hormones are known as gonadotrophins?**
A. LH and oxytocin B. LH and vasopressin
C. LH and FSH D. FSH and oxytocin

24. **An enlargement of thyroid gland is called ________.**
A. Oedema B. Goitre
C. Diabetes D. Dwarfism

25. **Islets of Langerhans are related to which of the following?**
A. Calcitonin B. Diabetes
C. Thyroxine D. Insulin

26. **__________ stimulates growth and activity of thyroid gland and secretion of T3 and T4.**
A. Growth hormone (GH)
B. Thyroid stimulating hormone (TSH)
C. Both A and B
D. None of the above

27. **The protein that controls metabolic activities of the cells is ________.**
A. Ligand B. Receptor
C. Hormone D. Neurotransmitter

28. **The production of which hormone is reduced to retain water when the body is dehydrated?**
A. Insulin B. Thyroxine
C. Oxytocin D. ADH

29. **ADH is also known as __________.**
A. Renin B. Vasopressin
C. Aldosterone D. Angiotensin

30. **Pituitary gland is situated in __________.**
A. Hypothalamus B. Medulla oblongata
C. Sella turcica D. None of the above

31. **Which of the following is an endocrine and exocrine gland of the body?**
A. Parathyroid gland B. Pancrease
C. Pineal D. Pituitary gland

32. **Which of the following hormones stimulates contraction of uterus?**
A. Prolactin B. Oxytocin
C. Vasopressin D. Renin

33. **The parathyroid glands are present on the poles of _________.**
A. Adrenal glands B. Pituitary gland
C. Thyroid gland D. All of the above

34. **Myxoedema is caused by the deficiency of a hormone secreted by _________.**
A. Parathyroid gland B. Hypothalamus
C. Thyroid gland D. Pineal body

35. **_________ means stunted growth of the body caused due to hypoactivity of pituitary gland.**
A. Gigantism B. Dwarfism
C. Goitre D. Diabetes

36. **Cretinism is caused by the deficiency of hormone ___________.**

A. Adrenaline B. Growth hormone
C. Parathormone D. Thyroxine

37. **Medulla and cortex are the parts of an endocrine gland called ___________.**

A. Pituitary B. Thymus
C. Adrenal D. Hypothalamus

38. **Calcitonin is a hormone secreted by __________.**

A. Pituitary gland B. Thyroid gland
C. Testis D. Adrenal glands

39. **A gland that disappears in the adult but is active during childhood is ___________.**

A. Hypothalamus B. Parathyroid
C. Adrenal cortex D. Thymus

40. **Renin is a hormone secreted by the __________.**

A. Pancreas B. Kidney
C. Liver D. Ovary

41. **___________ disease is caused by deficiency of hyper-activity of pituitary gland.**

A. Gigantism B. Dwarfism
C. Goitre D. Gout

42. **Deficiency of which of the following hormones produces cretinism?**

A. Adrenaline B. Growth hormone
C. Parathormone D. Thyroxine

43. **Which of the following diseases is not related to thyroid gland?**

A. Myxoedema B. Acromegaly
C. Cretinism D. Goitre

44. **Goitre is a disease caused by the deficiency of_________.**

A. Calcium B. Sodium
C. Chloride D. Iodine

45. **Hormone which helps in production of milk is_________.**

A. FSH B. LH
C. Prolactin D. Oxytocin

46. **Diabetes insipidus is caused due to hyposecretion of __________.**

A. Renin B. ADH
C. Aldosterone D. Oestrogen

47. **Parathormone increases blood __________.**

A. Sodium level
B. Chloride level
C. Potassium level
D. Calcium level

48. **Chemical messengers secreted by ductless glands are called __________.**

A. Lymph B. Hormones
C. Enzymes D. Plasma

49. **Which of the following is not an endocrine?**

A. Lacrimal gland
B. Pituitary gland
C. Adrenal gland
D. Pineal gland

50. **Which gland is located just superior to the kidneys?**

A. Thyroid gland
B. Ovaries
C. Pituitary gland
D. Adrenal gland

Answer Key

1 C	2 B	3 C	4 C	5 C	6 B	7 D	8 C	9 A	10 D
11 B	12 A	13 C	14 B	15 A	16 D	17 B	18 B	19 B	20 C
21 A	22 A	23 C	24 B	25 D	26 B	27 C	28 D	29 B	30 A
31 B	32 B	33 C	34 C	35 B	36 D	37 C	38 B	39 D	40 B
41 A	42 D	43 B	44 D	45 C	46 B	47 D	48 B	49 A	50 D

CHAPTER 15

The Reproductive System

1. **In adult males, sperms are produced in the ________**
   A. Testis B. Epididymis
   C. Vas deferens D. Scrotum

2. **Which of the following conditions means permanent cessation of the menses?**
   A. Menstruation B. Menopause
   C. Menstrual phase D. Dysmenorrhoea

3. **Each testis consists of ________ tubules.**
   A. Convoluted B. Uriniferous
   C. Seminiferous D. Renal tubule

4. **The following are accessory glands of the male reproductive system *except* ________.**
   A. Seminal vesicles B. Prostate glands
   C. Cowper's glands D. Ovary

5. **Menopause period occurs in women in between ages of ________.**
   A. 15 to 35 years B. 25 to 35 years
   C. 45 to 55 years D. 60 to 70 years

6. **________ is a fluid ejaculated from urethra of male during coitus.**
   A. Sebum B. Semen
   C. Sweat D. Mucus

7. **Menstruation/menstrual cycle is about ________ cycle.**
   A. 15 days B. 20 days
   C. 28 days D. 14 days

8. **In adult males, what are the cells which produce testosterone known as?**
   A. Spermatogonia B. Sertoli cells
   C. Spermatids D. Leydig cells

9. **Name the hormone produced by a corpus luteum after ovulation.**
   A. Prolactin B. Progesterone
   C. Testosterone D. Inhibin

10. **________ helps to regulate temperature of testis.**
    A. Prepuce B. Glans penis
    C. Epididymis D. Scrotum

11. **What is the name of tube through which both urine and semen leave a man's body called?**
    A. Epididymis
    B. Spermatic cord
    C. Urethra
    D. Seminiferous tubule

12. **What is the membrane that covers the opening of the vagina called?**
    A. The hymen B. The mons pubis
    C. The labia minora D. The labia majora

13. **The process of spermatogenesis is better when the temperature of testis is less than ________ than normal body temperature.**
    A. 1°C B. 2°C
    C. 3°C D. 4°C

14. **Which phase of the ovarian cycle is characterised by growth and development of follicles?**
    A. Luteal phase B. Ovulation
    C. Follicular phase D. Menstruation

15. **The testis secretes the hormone ________.**
    A. Oestrogen B. Testosterone
    C. Progesterone D. Aldosterone

16. **Fertilization it usually takes place in the ________.**
    A. Ovary
    B. Endometrium
    C. Fallopian tube (oviduct)
    D. Myometrium

17. **Which of the following is the largest accessory gland of the male reproductive system?**
    A. Seminal vesicle
    B. Prostate gland
    C. Cowper's gland
    D. Vestibular gland

18. **The fertilised egg is known as ________.**
    A. Blastocyst B. Zygote
    C. Morula D. Trophoblast

19. **An essential organ of reproduction is known as a ________.**
    A. Gamete B. Gender
    C. Gonad D. Gluteal

20. **The onset of reproductive maturity is known as _____.**
    A. Menstruation B. Menarche
    C. Climacteric D. Puberty

21. **Innermost layer of the uterus is ________.**
    A. Endometrium
    B. Endocardium
    C. Endopelvic
    D. None of the above

22. **________ gland is also known as bulbourethral gland.**
    A. Seminal vesicles
    B. Prostate gland
    C. Cowper's gland
    D. None of the above

23. **Colostrum is a thin fluid which is rich in ________.**
    A. Carbohydrates B. Proteins
    C. Fat D. None of the above

24. **Corpus luteum is formed of dead ________.**
    A. RBCs B. WBCs
    C. Graafian follicles D. Chorion

25. **Which one of the following is not a paired organ in the male reproductive system ________.**
    A. Prostate gland
    B. Seminal vesicle
    C. Epididymis
    D. Cowper's gland

26. **The cell formed by the process of meiosis after which sperm formation takes place is called ________.**
    A. Primary spermatocyte
    B. Spermatid
    C. Secondary spermatocyte
    D. Sperm mother cell

27. **Nourishment to the developing cells in the testes is provided by ________.**
    A. Leydig cells B. Sertoli cells
    C. Endometrium D. Germinal epithelium

28. **________ is the process of formation of sperms in the testis.**
    A. Oogenesis B. Spermatogenesis
    C. Spermatocytes D. Gametogenesis

29. **Proliferation of uterine wall is maximum when the blood contains high levels of ________.**
    A. Progesterone B. FSH
    C. LH D. Estrogen

30. **________ is a motile living male gamete.**
    A. Ovum B. Semen
    C. Penis D. Spermatozoon

31. **Fructose and prostaglandins are present in the secretion of ________.**
    A. Uterus B. Seminal vesicles
    C. Cowper's gland D. Prostate glands

32. **The fold of skin covering the penis is called ________.**
    A. Corpora cavernosa B. Prepuce
    C. Corpus spongiosum D. None of the above

33. **Location and secretion of Leydig's cell are ________.**
    A. Liver cholesterol B. Testis testosterone
    C. Ovary estrogens D. Pancreas glucagon

34. **The total length of spermatozoon is about ________.**
    A. 55 to 65 microns B. 20 to 30 microns
    C. 10 to 20 microns D. 80 to 100 microns

35. **Seminiferous tubules develop central lumen after ________.**
    A. Birth B. Puberty
    C. Prepuberal time D. Old age

36. **Sertoli cells in human testis are found in ________.**
    A. Leydig cells
    B. Seminiferous tubules
    C. Outside the seminiferous tubules
    D. None of the above

37. _________ is marked by onset of menstruation.
A. Menopause B. Reproduction
C. Fertilization D. Puberty

38. Testis produce __________.
A. Eggs B. Seeds
C. Sperms D. Spores

39. The seminiferous tubules of the testis are lined by the germinal epithelium consisting of _______.
A. Cells of Sertoli
B. Spermatogonium
C. Spermatocytes
D. Spermatids

40. Puberty usually occurs at the age of ________.
A. 5 to 7 years B. 10 to 14 years
C. 18 to 20 years D. 20 to 25 years

41. Supporting cells found in between the germinal epithelium of testes are called __________.
A. Interstitial cells of Leydig
B. Granular cells
C. Phagocytes
D. Sertoli cells

42. The nutritive medium for the ejaculated sperms is given by the ________.
A. Vaginal fluid B. Uterine lining
C. Seminal fluid D. Fallopian tube

43. ________ means absence of menses.
A. Dysmenorrhoea B. Galactorrhea
C. Amenorrhoea D. Leucorrhoea

44. Functions of seminal fluid is ________.
A. Provides proper pH and ionic strength
B. Maintains the viability of sperms
C. Maintains motility of sperms
D. All of the above

45. The narrow middle part of the epididymis is called ________.
A. Caput epididymis B. Corpus epididymis
C. Cauda epididymis D. All of the above

46. Painful menstruation means __________.
A. Amenorrhoea B. Leucorrhoea
C. Dysmenorrhoea D. Galactorrhea

47. In human male a single ejaculation may contain ______ million spermatozoa.
A. 300 B. 500
C. 200 D. 100

48. __________ is a process of giving birth.
A. Micturition B. Parturition
C. Mastication D. Deglutition

49. Seminal fluid contains __________.
A. Ascorbic acid B. Fructose
C. Citrate D. All of the above

50. The menstrual cycle in a normal adult woman is __________.
A. 48 days B. 28 days
C. 38 days D. 18 days

51. Which of the following structure helps in collection of ovum after ovulation?
A. Internal os B. Fimbriae
C. Ampulla D. Cervix

52. Parturition duct in females is called _________.
A. Uterus B. Oviduct
C. Cervix D. Vagina

53. The menstrual cycle begins with the casting off of __________.
A. Endometrial lining along with blood vessels
B. Placenta
C. Blood
D. All of the above

54. In human beings the median tube where the uterus opens independently is called __________.
A. Cervix B. Vagina
C. Clitoris D. Cloaca

55. Parturition is controlled by two hormones, namely __________.
A. Renin and aldosterone
B. ADH and TSH
C. Oxytocin and relaxin
D. ACTH and progesterone

56. Ovulation in mammals is caused by __________.
A. FSH and TSH B. FSH and LTH
C. FSH and LH D. LTH and LH

57. Which of the following is a female gamete?
A. Serum B. Sebum
C. Sperm D. Ovum

58. In females, the oviducts are cut or removed surgically to avoid the chances of fertilization. This is called __________.
A. Vasectomy B. Tubectomy
C. Ovariectomy D. Sterilization

59. __________ is a copulatory organ and the terminal part of urethra.
A. Testis B. Penis
C. Spermatic cord D. All of the above

60. The wider part of the fallopian tube is _________.
A. Infundibulum B. Isthmus
C. Ampulla D. Cervix

61. The phase of the menstrual cycle in humans that lasts for 7–8 days is _________.
A. Ovulatory phase
B. Follicular phase
C. Luteal phase
D. Menstruation

62. Female reproductive system does not include _______.
A. Ovaries B. Fallopian tubes
C. Uterus D. Cowper's gland

63. Parts of penis are __________.
A. Glans penis
B. Corpora cavernosa
C. Corpora spongiosum
D. All of the above

64. Secretion of progesterone by corpus luteum is initiated by __________.
A. TSH B. Testosterone
C. LH D. Thyroxine

65. Which hormone is decreased in the menstrual cycle causing menstruation?
A. Progesterone B. Luteinising hormone
C. Oestrogen D. None of the abcve

66. External genitalia of women are collectively called __________.
A. Labia B. Vulva
C. Clitoris D. Mons pubis

67. The sac of skin in which the testes are located is called __________.
A. Seminiferous tubules B. Vas deferens
C. Epididymis D. Scrotum

68. In which organ of the female reproductive system, the process of fertilization takes place?
A. Uterus B. Fallopian tubes
C. Ovary D. Vagina

69. Umbilical cord contains ___________.
A. Plenipotent cells
B. Cord blood stem cells
C. Blood stem cells
D. None of the above

70. __________ is an organ of sexual pleasure which is located above the vaginal opening.
A. Uterus B. Ovary
C. Clitoris D. Fallopian tubes

Answer Key

1 A	2 B	3 C	4 D	5 C	6 B	7 C	8 D	9 B	10 D
11 C	12 A	13 C	14 C	15 B	16 C	17 B	18 B	19 C	20 D
21 A	22 C	23 B	24 C	25 A	26 B	27 B	28 B	29 D	30 D
31 B	32 B	33 B	34 A	35 B	36 B	37 D	38 C	39 B	40 B
41 D	42 C	43 C	44 D	45 B	46 C	47 A	48 B	49 D	50 B
51 B	52 D	53 A	54 B	55 C	56 C	57 D	58 B	59 B	60 C
61 B	62 D	63 D	64 C	65 A	66 B	67 D	68 B	69 B	70 C

Section V

Social Pharmacy

1. Introduction to Social Pharmacy
2. Preventive Healthcare: Role of Pharmacist
3. Nutrition and Health
4. Introduction to Microbiology and Common Microorganisms
5. Introduction to Health System
6. Pharmacoeconomics

Syllabus (As per ER 2020) Social Pharmacy

Chapter	Topics
1	**Introduction to Social Pharmacy** ■ Definition and Scope. Social pharmacy as a discipline and its scope in improving the public health. Role of Pharmacists in Public Health ■ Concept of health—WHO definition, various dimensions, determinants, and health indicators ■ National Health Policy—Indian perspective ■ Public and private health system in India, National Health Mission ■ Introduction to Millennium Development Goals, Sustainable Development Goals, FIP Development Goals
2	**Preventive Healthcare: Role of Pharmacists in the following** ■ Demography and Family Planning ■ Mother and child health, importance of breastfeeding, ill-effects of infant milk substitutes and bottle feeding ■ Overview of vaccines, types of immunity and immunization ■ Effect of environment on health—water pollution, importance of safe drinking water, waterborne diseases, air pollution, noise pollution, sewage and solid waste disposal, occupational illnesses, environmental pollution due to pharmaceuticals ■ Psychosocial pharmacy: Drugs of misuse and abuse—psychotropics, narcotics, alcohol, tobacco products. Social impact of these habits on social health and productivity and suicidal behaviors
3	**Nutrition and Health** ■ Basics of nutrition: Macronutrients and micronutrients ■ Importance of water and fibers in diet ■ Balanced diet, malnutrition, nutrition deficiency diseases, ill effects of junk foods, calorific and nutritive values of various foods, fortification of food ■ Introduction to food safety, adulteration of foods, effects of artificial ripening, use of pesticides, genetically modified foods ■ Dietary supplements, nutraceuticals, food supplements—indications, benefits, drug–food interactions
4	**Introduction to microbiology and common microorganisms** **Epidemiology:** Introduction to epidemiology, and its applications. Understanding of terms such as epidemic, pandemic, endemic, mode of transmission, outbreak, quarantine, isolation, incubation period, contact tracing, morbidity, mortality **Causative agents, epidemiology and clinical presentations and role of pharmacists in educating the public in prevention of the following communicable diseases:** ■ Respiratory infections—chickenpox, measles, rubella, mumps, influenza (including Avian-Flu, H1N1, SARS, MERS, COVID-19), diphtheria, whooping cough, meningococcal meningitis, acute respiratory infections, tuberculosis, Ebola ■ Intestinal infections—poliomyelitis, viral hepatitis, cholera, acute diarrheal diseases, typhoid, amebiasis, worm infestations, food poisoning ■ Arthropod-borne infections—dengue, malaria, filariasis and, chikungunya ■ Surface infections—trachoma, tetanus, leprosy ■ STDs, HIV/AIDS
5	Introduction to health systems and all ongoing National Health Programs in India, their objectives, functioning, outcome, and the role of pharmacists.
6	Pharmacoeconomics—introduction, basic terminologies, importance of pharmacoeconomics

CHAPTER 1

Introduction to Social Pharmacy

1. __________ is defined as the science which deals with social aspects of the profession of pharmacy.
   A. Simple pharmacy
   B. Social pharmacy
   C. Similar pharmacy
   D. Symbolic pharmacy

2. The state of being free from illness or injury means?
   A. Happiness B. Fitness
   C. Disease D. Health

3. MDGs stand for _________.
   A. Mega Development Goals
   B. Main Development Goals
   C. Millennium Development Goals
   D. Millions Development Goals

4. All of the following indicators are used to measure disability rates in a community *except* _________.
   A. Health adapted life expectancy
   B. Human poverty index
   C. Sullivan's Index
   D. Disability adjusted life year

5. FIP is the global federation of National Associations of ___________.
   A. Physicians and Pharmacists
   B. Nurses and Physicians
   C. Pharmacists and Pharmaceutical Scientists
   D. Nurses and Pharmacists

6. The burden of disease is given by ________.
   A. Incidence
   B. Crude death rate
   C. Promotional mortality rate
   D. Cause-specific death rate

7. The pharmacy is an integral and essential part of _________.
   A. Computerized system
   B. Development system
   C. Diagnostic system
   D. Health care system

8. In a village with a population of 5000, 50 people have a disease and 10 of them died. What is the case fatality rate?
   A. 1% B. 2%
   C. 0.5% D. 20%

9. Which of the following is not a mental disorder?
   A. Neurosis B. Gout
   C. Depression D. Schizophrenia

10. The communicability of disease is assessed by ______.
    A. Serial interval
    B. Generation time
    C. Secondary attack rate
    D. Incubation period

11. NHP stands for ________.
    A. National Health Policy
    B. National Home Policy
    C. National Higher Policy
    D. National Hints Policy

12. Which one of the following is not a mortality indicator?
    A. Prevalence
    B. Life expectancy
    C. Years of potential life lost
    D. IMR

13. **Which of the following is not a National Health Policy?**
    A. Yatri Suraksha
    B. Nirbhaya Nari
    C. Loan Facility
    D. Control on air pollution

14. **The Health indicator characteristics include all *except* ________.**
    A. Validity **B.** Affordability
    C. Reliability **D.** Feasibility

15. **The health indicators are used to measure ________.**
    A. The requirement of health needs
    B. Assess the rate of infection
    C. Health status of the community
    D. To meet basic needs

16. **SDGs means ________.**
    A. Serial Development Goals
    B. Sustainable Development Goals
    C. Summer Development Goals
    D. Standard Development Goals

17. **The role of pharmacist is to take care of the patient care through ________.**
    A. Home care
    B. Hospitals
    C. Community pharmacy
    D. All of the above

18. **Which one of the following is known as "epidemiological triad"?**
    A. Host, water, environment
    B. Host, agent, environment
    C. Host, air, water
    D. Host, water, animal

19. **Which of the following are determinants of health?**
    A. Environment **B.** Heredity
    C. Lifestyle **D.** All of the above

20. **________ is a disorder or bad functioning (malfunction of mind or body) which leads to departure of good health.**
    A. Diet **B.** Disease
    C. Exercise **D.** Immunity

21. **Which of the following is not principle of National Health Policy?**
    A. Education
    B. Professionalism, integrity and ethics
    C. Universality
    D. Accountability

22. **The time interval from the entry of agent in the host to the appearance of disease is termed ________.**
    A. Inhibition period
    B. Incubation period
    C. Intermittent period
    D. Interval period

23. **The hereditary traits means ________.**
    A. Profession continued from the days of parents
    B. Social relationship continued from the days of parents
    C. Physical characteristics similar to friends
    D. Physical characteristics transferred from parents

24. **Which of the following is the dimension of health?**
    A. Spiritual **B.** Mental
    C. Physical **D.** All of the above

25. **All are the concepts of prevention of diseases *except* ________.**
    A. Secondary prevention
    B. Quaternary prevention
    C. Primary prevention
    D. Tertiary prevention

26. **The main determinants of health are ________.**
    A. Socioeconomic conditions
    B. Lifestyle
    C. Genetic makeup
    D. All of the above

27. **The action taken prior to the onset of disease come under ________.**
    A. Tertiary prevention
    B. Primary prevention
    C. Secondary prevention
    D. None of the above

28. **The long form of WHO is ________.**
    A. World Hospital Committee
    B. World Heart Organization
    C. World Health Organization
    D. None of the above

29. **Physical health depends on ________.**
    A. Healthy food
    B. Coordination of all organs of the body
    C. Regular exercise
    D. All of the above

30. **In which year National Health Policy in India was implemented?**
    A. 2001 **B.** 2002
    C. 2003 **D.** 2004

31. ________ indicators give information regarding the disease situation in the community.

A. Morbidity B. Mortality
C. Disability D. Sanitation

32. What are the dimensions of public health?

A. Health promotion B. Disease prevention
C. Rehabilitation D. All of the above

33. AYUSH stands for ________.

A. All Youth and Usual Health Status
B. Ayurveda, Yoga and Naturopathy, Unani, Siddha and Homeopathy
C. Accredited Youth and Usual Special Health Care
D. None of the above

34. Social pharmacy deals with the role of medicines from ________.

A. Social perspective
B. Humanistic perspective
C. Scientific perspective
D. All of the above

35. ________ means interruption of the natural sequence of disease.

A. Infection
B. Invading
C. Intervention
D. Incubation

36. The factors that affect various aspects of health are considered as ________ .

A. Determinants of health
B. Indicators of health
C. Protectors of health
D. All of the above

37. The millennium development goals are ________.

A. Promote gender equality
B. Combat HIV/AIDS
C. Ensure environmental sustainability
D. All of the above

38. Death rate is defined as the number of deaths ________.

A. Per 100 population
B. Per 1000 population
C. Per one lakh population
D. All of the above

39. Full form of FIP is ________.

A. Federation of Indian Pharmacy
B. Federation of Italian Pharmacy
C. International Pharmaceutical Federation
D. All of the above

40. ________ is the process of returning to a healthy or good way of life.

A. Compulsion
B. Rehabilitation
C. Addiction
D. Expulsion

41. A mentally healthy person has the following qualities ________.

A. Arrogance B. Self control
C. Jealous D. Gets easily upset

42. All are indicators of health *except* ________.

A. Mortality B. Morbidity
C. Visibility D. Utilization

43. The achievement of optimum health requires adoption of ________.

A. Bad lifestyles
B. Good lifestyles
C. Both A and B
D. None of the above

44. The Sustainable Development Goals adopted by United Nation in the year ________.

A. 2016 B. 2017
C. 2018 D. 2015

45. Essential requirements for maintaining a good health are ________.

A. Exercise and rest B. Balanced diet
C. Both A and B D. None of the above

46. How many goals and targets are there in SDGs?

A. 15 and 129 B. 16 and 149
C. 17 and 169 D. 18 and 189

47. Public health means the health of people in terms of ________.

A. Mental and spiritual health
B. Physical and social health
C. Both A and B
D. None of the above

48. The services provided by public health pharmacists to achieve health are ________.

A. Preventive and curative
B. Promotive
C. Rehabilitative
D. All of the above

49. ________ rate means death rate.

A. Mortality B. Morbidity
C. Disability D. Modality

50. What is the first goal of Sustainable Development Goal?
A. Zero hunger
B. End poverty
C. Good health and well being
D. Gender equality

51. Health promotional activities include ________.
A. Inadequate health system
B. Information, communication, education.
C. Poor environment
D. Unhealthy lifestyle

52. Health maintenance requires the measures to achieve health by ________.
A. Unsafe environment
B. Increasing stress
C. Health services
D. Unhygienic conditions

53. India's largest National Health Protection scheme has been implemented under the scheme ________.
A. Adarsh Bharat
B. Sanman Bharat
C. Ayushman Bharat
D. Nirman Bharat

54. Which of the factors are responsible for good health?
A. Genetic inheritance
B. Social support system
C. External environment
D. All of the above

55. The physiological functioning of the body is known as ________.
A. Physical health B. Illness
C. Disease D. Sickness

56. The way of thinking and expression of feelings is also known as ________.
A. Social health B. Physical health
C. Mental/emotional health D. None of the above

57. External environment can be divided into ________.
A. Biological
B. Physical
C. Psychological environment
D. All of the above

58. Natural history of disease consists of two phases, namely ________.
A. Pathogenesis and oogenesis
B. Gametogenesis and pathogenesis
C. Pathogenesis and pre-pathogenesis
D. Pre-pathogenesis and gametogenesis

59. Which of the following is a sign of good health?
A. Having sickness
B. Free from unnecessary anxiety
C. Feeling sad
D. Having social tension

60. Exercise is helpful in maintaining health by ________
A. Improving the immune system
B. Strengthening the heart muscles
C. Strengthening the body muscles and bones
D. All of the above

Answer Key

1 B	2 D	3 C	4 B	5 C	6 C	7 D	8 D	9 B	10 C
11 A	12 A	13 C	14 B	15 C	16 B	17 D	18 B	19 D	20 B
21 A	22 B	23 B	24 D	25 B	26 D	27 B	28 C	29 D	30 B
31 B	32 D	33 B	34 D	35 C	36 A	37 D	38 B	39 C	40 B
41 B	42 C	43 B	44 D	45 C	46 C	47 C	48 D	49 A	50 B
51 B	52 C	53 C	54 D	55 A	56 C	57 D	58 C	59 B	60 D

CHAPTER 2

Preventive Healthcare: Role of Pharmacist

1. **The objective of demography is to study _________.**
   A. The change in population size
   B. The composition of population
   C. The distribution of population in space
   D. All of the above

2. **The following is an important determinant of population change _________.**
   A. Morbidity
   B. Life expectancy
   C. Migration
   D. Human development rate

3. **Which one of the following is a fertility reduction practice?**
   A. Reproduction
   B. Contraception
   C. Ovulation
   D. Puberty

4. **_________ suggests the population growth of the nation.**
   A. Cardiac cycle
   B. Respiratory cycle
   C. Demographic cycle
   D. Reproductive cycle

5. **Breast fed children are less likely to have _________.**
   A. Pneumonia
   B. Diarrhoea
   C. Ear infections
   D. All of the above

6. **There are _________ stages of demographic cycle.**
   A. 02 **B.** 03
   C. 05 **D.** 04

7. **The milk made by the body in the last days after birth is named _________.**
   A. Lactose
   B. Colostrum
   C. Acidophil
   D. None of the above

8. **Breastfeeding is not recommended for mothers who have _________.**
   A. Hepatitis **B.** Untreated TB
   C. HIV **D.** Diabetes

9. **_________ means actual child bearing period.**
   A. Menopause
   B. Puberty
   C. Fertility
   D. Ovulation

10. **The process of introduction of weakened pathogen into human body is called _________.**
    A. Vaccination
    B. Immunization
    C. Attenuation
    D. None of the above

11. **The woman's reproductive period is from _________.**
    A. 5–10 years
    B. 15–45 years
    C. 50–60 years
    D. 60–70 years

12. **A vaccine can be _________.**
    A. Live attenuated pathogen
    B. An antigenic protein
    C. Weakened pathogen
    D. All of the above

13. **The unit of measurement of noise is __________.**
A. Grams B. Decibels
C. Millilitres D. Milligrams

14. **Active immunity can be gained by __________.**
A. Toxoids B. Natural infection
C. Vaccines D. All of the above

15. **__________ is an unwanted waste material from the industries, houses, streets and agricultural activities.**
A. Diffuse B. Refuse
C. Perfuse D. Reuse

16. **The area draining into the reservoir is called ________.**
A. Draining area
B. Collection area
C. Attached area
D. Catchment area

17. **Water Prevention and Control of Pollution Acts was passed in the year __________.**
A. 1964 B. 1974
C. 1978 D. 1968

18. **Which one of the following is not a method of solid disposal of waste?**
A. Dumping B. Compositing
C. Scattering D. Burial

19. **Which is the most common method used to dump solid wastes?**
A. River B. Landfill
C. Ocean D. None of the above

20. **Which of the following is not an occupational disease?**
A. Diabetes B. Silicosis
C. Asbestosis D. COPD

21. **_________ is a key indicator of good reproductive health of the community.**
A. Total mortality rate
B. Total fertility rate
C. The glomerular filtration rate
D. Total respiratory rate

22. **The risks associated with cigarette smoking are_______.**
A. Emphysema B. Lung cancer
C. CAD D. All of the above

23. **The systematic and scientific study of human populations is known as __________**
A. Census B. Fertility
C. Demography D. Family planning

24. **Which of the following is an occupational illness?**
A. Silicosis B. Asbestosis
C. Byssinosis D. Amoebiasis

25. **Which one of the following is not an example of a spacing method of family planning?**
A. Intrauterine contraceptive devices
B. Condom
C. Laparoscopy
D. Oral contraceptive pills

26. **_________ is the best way to satisfy the nutritional and psychological needs of the baby.**
A. Spoon feeding
B. Khimati feeding
C. Boost powder feeding
D. Breast feeding

27. **Vaccines produced by modifying disease-producing viruses or bacteria in a laboratory are known as _________.**
A. Inactivated vaccines
B. Surface protein
C. Live attenuated vaccines
D. Monoclonal antibodies

28. **_________ is the mother's first milk.**
A. Nutrients B. Colostrum
C. Food D. Collagen

29. **Resistance to the infections which an individual exhibits by virtue of his or her genetic and constitutional make up is known as __________.**
A. Acquired immunity B. Herd immunity
C. Infection D. Innate immunity

30. **Following one is not a waterborne disease ________.**
A. Cholera B. Typhoid
C. Arthritis D. Malaria

31. **Mini laparotomy is an example of ________.**
A. Spacing method of family planning
B. Permanent method of family planning
C. Reproduction
D. Castration

32. **__________ is the power of the body to resist the effect of invasion of pathogenic micro-organisms in the body.**
A. Invasion B. Interruption
C. Immunity D. Invading

33. **Population explosion is defined as the population growth rate of more than __________ per year**
A. 1.75 B. 2
C. 15 D. 1.23

34. **Family size is __________.**
    A. Total number of children in the family
    B. Total number of family members in the family
    C. Total number of female children born in the family
    D. Total number of female children in the family considering the mortality

35. **"The Infant Milk Substitute, Feeding Bottles and Infants Food Act" was passed in __________.**
    A. 1985 B. 1992
    C. 1997 D. 2002

36. **Most significant indicator of fertility is __________.**
    A. Family size
    B. Gross reproduction rate
    C. Net reproductive rate
    D. General fertility rate

37. **Hormonal pills/oral contraceptives contains ________.**
    A. Oestrogens and progesterone
    B. Testosterone and oestradiol
    C. Oestrogen and aldosterone
    D. Aldosterone and testosterone

38. **General fertility rate is the __________.**
    A. Indicator of complete family size
    B. Not better than crude birth rate
    C. Measure of fertility
    D. All of the above

39. **Which of the following is an example of Hallucinogens?**
    A. PAS B. INH
    C. DEC D. LSD

40. **__________ is an operation in female.**
    A. Vasectomy B. Tubectomy
    C. Laparectomy D. Anatomy

41. **Explosive growth rates occur when the annual rate of growth % is __________.**
    A. 0.5–1.0 B. >2.0
    C. 10–15 D. 15–20

42. **The immune system comprises __________.**
    A. Humoral and fibrous systems
    B. RBCs
    C. Humoral and cell-mediated systems
    D. Lymphocytes

43. **The programs to get total reproductive health as a social goal of national level are called __________.**
    A. Family organization B. Family care
    C. Reproductive care D. Family planning

44. **Establishment of __________ between industrial and residential areas is essential to prevent air pollution.**
    A. Red belt B. Green belt
    C. Yellow belt D. Orange belt

45. **Which is the first country to initiate a family planning program in the world?**
    A. Brazil B. India
    C. Pakistan D. France

46. **Lippes loop is __________ IUCD.**
    A. First generation
    B. Second generation
    C. Third generation
    D. Fourth generation

47. **Which of the following is derived from the hemp plant?**
    A. Opium B. Marijuana
    C. MDMA D. Coffee

48. **Which of the following is an addictive drug found in tobacco?**
    A. Ethanol B. Ammonia
    C. Nicotine D. Tar

49. **Which of the following are methods for contraception?**
    A. Sterilization
    B. Diaphragm
    C. Intrauterine device (IUD)
    D. All of the above

50. **Copper-T is __________ IUCD.**
    A. First generation
    B. Second generation
    C. Third generation
    D. Fourth generation

51. **What is the recommended duration for exclusive breastfeeding?**
    A. 2 months B. 4 months
    C. 6 months D. 12 months

52. **Lysergic acid diethylamide (LSD) starts to take effect around 30 to 90 minutes after taking it and physical effects include:**
    A. Raised body temperature
    B. Increased heart rate and BP
    C. Sleeplessness
    D. All of the above

53. **The Worlds Health Day is celebrated on __________.**
    A. 1st March B. 7th April
    C. 6th October D. 10th December

54. **A long-term user of cocaine may develop symptoms of other psychological disorders such as ________.**
A. Major depression
B. Social problems
C. Eating disorders
D. All of the above

55. **________ is a permanent sterilization surgery meant for men.**
A. Hysterectomy
B. Pelvic organ prolapses
C. Vasectomy
D. None of the above

56. **What are the two hormones combined in oral contraceptives, or "the pill"?**
A. Oestrogens and progestin
B. Dopamine and serotonin
C. Prolactin and oxytocin
D. Oestrogen and testosterone

57. **The concept of vaccination was first developed by ________.**
A. Louis Pasteur
B. Carl Landsteiner
C. Edward Jenner
D. Joseph Miester

58. **What is the purpose of breastfeeding on demand?**
A. To established a feeding routine
B. To increase milk supply
C. To decrease milk supply
D. To promote bonding and meet the babies' needs

59. **The process of weakening a pathogen is called ______.**
A. Attenuation
B. Vaccination
C. Immunization
D. Virulence reduction

60. **The first vaccine developed by Louis Pasteur was against ________.**
A. Poxvirus B. Rabies virus
C. Hepatitis virus D. None of the above

61. **The disease of heart, joints and nervous system are called ________.**
A. Communicable diseases
B. Mental diseases
C. Degenerative diseases
D. Deficiency diseases

62. **Passive immunization includes ________.**
A. Transfer of lymphocyte directly
B. Introduction of antibodies directly
C. Transfer of maternal antibodies across placenta
D. All of the above

63. **Which of the following is a combined vaccine ______.**
A. DPT vaccine
B. Hepatitis B vaccine
C. Hib vaccine
D. Var vaccine

64. **Which of the following cause harm to human health?**
A. Organic farming
B. Using pesticides
C. Using solar vehicles
D. Protecting forests

65. **The first recombinant antigen vaccine approved for human use is ________.**
A. Hib vaccine B. Var vaccine
C. Hepatitis B vaccine D. DPT vaccine

66. **Which of the following statements are true regarding polio vaccines?**
A. Sabin is live attenuated polio vaccine
B. Salk and Sabin are polio vaccines
C. Salk is an inactivated polio vaccine
D. All of the above

67. **Which of the following can cause breast cancer in women?**
A. Breast feeding
B. Being physically fit
C. Using antiperspirants
D. Eating healthy food

68. **Which of the following is a polysaccharide vaccine?**
A. Anthrax vaccine
B. Rabies vaccine
C. Hib vaccine
D. Hepatitis A

69. **Highest percentage of air consists of ________.**
A. Nitrogen B. Oxygen
C. Carbon dioxide D. Argon

70. **________ is a process of prevention of pregnancy.**
A. Reproduction
B. Contraception
C. Fertilization
D. Ovulation

71. The Taj Mahal is being affected by ________.
A. Noise pollution
B. Water pollution
C. Air pollution
D. None of the above

72. Which is a permanent method of family planning?
A. Vasectomy B. Abstinence
C. Abortion D. IUCD

73. Air pollution causes ________.
A. Global warming
B. Soil erosion
C. Respiratory problems
D. None of the above

74. IUCD stands for ________.
A. Intrauterine contraceptive device
B. Intrauterine conventional device
C. Internal ureter device
D. Intraunique device

75. Greenhouse gas is ________.
A. Carbon dioxide B. Nitrogen
C. Oxygen D. Methane

76. ________ is an operation in male.
A. Vasectomy B. Tubectomy
C. Laparotomy D. Anatomy

77. CNG is a ________.
A. Polluted fuel
B. Harmful fuel
C. Clean fuel
D. None of the above

78. ________ is also known as calender method used in contraception.
A. Safe period
B. Abstinence
C. Coitus interruption
D. All of the above

79. All are the causes of air pollution *except* ________.
A. By combustion
B. By dust
C. By decomposition
D. By filtration

80. ________ is a contraceptive device used by male.
A. Diaphragm B. Cap
C. Condom D. Foam tablet

Answer Key

1 D	2 C	3 B	4 C	5 D	6 C	7 B	8 C	9 C	10 A
11 B	12 D	13 B	14 D	15 B	16 D	17 B	18 C	19 B	20 A
21 B	22 D	23 C	24 D	25 C	26 D	27 C	28 B	29 D	30 C
31 B	32 C	33 B	34 A	35 B	36 C	37 A	38 C	39 D	40 B
41 B	42 C	43 D	44 B	45 B	46 A	47 B	48 C	49 D	50 B
51 C	52 D	53 B	54 D	55 C	56 A	57 C	58 D	59 A	60 B
61 C	62 D	63 B	64 B	65 C	66 B	67 C	68 C	69 A	70 B
71 C	72 A	73 C	74 A	75 A	76 A	77 C	78 A	79 D	80 C

CHAPTER 3

Nutrition and Health

1. **A substance needed by the body for growth, energy, repair and maintenance is called __________.**
   A. Immunity
   B. Nutrient
   C. Energy
   D. Caloric value

2. **What is the main action of dietary fibres?**
   A. To ensure proper functioning of the liver
   B. To secrete hormones
   C. To maintain pH
   D. To make changes to how nutrients and chemicals are absorbed.

3. **Glycoprotein is a type of __________.**
   A. Simple protein
   B. Conjugated protein
   C. Derived protein
   D. None of the above

4. **Vitamin C is also known as _________.**
   A. Ascorbic acid
   B. Pyridoxine
   C. Cyanocobalamin
   D. None of the above

5. **__________ are the building blocks of proteins.**
   A. Acetic acid
   B. Lactic acid
   C. Pyruvic acid
   D. Amino acids

6. **Which of the following vitamin is fat soluble?**
   A. Vitamin B_6
   B. Vitamin C
   C. Vitamin A
   D. Vitamin B_{12}

7. **Which of the following vitamin is water soluble?**
   A. Vitamins B_3 and B_4
   B. Vitamin C
   C. Vitamins B_1 and B_2
   D. All of the above

8. **__________ are the examples of complete proteins.**
   A. Gelatine and zein of maize
   B. Milk and egg protein
   C. Soya and gelatine
   D. Soya and zein of maize

9. **Milk contains _________ % of calories.**
   A. 83
   B. 100
   C. 200
   D. 800

10. **The science of food and its relationship to health means ________**
    A. Disease
    B. Immunity
    C. Nutrition
    D. Psychology

11. **Which of the following is rich source of calcium?**
    A. Milk
    B. Cheese
    C. Fish
    D. All of the above

12. **_______________ are the protein deficiency disorders occurring commonly in children.**
    A. Goitre and Graves disease
    B. Thyrotoxicosis and hypertension
    C. Kwashiorkor's and marasmus disease
    D. Anaemia and egg white injury

13. **The balanced diet includes some important nutrients such as __________.**
    A. Proteins
    B. Carbohydrates
    C. Vitamins
    D. All of the above

14. **Which of the following are essential amino acids?**
    A. Leucine and phenylalanine
    B. Cysteine and proline
    C. Tyrosine and cysteine
    D. Serine and alanine

15. **Good source of carbohydrates is _________.**
    A. Milk B. Soft drinks
    C. Popcorn D. All of the above

16. **PEM means _________.**
    A. Pure energy nutrition
    B. Protein energy nutrition
    C. Protein electrolyte nutrition
    D. Protected energy nutrition

17. **Which of the following conditions are related to over nutrition?**
    A. Obesity
    B. Type 2 diabetes
    C. CVS disorders
    D. All of the above

18. **The parameter used for grading protein energy malnutrition is _________.**
    A. Bishop scoring
    B. Ballard's scale
    C. Gomez scale
    D. Cramer's rule

19. **The food rich in omega-3 fatty acids is ________.**
    A. Egg B. Oily fish
    C. Chicken D. Pork

20. **The glycogen reserve of human adult is _________.**
    A. 100 gm B. 500 gm
    C. 300 gm D. 400 gm

21. **The mineral essential for preventing dental caries is _________.**
    A. Fluorine B. Iodine
    C. Iron D. Zinc

22. **Which of the following mineral is necessary for the maturation of sperms?**
    A. Iodine B. Calcium
    C. Zinc D. Iron

23. **________ necessary for coagulation of blood.**
    A. Vitamin B
    B. Vitamin C
    C. Vitamin E
    D. Vitamin K

24. **The mineral essential for the transmission of nerve impulses in the nerve fibres of human body is ______.**
    A. Calcium B. Cobalt
    C. Sodium D. Iodine

25. **All are nutrition related programs developed by Government of India *except* ________.**
    A. Balwadi Nutrition Program
    B. Mid-Day Meal Program
    C. Vitamin A Prophylaxis Program
    D. Leprosy Eradication Program

26. **Which one of the following mineral elements is required for muscle contraction?**
    A. Iron B. Sodium
    C. Calcium D. Zinc

27. **________ deficiency causes egg white injury.**
    A. Vitamin D B. Vitamin A
    C. Biotin D. Vitamin C

28. **Which of the following is not an artificial sweetener?**
    A. Aspartame B. Saccharin
    C. Neotame D. Sucrose

29. **Which of the following food constituents is not digested but is still important for us?**
    A. Fibre B. Vitamins
    C. Proteins D. Minerals

30. **ORS stands for __________.**
    A. Onset rehydration salt
    B. Oral rehydration salt
    C. Oval rehydration salt
    D. Only rehydration salt

31. **Nutritionist is a synonym for __________.**
    A. Dietologist B. Dietician
    C. Diet expert D. All of the above

32. **Beriberi is caused due to deficiency of _________.**
    A. Vitamin B_1 B. Vitamin B_2
    C. Vitamin B_3 D. Vitamin B_{12}

33. **Which foods are also called anabolic foods?**
    A. Protective foods
    B. Energy supplying foods
    C. Body building foods
    D. None of the above

34. **Carbohydrates and fat rich food are classified as ________.**
    A. Energy supplying food B. Body building food
    C. Protective food D. None of the above

35. The daily intake of iron in an adult is ________.

A. 0.5 to 1 gm B. 10 to 12 gm
C. 2 to 6 gm D. 1 to 2 gm

36. Deficiency of iodine may lead to development of ________.

A. Anaemia B. Goitre
C. Night blindness D. Arthritis

37. Which one of the following is not an example of water-soluble vitamin?

A. Biotin B. Vitamin D
C. Folic acid D. Niacin

38. Scurvy is a deficiency disorder caused due to ________.

A. Vitamin K B. Vitamin D
C. Vitamin A D. Vitamin C

39. Limit of per day salt consumption as per WHO recommendation is ________.

A. More than 5 gm
B. More than 8 gm
C. Less than 5 gm
D. More than 10 gm

40. Marasmus is a type of ________.

A. Iodine deficiency disorder
B. Iron deficiency disorder
C. Vitamin A deficiency disorder
D. Protein energy malnutrition

41. ________ is a deficiency disorder caused due to calcium.

A. Rickets B. Rheumatism
C. Goitre D. Hyponatremia

42. Full form of FSSAI is ________.

A. Food Security and Standards Authority of India
B. Food Safety and Standards Authority of India
C. Functional Safety and Standards Authority of India
D. Food Safety and Standards Autonomy of India

43. Fortification food involves ________.

A. Supplementary food
B. Intermediate food
C. Adulterated food
D. Miscellaneous food

44. Presence of pesticides in food grains is an example of ________.

A. Intentional adulteration
B. Metallic adulteration
C. Incidental adulteration
D. Packaging hazard

45. ________ is popularly known as "Masala".

A. Calcium carbide
B. Sodium carbonate
C. Calcium phosphate
D. Sodium phosphate

46. A substance needed by the body for growth, energy repair and maintenance is called ________.

A. Carbohydrate B. Calorie
C. Fatty acid D. Nutrients

47. Which one of the following is not a method of fortification of food?

A. Commercial fortification
B. Natural fortification
C. Bio fortification
D. Home fortification

48. About half of the human diet should be made up of ________.

A. Fruits and milk
B. Milk and cheese
C. Grains and vegetables
D. Fats and sugars

49. A mineral that the body needs to work properly is ________.

A. Calcium B. Gold
C. Silver D. Lead

50. Which of the following is not an artificial ripener?

A. Ethylene oxide
B. Sulphur dioxide
C. Calcium carbide
D. Acetylene gas

51. Citrus fruits are excellent source of ________.

A. Vitamin B B. Calcium
C. Vitamin C D. Sodium

52. ________ are the substances used for destroying insects or other organisms harmful to cultivated plant or animals.

A. Fungicide B. Pesticide
C. Amoebicide D. Helmithicide

53. Which of the following is known as the sunshine vitamin?

A. Vitamin B B. Vitamin D
C. Vitamin K D. Vitamin C

54. GMF stands for ________.

A. Generally Modified Food
B. Good Modified Food
C. Genetically Modified Food
D. Genetically Minimum Food

55. Which of the following is the best source of omega 3-fatty acids?

A. Sardines B. Corn oil
C. Wheat products D. Pork

56. Genetically modifications involve alteration of an organism ________.

A. RNA B. m-RNA
C. t-RNA D. DNA

57. Which nutrient is most important for healthy vision?

A. Vitamin K B. Vitamin A
C. Iron D. Calcium

58. Fruits and vegetables are usually considered as good sources of ________.

A. Protein
B. Unsaturated fats
C. Vitamin and minerals
D. None of the above

59. Which one of the following is not an advantage of genetically modified foods?

A. It contains more nutrients
B. They grow faster
C. Increases crop production
D. Easily damaged by pests

60. A person who had a renal transplant should regulate the intake of ________.

A. Carbohydrates B. Fats
C. Proteins D. Vitamins

61. ________ are biologically active phytochemicals that possess health benefits.

A. Chemicals
B. Biological
C. Nutraceuticals
D. Pharmaceuticals

62. A person suffering from high blood pressure should cut down as ________.

A. Potassium B. Calcium
C. Magnesium D. Sodium

63. Ascorbic acid is an example of a nutraceuticals substances grouped by the following food source ________.

A. Plants B. Animals
C. Microbial D. Minerals

64. Junk food affects the ability of the body to use one of the following in the body ________.

A. Calcium B. Sodium
C. Insulin D. Zinc

65. Which one of the following is an example of water-soluble fibres?

A. Oats
B. Whole grains cereals
C. Whole wheat products
D. Brown rice

66. Genetically modified foods are ________.

A. More tasty B. More nutritious
C. Cheaper D. All of the above

67. The mode of obtaining food for growth, energy, repair, and maintenance is called ________.

A. Carbohydrate B. Calorie
C. Nutrition D. Fatty acids

68. Pellagra is a deficiency disease of ________.

A. Thiamine
B. Niacin
C. Riboflavin
D. Biotin

69. Which one of the following are called macronutrients?

A. Carbohydrates, proteins, and vitamins
B. Carbohydrates, proteins, and dats
C. Minerals, proteins, and vitamins
D. Proteins, fats, and minerals

70. Which of the following is used for artificial ripening of banana fruits?

A. Auxin B. Ethylene
C. Cytokinin D. Gibberlins

71. ________ components of food are called body builder.

A. Carbohydrate B. Vitamins
C. Protein D. Minerals

72. A diet containing right amount of energy, carbohydrates, proteins, fats, fibre, vitamins, minerals, and water to fulfil requirement of body is called ________.

A. Nutrition B. Balanced diet
C. Perfect diet D. Food pyramid

73. IPM stands for ________.

A. International Population Management
B. Integrated Pest Management
C. International Plant Management
D. Integrated Plant Management

74. Recommended daily intake of water is ________.

A. 0.5 litre per day
B. 0.75 litre per day
C. 1 litre per day
D. 2–3 litres per day

75. ________ nutrient is most important for building and repairing the cells in your body.

A. Carbohydrates B. Vitamins
C. Fats D. Proteins

76. __________ nutrients are referred to as micronutrients.

A. Proteins
B. Minerals
C. Fats
D. Carbohydrates

77. The insecticide obtained from the plant Neem is______.

A. Pyrethrin
B. Pyrethroid
C. Thiocarbamate
D. Azadirachtin

78. __________ are methods of food adulteration.

A. Artificial ripening
B. Using decomposed food
C. Additions of toxic substances
D. All of the above

79. Scurvy is deficiency disease of __________.

A. Vitamin A B. Vitamin C
C. Vitamin B D. Vitamin D

80. A diet high in saturated fats can be linked to which of the following ________.

A. Kidney failure
B. Bulimia
C. Anorexia
D. Cardiovascular diseases

Answer Key

1 B	2 D	3 B	4 A	5 D	6 C	7 D	8 B	9 A	10 C
11 D	12 C	13 D	14 A	15 D	16 B	17 D	18 C	19 B	20 B
21 A	22 C	23 D	24 C	25 D	26 C	27 C	28 D	29 A	30 B
31 D	32 A	33 C	34 A	35 C	36 B	37 B	38 D	39 C	40 D
41 A	42 B	43 A	44 C	45 A	46 D	47 B	48 C	49 A	50 B
51 C	52 B	53 B	54 C	55 A	56 D	57 B	58 C	59 D	60 C
61 C	62 D	63 A	64 C	65 A	66 D	67 C	68 B	69 B	70 B
71 C	72 B	73 B	74 D	75 D	76 B	77 D	78 D	79 B	80 D

CHAPTER 4

Introduction to Microbiology and Common Microorganisms

1. _________ is the study of all living organisms that are excessively small to be visible with the bare eye.

A. Biology
B. Microbiology
C. Zoology
D. Pathophysiology

2. Who developed differential staining technique (Gram staining)?

A. Gram Bell
B. Gram Stain
C. Christine Gram
D. Alvord Gram

3. Which of the following is a gram +ve bacterium?

A. Clostridium
B. Actinomyces
C. Rhizobium
D. Actinomyces

4. _________ is a contagious disease.

A. Cholera
B. Typhoid
C. Scabies
D. Gout

5. Which of the following types of microorganisms is photosynthetic?

A. Yeast
B. Algae
C. Virus
D. Fungi

6. Ziehl-Neelsen acid fast staining is used for separation of _________ group of members form others.

A. Fungi
B. Algae
C. Mycobacterium
D. Virus

7. The diseases that spread from one person to another are called _________.

A. Degeneration diseases
B. Communicable diseases
C. Non-communicable diseases
D. None of the above

8. Which of the following is the method of isolation of micro-organisms?

A. Streak plate method
B. Pour plate method
C. Serial dilution method
D. All of the above

9. AIDS, common cold, dengue are example of________.

A. Bacterial diseases
B. Viral diseases
C. Fungal diseases
D. Protozoal diseases

10. The most vulnerable age for chickenpox disease is _________.

A. 10 years onwards
B. 1 year onwards
C. 15 years
D. 72 years

11. The SARS coronavirus was first identified in the year ________.

A. 2009
B. 2007
C. 2003
D. 2015

12. Which one of the following is a gram –ve bacteria?

A. Staphylococci
B. Streptococci
C. Gonococci
D. *B. anthracis*

13. COVID-19 is ________.

A. Viral disease
B. Bacterial disease
C. Fungal disease
D. None of the above

14. Polio virus mainly replicates in ________.

A. Liver
B. GIT
C. Lungs
D. None of the above

15. _________ is a restriction on the movement of people, animal and goods which is intended to prevent the spread of disease.
A. Isolation B. Contamination
C. Quarantine D. Eradication

16. _________ are eukaryotic cells.
A. Minerals B. Virus
C. Bacteria D. Fungi

17. Hepatitis is a systemic infection of ________.
A. Lungs B. Liver
C. Kidneys D. None of the above

18. AIDS and COVID-19 are the ________.
A. Sporadic diseases B. Endemic diseases
C. Pandemic diseases D. Bacterial diseases

19. Dengue is also called ________.
A. Headache fever B. Break bone fever
C. Mosquito fever D. None of the above

20. Malaria spreads by ________.
A. Bite of dogs
B. Bite of female anopheles mosquito
C. Flies
D. All of the above

21. ____________ is a sudden increase in occurrence of a disease than normal.
A. Outbreak B. In-break
C. Mid-break D. Decline

22. Rabies is a _________.
A. Fungal disease B. Viral disease
C. Bacterial disease D. None of the above

23. Trachoma is a serious and contagious disease that affects __________.
A. Lungs B. Liver
C. Eyes D. All of the above

24. _________ is an infection appearing in a patient when he or she visited the hospital or other healthcare facility.
A. Hypertension B. Diabetes
C. Gout D. Nosocomial infection

25. Which is the most common STD caused by bacteria?
A. Syphilis B. Genital warts
C. Chlamydia D. Gonorrhoea

26. When HIV was first recognized in the US?
A. 1975 B. 1970
C. 1981 D. 1986

27. Which of these is a symptom of AIDS?
A. Tiredness B. Swollen lymph nodes
C. Fever D. All of the above

28. A virus can be composed of ________.
A. Envelope B. Nucleic acid
C. Capsid D. All of the above

29. SARS and MARS are _________.
A. Intestinal infections
B. Respiratory infections
C. Arthropod borne infections
D. Surface infections

30. Which of the following is not true for Gram-negative bacteria?
A. They contain a thick peptidoglycan cell wall
B. They contain a thin peptidoglycan cell wall
C. They possess an outer membrane
D. They possess Braun's lipoproteins

31. Gram-positive bacteria possess _________.
A. Cytoplasmic membrane
B. Thick peptidoglycan cell wall
C. Teichoic acids
D. All of the above

32. Which of the following is an example of vertical/trans-placental transmission?
A. Leprosy B. Hepatitis
C. Eye infection D. Chickenpox

33. Hospital acquired infections are also known as ________.
A. Fungal infections
B. Epidemic diseases
C. Nosocomial infections
D. Contagious infections

34. Gram-negative bacteria do not possess ___________.
A. Teichoic acids
B. Bayer's patches
C. Braun's lipoproteins
D. Intermembranous space

35. Which of the following is multicellular?
A. Protozoa B. Mould
C. Bacteria D. Yeast

36. All are methods of epidemiological studies *except* ____________.
A. Retrospective studies
B. Prospective studies
C. Uniform studies
D. Experimental studies

37. Who is the Father of Microbiology?
- **A.** Robert Koch
- **B.** Joseph Lister
- **C.** Louis Pasteur
- **D.** Antonie van Leeuwenhoek

38. All are venereal diseases *except* _________.
- **A.** Dengue **B.** Syphilis
- **C.** Gonorrhoea **D.** AIDS

39. In simple negative staining ________.
- **A.** Bacterial cells are coloured, the background is not coloured
- **B.** More than one stain is used
- **C.** Bacterial cells are not coloured; the background is coloured
- **D.** A de-colonizer is used between the primary and counter stains

40. Rubella is another name of __________.
- **A.** Chickenpox **B.** Smallpox
- **C.** Measles **D.** Mumps

41. Acid-fast staining is used for which bacterial species?
- **A.** Streptococcus
- **B.** *Escherichia coli*
- **C.** Mycobacteria
- **D.** Staphylococcus

42. The causative agent for chickenpox is ________
- **A.** Non-enveloped DNA virus
- **B.** Chickenpox virus
- **C.** Varicella-zoster virus
- **D.** RNA virus

43. __________ is normally known as "bird flu".
- **A.** Avian flu **B.** Malarial flu
- **C.** Typhoid flu **D.** Dengue flu

44. COVID-19 is caused by a __________
- **A.** ssRNA virus
- **B.** SARS-CoV-2 virus
- **C.** Coronavirus
- **D.** All of the above

45. MERS was first identified in _________ 2012.
- **A.** India **B.** China
- **C.** Russia **D.** Saudi Arabia

46. Whooping cough is caused by __________
- **A.** Mycobacterium
- **B.** Corynebacterium
- **C.** *Bordetella pertussis*
- **D.** Neisseria

47. Amebiasis is caused by a __________.
- **A.** Virus **B.** Bacterium
- **C.** Protozoan **D.** None of the above

48. COVID-19 was first identified in _________ district of China in December 2019.
- **A.** Yunan **B.** Wuhan
- **C.** Hainan **D.** Fujian

49. The parasite species that cause malaria in humans is/are __________.
- **A.** *P. vivax* **B.** *P. falciparum*
- **C.** *P. ovale* **D.** All of the above

50. Filariasis is caused by __________.
- **A.** *Brugia timori*
- **B.** *Wuchereri banocrofti*
- **C.** *Brugia malayi*
- **D.** All of the above

51. Mode of transmission of filariasis is ________.
- **A.** Through close contact with bodily fluids
- **B.** Faecal-oral route
- **C.** Through arthropod
- **D.** Through air droplets

52. ________ is a fatal form of food poisoning.
- **A.** Embolism **B.** Botulism
- **C.** Cinchonism **D.** Endemism

53. Influenza viruses are __________.
- **A.** Double-stranded RNA virus
- **B.** Double-stranded DNA virus
- **C.** Single-stranded DNA virus
- **D.** Single-stranded RNA virus

54. HIV belongs to __________.
- **A.** Picornaviridae **B.** Retroviridae
- **C.** Flaviviridae **D.** Hepadnaviridae

55. Incubation period of dengue is _________.
- **A.** 1 to 2 days **B.** 2 to 3 days
- **C.** 4 to 10 days **D.** 15 to 20 days

56. Which poliovirus has been eradicated?
- **A.** Poliovirus type 1
- **B.** Poliovirus type 2
- **C.** Poliovirus type 3
- **D.** Both B and C

57. Following are zoonotic diseases *except* __________.
- **A.** Rabies **B.** Plague
- **C.** Cholera **D.** Brucellosis

58. The disease present almost in all countries (at Global level) is referred to as __________.
A. Spanish flu
B. Pandemic disease
C. Hyperendemic disease
D. All of the above

59. HIV is caused by _________.
A. Fungi B. Virus
C. Bacteria D. Protozoa

60. Leprosy is also known as _________.
A. Crones disease
B. Graves disease
C. Addison disease
D. Hansen's disease

61. TB is caused by _________.
A. Protozoa B. Virus
C. Bacteria D. Fungi

62. *Vibrio cholera* is a motile bacterium belongs to the group of __________.
A. Amphitrichous
B. Lophotrichous
C. Peritrichous
D. Monotrichous

63. Trophozoites, schizonts and gametocytes of all the malarial parasites are seen in the peripheral blood smear *except* __________
A. *P. ovale* B. *P. falciparum*
C. *P. malariae* D. *P. vivax*

64. Mosquito responsible for malaria transmission ______
A. Haemagogus B. Aedes aegypti
C. Aedes albopictus D. Anopheles

65. Chikungunya is primarily spread by ________
A. Protozoa B. Bacteria
C. Viruses D. Mollusc

66. What is the full form of SARS?
A. Severe actual respiratory symptoms
B. Severe acute respiratory syndrome
C. Severe acute respiratory symptoms
D. Serious acute respiratory syndrome

67. Which of the following is a set of bacterial diseases?
A. Measles, tuberculosis, tetanus
B. Malaria, polio, mumps
C. Plague, leprosy, diphtheria
D. Mumps, cholera, typhoid

68. What are the microvascular complications of uncontrolled diabetes?
A. Acidosis
B. Delay gastric emptying
C. Retinopathy
D. Vomiting

69. Malaria is caused by __________.
A. Clostridium
B. *Endameba histolytica*
C. Plasmodium
D. Leishmania

70. First line drug for falciparum malaria is __________.
A. Tetracycline B. Chloroquine
C. Primaquine D. Quinine

71. Pneumonia is commonly infection of _________.
A. Stomach B. Heart
C. Lung D. Intestine

72. ALRI stands for _________.
A. Acute Left Respiratory Infection
B. Acute Lower Respiratory Infection
C. Acute Linear Respiratory Infection
D. None of the above

73. Hepatitis D is caused by_________.
A. HDC
B. Hepatitis delta virus
C. HDV
D. Both B and C

74. AURI stands for ___________.
A. Acute Upper Resistant Infection
B. Agricultural Utilization Research Institute
C. Acute Upper Respiratory Infection
D. None of the above

75. Chikungunya is spread by_________.
A. Birds B. Mosquito
C. Chicken D. Both A and C

76. Diagnosis of chikungunya can be confirmed by________.
A. Serological test
B. Sputum test
C. X-ray of joints
D. All of the above

77. Cancer is caused by __________.
A. Loss of immunity of cells
B. Uncontrolled mitosis
C. Uncontrolled meiosis
D. Rupturing of cells

78. Cancer cells are ________.

A. Beta cells B. Delta cells
C. Hela cells D. Alpha cells

79. Ebola virus particle contains ________.

A. Negative sense dsRNA
B. Negative sense ssRNA
C. Positive sense dsRNA
D. Negative sense ssDNA

80. Tuberculosis is indicated by?

A. Hemoptysis
B. Edema
C. Runny nose (Rhinitis)
D. Strider

81. Bacteria are called ________ organisms.

A. Granular
B. Multicellular
C. Unicellular
D. None of the above

82. ________ are a type of protein.

A. Bacteria B. Prions
C. Fungi D. Algae

83. _________ is a medical science that involves the study of the incidence and distribution of diseases in large population.

A. Physiology
B. Zoology
C. Biology
D. Epidemiology

84. ________ can cause communicable diseases.

A. Parasites B. Virus
C. Bacteria D. All of the above

85. The causative agent for tuberculosis is _________.

A. *Treponema palladium*
B. *Plasmodium vivax*
C. *Salmonella typhi*
D. *Mycobacterium tuberculosis*

86. ____________ is an infection caused by the Varicella-zoster virus.

A. Rubella B. Measles
C. Chickenpox D. Mumps

87. _______________ is an example of arthropod borne diseases.

A. Measles B. Dengue
C. Chickenpox D. Mumps

88. _______ is the main risk of gastrointestinal infections.

A. Rehydration B. Nausea
C. Dehydration D. Vomiting

89. Hepatitis means inflammation of the _________.

A. Muscles B. Kidney
C. Liver D. Brain

90. The main symptoms of cholera are _______.

A. Diarrhoea
B. Vomiting
C. Both A and B
D. None of the above

91. _______ infections are caused by the bite of infected mosquitoes and ticks.

A. Intestinal
B. Arthropod borne
C. Respiratory
D. Surface

92. Filariasis is also known as Filarial ________.

A. Amoebiasis
B. Elephantiasis
C. Typhi
D. None of the above

93. Chikungunya is an infection caused by the ________. virus.

A. CHAK
B. CHBKV
C. CHIKV
D. None of the above

94. Trachoma is an infectious disease caused by bacterium _______.

A. *M. leprae*
B. *Chlamydia trachomatis*
C. *Clostridium tetani*
D. None of the above

95. Tetanus is an infectious disease caused by bacterium _______.

A. *M. leprae*
B. *Chlamydia trachomatis*
C. *Clostridium tetani*
D. None of the above

96. STD may also be called _________.

A. Waterborne diseases
B. Venereal diseases
C. Fungal diseases
D. None of the above

97. __________ is the shortened name for HSV.

A. Gonorrhoea
B. Herpes
C. Syphilis
D. None of the above

98. Another name for Tetanus is __________

A. Tetani
B. German measles
C. Lockjaw
D. Clostridium

99. Trichomoniasis is caused by infection with a ________ parasite.

A. Virus
B. Bacteria
C. Protozoan
D. All of the above

100. The long form of HPV is __________

A. Human Papillomavirus
B. Human Population Virus
C. Human Papilloma Virology
D. All of the above

Answer Key

1 B	2 C	3 A	4 C	5 B	6 C	7 B	8 D	9 B	10 B
11 C	12 C	13 A	14 B	15 C	16 D	17 B	18 C	19 B	20 B
21 A	22 B	23 C	24 C	25 D	26 B	27 D	28 D	29 B	30 A
31 D	32 B	33 C	34 A	35 B	36 C	37 C	38 A	39 C	40 C
41 C	42 C	43 A	44 D	45 D	46 C	47 C	48 B	49 D	50 D
51 C	52 B	53 D	54 B	55 C	56 D	57 C	58 B	59 B	60 D
61 C	62 D	63 B	64 D	65 C	66 B	67 D	68 C	69 C	70 B
71 C	72 B	73 D	74 C	75 B	76 D	77 B	78 C	79 B	80 D
81 C	82 B	83 D	84 D	85 D	86 C	87 B	88 C	89 C	90 C
91 B	92 B	93 C	94 B	95 C	96 B	97 B	98 C	99 C	100 A

CHAPTER 5

Introduction to Health System

1. **Health means ________.**
   A. Our ability to remaining free from fever
   B. Our ability of not having any disease
   C. Our ability to remain free of illness
   D. Our ability of remaining free from any injury

2. **NGO stands for __________.**
   A. National Government Organization
   B. Non-Governmental Organization
   C. Native Governmental Organization
   D. Notable Governmental Organization

3. **PHC stands for ________.**
   A. Primary Hospital Centres
   B. Prime Human Centre
   C. Primary Healthcare Centre
   D. Public Health Centre

4. **_________ care is specialized medical care for people living with serious illness.**
   A. Malarial B. Executive
   C. Palliative D. Affordable

5. **Which of the following is not the communicable disease?**
   A. Tuberculosis B. Diabetes
   C. Cold D. Malaria

6. **National Vector Borne Disease Control Programme launched in _________.**
   A. 2005–06 B. 2001–02
   C. 2003–04 D. 2007–08

7. **DGHS stands for _________.**
   A. Director General of Hospital Services
   B. Director General of Health Services
   C. Dean General of Hospital Administrative Services
   D. Director General of HIV Services

8. **NAMP is _________.**
   A. National AIDS Management Programme
   B. National Anti-Malarial Process
   C. National Anti-malarial Programme
   D. National Anti-angina Management Programme

9. **National Filaria Control Programme was launched in __________.**
   A. 1956 B. 1958
   C. 1955 D. 1952

10. **National Oral Health Programme was launched in**
    A. 2011–2012
    B. 2016–2017
    C. 2009–2010
    D. 2014–2015

11. **NACP stands for _________.**
    A. National AIDS Contract Process
    B. National AIDS Control Programme
    C. National AIDS Control Process
    D. National AIDS Control Parts

12. **What is ASHA?**
    A. Additional Social Health Activist
    B. Accredited Social Health Activist
    C. Additional Socio-Health Activist
    D. None of the above

13. **Pulse Polio Inoculation Programme was launched in __________.**
    A. 1995 B. 1997
    C. 1998 D. 1955

14. AIDS can be transmitted by _______.

A. Courtship
B. Blood transfusion
C. Handshake
D. All of the above

15. What is the IDSP?

A. Integrated development standard programme
B. Integrated disease surveillance programme
C. Integrated development statement programme
D. Integrated disease surveillance project

16. WHO launched a global immunization programme in _________.

A. 1973
B. 1971
C. 1974
D. 1972

17. BCG stands for __________.

A. Bacteria Calmette Gram
B. Bacillus Calmette-Guérin
C. Bacillus Cardio Graph
D. Best Closely Guerin

18. IEC stands for _________.

A. In Education, Communication
B. Irreversible Eye Contact
C. Information, Education, Communication
D. None of the above

19. MDT stands for _________.

A. Multi Drug Therapy
B. Most Moderate Therapy
C. Most Drug Therapy
D. Both B and C

20. NHM stands for _________.

A. National Higher Mission
B. National Health Mission
C. Neither Higher Mission
D. National Highest Mission

21. In which year National Programme for control of blindness was introduced?

A. 1977
B. 1975
C. 1974
D. 1976

22. World's AIDS day was celebrated on which day?

A. 2nd December
B. 1st December
C. 30th November
D. 3rd December

23. Which body is responsible for formulating policy and implementing programs for prevention and control of HIV in India?

A. NACO
B. NEPL
C. NRCP
D. NPPCD

24. National mental health program was launched in ______.

A. 1985
B. 1980
C. 1982
D. 1990

25. Full form of NLEP _________.

A. National leprosy eradication process
B. National leprosy eradication program
C. National leprosy enrolment program
D. None of the above

26. When India Government has adopted Family Planning Programme?

A. 1951
B. 1953
C. 1952
D. 1949

27. In which year, the Government of India launched the Reproductive and Child Health (RCH) Programme?

A. 1994
B. 1996
C. 1993
D. 1995

28. Which one amongst the following is not a Millennium Development Goal?

A. Improve maternal health
B. Develop a local partnership for development
C. Combat HIV/AIDS, malaria, and other diseases
D. Ensure environmental sustainability

29. In which year the Government of India conceived the Annual Health Survey?

A. 2005
B. 2006
C. 2004
D. 2007

30. DOTS is a national program to address ________.

A. Malaria
B. Tuberculosis
C. Filaria
D. Japanese encephalitis

31. The NACO is _________

A. National AIDS Care Official Persons
B. National AIDS Control Organization
C. National AIDS Case organization
D. National AIDS Control Office

32. NACO was initiated in the year __________.

A. 1989
B. 1990
C. 1992
D. 1991

33. NLEP functions for the control and prevention of _________.

A. AIDS
B. Tuberculosis
C. Leprosy
D. None of the above

34. National Leprosy Control Programme was launched by Government of India in the year ________.

A. 1955–56
B. 1956–57
C. 1954–55
D. 1957–58

35. Directly Observed Treatment-Short Course (DOTS) was launched in India for the treatment of ________.

A. AIDS
B. Leprosy
C. Tuberculosis
D. None of the above

36. OPD stands for ________.

A. Out Private Department
B. Outpatient Department
C. Out Primary Department
D. Out Public Department

37. Which of the following organizations provides blood to all the patients?

A. Medical store
B. Dispensary
C. Blood bank
D. Hospital

38. Healthcare facilities are divided into two categories ________.

A. Rural and urban
B. Public and private
C. Primary and secondary
D. Small and large

39. AIIMS stands for ________.

A. All India Institutes of Methodology Science
B. All India Institute of Medical Sciences
C. Both A and B
D. None of the above

40. Who is the chief technical advisor to the Government on all matters relating to medical use and public health at the centre?

A. Health Secretary
B. Health Minister
C. Director of Health Sciences
D. Director General of Health Sciences

Answer Key

1 C	2 B	3 C	4 C	5 B	6 C	7 B	8 C	9 C	10 D
11 B	12 B	13 A	14 B	15 B	16 C	17 B	18 C	19 A	20 B
21 D	22 B	23 A	24 C	25 B	26 C	27 D	28 B	29 A	30 B
31 B	32 C	33 C	34 C	35 C	36 B	37 C	38 B	39 B	40 D

CHAPTER 6

Pharmacoeconomics

1. **All of the following are costs involved in pharmacoeconomic evaluation *except* ________.**
   A. Financial cost
   B. Ordering cost
   C. Economic cost
   D. Opportunity cost

2. **Components of pharmacoeconomics are __________.**
   A. Humanistic
   B. Economic
   C. Both A and B
   D. None of the above

3. **CMA stands for __________.**
   A. Cost minimization analysis
   B. Cost measurement analysis
   C. Cost maximization analysis
   D. None of the above

4. **All are the stakeholders of pharmacoeconomic *except* __________.**
   A. Pharmaceutical manufacturers
   B. Healthcare practitioners
   C. Patients
   D. Food industries

5. **CUA stands for __________.**
   A. Cost uncertainty analysis
   B. Cost utility analysis
   C. Cost understanding analysis
   D. None of the above

6. **Pharmacoeconomics analyses the cost of drug therapy to __________.**
   A. Pharmacist
   B. Hospital
   C. Healthcare system and society
   D. Doctors

7. **QALY means __________.**
   A. Quality-adjusted life years
   B. Quantity-adjusted life years
   C. Quality-added life years
   D. Quantity-added life years

8. **The full form of HMO is _________.**
   A. Height Maintenance Organization
   B. Habit Maintenance Organization
   C. Health Maintenance Organization
   D. None of the above

9. **A QALY of 1 means ________.**
   A. Coma
   B. Death
   C. Perfect death
   D. Living being

10. **The amount paid by customers to get health insurance is called ________.**
    A. Premium
    B. Co-payment
    C. Rent
    D. Out-of-pocket expenses

11. **Which one of the following is not considered as phases of disaster management?**
    A. Preparedness
    B. Research
    C. Prevention
    D. Response

12. The term used to refer to the commonly charged or prevailing fees for health services that the patient pays is ________.

A. Cost B. Opportunity cost
C. U and C charges D. Reimbursed value

13. CBA in pharmacoeconmics stands for _______.

A. Cost benefit analysis
B. Cost below analysis
C. Cost billing analysis
D. Cost before analysis

14. Pharmacists can contribute in management of Covid-19 at the following levels, which one is inappropriate?

A. At community level pharmacy
B. Counterfeiting
C. Hospital pharmacist
D. Drug regulatory activities

15. The measurement of unit of CUA is _________.

A. Dollars B. Natural units
C. QALY D. Perfect life

16. Which one of the following is severe acute respiratory syndrome inflicted by the novel coronavirus?

A. Bird flu B. HIV
C. SARS-Cov-2 D. Herpes

17. Which of the following is a direct non-medical cost?

A. Prescription medications
B. Cost of diagnosis
C. Taking the bus to get to the hospital
D. X-ray cost

18. Being the producer, quality controller, and dispenser, who could be a vital member research team?

A. Pharmacist B. Pilot
C. Designer D. Engineer

19. Which of the following seeks to measure the benefits to individuals of additional life years following a medical intervention?

A. Cost minimization
B. Cost-utility
C. Quality-adjusted life years
D. Profit maximization

20. ____________ country became the first country to use pharmacoeconomics analysis.

A. India
B. United State of America
C. China
D. Australia

21. CEA in pharmacoeconomics stands for ________.

A. Cash effective analysis
B. Cost effective analysis
C. Common effective analysis
D. Coat easier analysis

22. Economic valuations are _________ which attempts to capture and summarize reality.

A. Organisms
B. Facts
C. Graphics
D. Models

23. The increase in life expectancy is closely correlated with which of the following?

A. Reduction in exercise
B. Reduction in spending on drug research
C. Fall in educational aspect
D. Increased health spending per capita

24. GDP stands for __________.

A. Government Document Process
B. Gross Domestic Product
C. Gross Document Product
D. Government Domestic Process

25. Health insurance helps to __________.

A. Prevent adverse situations from occurring
B. Neglect all consequences of adverse situations
C. Reduce the financial consequences of adverse situations
D. Make assets continuously productive

26. DALY stands for ________.

A. Development-adjusted life years
B. Disability-adjusted life years
C. Distant-adjusted life years
D. Deviated-adjusted life years

27. HMO stands for ___________.

A. Health majority organization
B. Human maintenance organization
C. Health monotonous organization
D. Health maintenance organization

28. The increase life expectancy is closely correlated with which of the following?

A. Reduction in exercise
B. Increased health spending per capita
C. Reduction in spending on drug research
D. Fall in educational aspect

29. The document which embodies the contract in health insurance is called __________.

A. Certificate
B. Security
C. Policy
D. None of the above

30. ____________ study evaluates the cost and effect of a pharmaceutical product.

A. Economics
B. Chemoeconomics
C. Pharmacoeconomics
D. Bioeconomics

Answer Key

1 B	2 C	3 A	4 D	5 B	6 C	7 A	8 C	9 C	10 A
11 C	12 C	13 A	14 B	15 C	16 C	17 C	18 A	19 C	20 D
21 B	22 B	23 D	24 B	25 C	26 B	27 D	28 B	29 C	30 C

Part 2

Second Year Diploma in Pharmacy Subjects

VI. Pharmacology
VII. Community Pharmacy
VIII. Biochemistry and Clinical Pathology
IX. Pharmacotherapeutics
X. Hospital and Clinical Pharmacy
XI. Pharmacy Law and Ethics

Section VI

Pharmacology

1. General Pharmacology
2. Drugs Acting on Peripheral Nervous System
3. Drugs Acting on the Eye
4. Drugs Acting on the Central Nervous System
5. Drugs Acting on the Cardiovascular System
6. Drugs Acting on Blood and Blood Forming Organs
7. Drugs Acting on Respiratory System
8. Drugs Acting on Gastrointestinal Tract
9. Drugs Acting on the Kidney
10. Hormones and Hormone Antagonists
11. Autocoids
12. Chemotherapeutic Agents

Syllabus (As Per ER 2020) Pharmacology

Chapter	Topics
1	**General Pharmacology** ■ Introduction and scope of Pharmacology ■ Various routes of drug administration—advantages and disadvantages ■ Drug absorption—definition, types, factors affecting drug absorption ■ Bioavailability and the factors affecting bioavailability ■ Drug distribution—definition, factors affecting drug distribution ■ Biotransformation of drugs—definition, types of biotransformation reactions, factors influencing drug metabolisms ■ Excretion of drugs—definition, routes of drug excretion ■ General mechanisms of drug action and factors modifying drug action
2	**Drugs Acting on the Peripheral Nervous System** ■ Steps involved in neurohumoral transmission ■ Definition, classification, pharmacological actions, dose, indications, and contraindications of: a. Cholinergic drugs b. Anti-cholinergic drugs c. Adrenergic drugs d. Anti-adrenergic drugs e. Neuromuscular blocking agents f. Drugs used in myasthenia gravis g. Local anaesthetic agents h. Non-steroidal anti-inflammatory drugs (NSAIDs)
3	**Drugs Acting on the Eye** Definition, classification, pharmacological actions, dose, indications and contraindications of: ■ Miotics ■ Mydriatics ■ Drugs used in Glaucoma
4	**Drugs Acting on the Central Nervous System** Definition, classification, pharmacological actions, dose, indications, and contraindications of: ■ General anesthetics ■ Anti-convulsant drugs ■ Anti-depressant drugs ■ Nootropic agents ■ Opioid analgesics ■ Hypnotics and sedatives ■ Anti-anxiety drugs ■ Anti-psychotics ■ Centrally acting muscle relaxants
5	**Drugs Acting on the Cardiovascular System** Definition, classification, pharmacological actions, dose, indications, and contraindications of: ■ Anti-hypertensive drugs ■ Anti-anginal drugs ■ Anti-arrhythmic drugs ■ Drugs used in atherosclerosis and congestive heart failure ■ Drug therapy for shock
6	**Drugs Acting on Blood and Blood Forming Organs** Definition, classification, pharmacological actions, dose, indications, and contraindications of: ■ Hematinic agents ■ Anti-coagulants ■ Anti-platelet agents ■ Thrombolytic drugs
7	**Drugs Acting on Respiratory System** Definition, classification, pharmacological actions, dose, indications, and contraindications of: ■ Bronchodilators ■ Expectorants ■ Anti-tussive agents ■ Mucolytic agents

Contd...

8	**Drugs Acting on the Gastrointestinal Tract** Definition, classification, pharmacological actions, dose, indications, and contraindications of: ■ Anti-ulcer drugs ■ Anti-emetics ■ Laxatives and purgatives ■ Anti-diarrheal drugs
9	**Drugs Acting on the Kidney** Definition, classification, pharmacological actions, dose, indications, and contraindications of: ■ Diuretics ■ Anti-diuretics
10	**Hormones and Hormone Antagonists** Physiological and pathological role and clinical uses of: ■ Thyroid hormones ■ Parathormone ■ Vitamin D ■ Oral hypoglycemic agents ■ Progesterone ■ Oxytocin ■ Anti-thyroid drugs ■ Calcitonin ■ Insulin ■ Estrogen ■ Corticosteroids
11	**Autocoids** ■ Physiological role of Histamine, 5 HT and Prostaglandins ■ Classification, clinical uses, and adverse effects of antihistamines and 5 HT antagonists
12	**Chemotherapeutic Agents** Introduction, basic principles of chemotherapy of infections, infestations and neoplastic diseases, classification, dose, indication and contraindications of drugs belonging to following classes: ■ Penicillins ■ Cephalosporins ■ Aminoglycosides ■ Fluoroquinolones ■ Macrolides ■ Tetracyclines ■ Sulphonamides ■ Anti-tubercular drugs ■ Anti-fungal drugs ■ Anti-viral drugs ■ Anti-amoebic agents ■ Anthelmintics ■ Anti-malarial agents ■ Anti-neoplastic agents
13	**Biologicals** Definition, types, and indications of biological agents with examples

CHAPTER 1

General Pharmacology

1. **The science which deals with the drug and their actions on human body is called __________.**
   A. Physiology B. Pharmacology
   C. Pathology D. Microbiology

2. **Pharmacokinetic decides the __________ in the body.**
   A. Toxicity B. Fate of drug
   C. Adverse effect D. Side effect

3. **__________ is the branch of pharmacology that defines fates of drug and deals with absorption, distribution, metabolism, and excretion of drug.**
   A. Pharmacodynamics
   B. Therapeutics
   C. Pharmacokinetics
   D. None of the above

4. **Total volume of drug injected by IM route is restricted up to __________.**
   A. 5 ml B. 10 ml
   C. 20 ml D. 30 ml

5. **Which of the following branch deals with the study of poison?**
   A. Biology B. Posology
   C. Microbiology D. Toxicology

6. **Aspirin is the drug which is obtained from the sources of __________.**
   A. Synthetic B. Mineral
   C. Microorganism D. Animal

7. **__________ means the drug goes to the liver first and then into the blood stream.**
   A. Cumulative effect B. First pass effect
   C. Synergistic effect D. Antagonistic effect

8. **The nature of eucalyptus oil is __________.**
   A. Alkaloid B. Volatile oil
   C. Fixed oil D. Glycosides

9. **BBB stands for __________.**
   A. Blood–brain barrier B. Blood–bone barrier
   C. Bone–blood barrier D. Blue–brain barrier

10. **The commonly used route of drug administration is __________.**
    A. Parenteral route B. Oral route
    C. Sublingual route D. Local route

11. **__________ indicates margin of safety of drug.**
    A. Cumulative index B. Therapeutic index
    C. Toxicity index D. Body mass index

12. **How much quantity of drug can be administered by subcutaneous route?**
    A. 1 ml B. 2 ml
    C. 3 ml D. 1.5 ml

13. **Simple diffusion is __________.**
    A. One direction B. Bidirectional
    C. Unidirectional D. Tridirectional

14. **Which one of the following is the costly route of drug administration?**
    A. Local route B. Parenteral route
    C. Enteral route D. Sublingual route

15. **In which route the drug is placed below the tongue?**
    A. Intramuscular route
    B. Rectal route
    C. Sublingual route
    D. Intravenous route

16. **Which one of the following is risky route of drug administration?**
A. Parenteral route B. Oral route
C. Sublingual route D. Topical route

17. **100% bioavailability is possible only by __________.**
A. Intramuscular route
B. Rectal route
C. Sublingual route
D. Intravenous route

18. **In intramuscular administration the small volume is injected in __________.**
A. Vastus muscle B. Deltoid muscle
C. Gluteal muscle D. All of the above

19. **Pharmacodynamics includes __________.**
A. Drug elimination
B. Drug excretion
C. Drug absorption
D. Mechanism of action

20. **In intradermal injection the drug is injected in ______.**
A. Layer of muscle tissue
B. Tissue under the skin
C. Layers of the skin
D. Lumen of the vein

21. **Major mechanism of transport of drugs across biological membranes is by _________.**
A. Passive diffusion B. Facilitated diffusion
C. Active transport D. Endocytosis

22. **The drugs are excreted from the body through ______.**
A. Kidney
B. Breast milk, saliva, sweat
C. Bile, intestine
D. All of the above

23. **Putting a drug in liquid form into the body cavity or body orifice is known as __________.**
A. Inhalation B. Instillation
C. Insufflation D. Insertion

24. **Which of the following is complication of injections?**
A. Infection
B. Pyrogenic reactions
C. Tissue trauma
D. All of the above

25. **Majority of drugs cross biological membranes primarily by __________ .**
A. Facilitated diffusion B. Passive diffusion
C. Active diffusion D. All of the above

26. **Application of drug to the skin usually by a friction is known as __________.**
A. Insertion B. Insufflation
C. Instillation D. Inunction

27. **After the dissolution of drug which process occurs?**
A. Absorption B. Transpiration
C. Disintegration D. All of the above

28. **Disposition of drug is also known as __________.**
A. Absorption B. Distribution
C. Excretion D. Hydrolysis

29. **Test dose of penicillin is administered by which of the following routes?**
A. Subcutaneous B. IV route
C. IM route D. Intradermal route

30. **Drug like synthetic drug steroids and hormones are absorbed by which route?**
A. Passive transport
B. Active transport
C. Facilitated diffusion
D. Both A and B

31. **In intra-articular route of the drug administration, the drug is injected into __________.**
A. Arteries B. Atria
C. Areolar tissue D. Joints

32. **__________ means the delivery of drug molecule between the water, lipid and protein contents of the body.**
A. Excretion B. Metabolism
C. Distribution D. Absorption

33. **In unconscious patient which route is preferred for administration of drug?**
A. Inhalation route
B. Intramuscular route
C. Intravenous route
D. Oral route

34. **Specialized transport includes __________.**
A. Facilitated transport B. Active transport
C. Pinocytosis D. All of the above

35. **Xenobiotics mean __________.**
A. Another form of antibiotics
B. A form of nutrient
C. Anything that is not nutrients and enters the body through different routes
D. Nutrients which kill the gut harmful microbes

36. ___________ is a microsomal enzyme involved in biotransformation reactions.

A. Cytochrome P450
B. Calcium P120
C. Sodium P150
D. Chromate 160

37. High plasma protein binding __________.

A. Increases volume of distribution of drug
B. Generally makes the drug long acting
C. Facilitates the glomerular filtration
D. Minimise the drug interaction

38. What is the mechanism of drug excretion for skin excretion?

A. Passive diffusion
B. Active secretion
C. Glomerular secretion
D. Passive reabsorption

39. Which of the following routes has the highest bioavailability?

A. Oral route B. IM route
C. IV route D. SC route

40. When two or more drugs administered together act on same physiological system, they try to oppose each other's pharmacological action. The phenomenon is termed _________.

A. Addition B. Synergism
C. Antagonism D. Additive effects

41. Acetylcholine and atropine are the examples of which antagonism?

A. Chemical antagonism
B. Reversible antagonism
C. Competitive antagonism
D. Both B and C

42. __________ is the phenomenon if an individual initially develops tolerance to a drug belonging to particular group, he shows tolerance to other drug belonging to the same group.

A. Tolerance B. Drug interaction
C. Cross tolerance D. Tachyphylaxis

43. The most common phase-2 reaction of biotransformation is _________.

A. Sulphate conjugation
B. Glucuronide conjugation
C. Amino acid conjugation
D. Methylation

44. Drug administered through the _________ is most likely to be subjected to the first-pass metabolism.

A. Rectal route
B. Oral route
C. Sublingual route
D. Subcutaneous route

45. Pharmacodynamics involves the study of

A. Biotransformation of drugs in the organism
B. Mechanisms of drug action
C. Distribution of drugs in the organism
D. Excretion of drug from the organism

46. Which of the following is not a pharmacokinetics process?

A. Absorption B. Distribution
C. Side effects D. Metabolism

47. The science that deals with drug and their action is called __________.

A. Physiology B. Pathology
C. Pharmacology D. Microbiology

48. When two or more drugs administered together and act on different receptors, but produces same physiological action, which is greater than some of their individual action. This phenomenon is termed _________.

A. Addition
B. Synergism
C. Antagonism
D. Additive effects

49. Drugs are excreted from body through __________.

A. Skin, saliva, mouth
B. Bile
C. Liver
D. All of the above

50. The rate of absorption of drug affected by ___________.

A. Site of administration
B. Route of drug administration
C. Solubility
D. All of the above

51. Biotransformation of the drugs is to render them ______.

A. Less lipid soluble
B. Less ionized
C. More pharmacologically active
D. More lipid soluble

52. What phenomenon can occur in case of using a combination of drugs?

A. Tolerance B. Synergism
C. Accumulation D. Antagonism

53. There are some undesirable but unavoidable pharmacodynamic effects of a drug known as _______.

A. Side effects
B. Toxic effects
C. Pharmacological effects
D. Intolerance

54. An antagonist is a drug that has __________.

A. No affinity and intrinsic activity
B. Affinity but not intrinsic activity
C. No affinity but has an intrinsic activity
D. Both affinity and intrinsic activity

55. The study of movement or passage of drug across the body is __________.

A. Emetics
B. Vermifuge
C. Carminatives
D. Pharmacokinetics

56. The advantages to the oral route of administration is __________.

A. It is simple and most convenient
B. Self-medication is possible
C. No complications
D. All of the above

57. Pharmacokinetics deals with the study of __________.

A. Rate of metabolism of drug
B. Rate of drug action
C. Rate of absorption, distribution, metabolism, and excretion of drug
D. Rate of distribution of drug

58. Idiosyncratic reactions are related to __________.

A. Clinical pharmacology
B. Toxicity
C. Pharmacogenetics
D. None of the above

59. The ____________ route in which the medication is taken in the mouth and swallowed is

A. Inhalation
B. Subcutaneous
C. Oral
D. Nasal

60. IM route stands for __________

A. Intermuscle route
B. Intramuscular route
C. Intramouth route
D. None of the above

61. The process which refers to the passage of a drug dose over cell membranes from the point of delivery to the bloodstream is called __________

A. Bioavailability
B. Metabolism
C. Absorption
D. Excretion

62. Most drugs and metabolites are excreted by ________.

A. The bile
B. The lungs
C. The kidneys
D. Perspiration, saliva, and tears

63. Weak acids are rapidly excreted in ____________ urine and weak bases are rapidly excreted in ___________ urine.

A. Acidic, alkaline
B. Acidic, acidic
C. Alkaline, acidic
D. None of the above

64. Simple diffusion is also called __________.

A. Passive diffusion
B. Active diffusion
C. Facilitated diffusion
D. None of the above

65. The macromolecules with which medicines bind to elicit their specific biological effects are called __________.

A. Synergism
B. Receptors
C. Antagonism
D. None of the above

66. The phenomenon of two medications being used at the same time to facilitate pharmacological reaction is called _________.

A. Antagonism
B. Additive effect
C. Synergism
D. Bioavailability

67. Which of the following is parenteral route of drug administration?

A. Rectal route
B. Inhalation route
C. Oral route
D. Sublingual route

68. The biological activity of the drug totally abolished or reduced by chemical reaction between the two drugs is called ________.

A. Chemical antagonism
B. Drug receptor
C. Synergistic effect
D. Physiological antagonism

69. _________ can occur when a drug progressively departs from its receptor combinations leading in continual receptor blockage and a diminished pharmacological action.

A. Drug tolerance
B. Antagonism
C. Tachyphylaxis
D. Additive effect

70. Biotransformation of the drugs is to render them _____.

A. Less lipid soluble
B. Less ionized
C. More pharmacologically active
D. More lipid soluble

71. The alteration of impact of one drug by the presence of another substance is called __________.

A. Pharmacovigilance
B. Drug interaction
C. Adverse drug reaction
D. None of the above

72. ADR stands for __________.

A. Adverse dosage regimen
B. All drug reaction
C. Adverse drug reaction
D. Adverse dose reaction

73. Direct interactions between medications, drug effects, or interactions at the receptor level are called _____.

A. Miscellaneous drug interaction
B. Pharmacokinetic interactions
C. Pharmacodynamic interactions
D. None of the above

74. The therapeutic index of a drug is a measure of its _____.

A. Potency B. Efficacy
C. Dose variability D. Safety

75. The phase I reaction is ________.

A. Conjugation B. Precipitation
C. Hydroxylation D. Sulfation

76. The primary site of drug metabolism is ________.

A. Liver B. Kidney
C. Stomach D. Brain

77. In which route of administration, the medications are delivered either as an aerosol system or as vapours?

A. Inhalation B. Subcutaneous
C. Parenteral D. Injections

78. ___________ is the branch of science that deals with study of harmful effects of drugs on the foetus.

A. Toxicology
B. Teratogenicity
C. Posology
D. Entomology

79. The drugs having __________ therapeutic index are safer.

A. Neutral B. Lesser
C. Larger D. Moderate

80. Which of the following is a pathway of biotransformation of drugs?

A. Conjugation B. Hydrolysis
C. Oxidation D. All of the above

Answer Key

1 B	2 B	3 C	4 B	5 D	6 A	7 B	8 B	9 A	10 B
11 B	12 B	13 B	14 B	15 C	16 A	17 D	18 B	19 D	20 C
21 A	22 D	23 B	24 D	25 B	26 D	27 A	28 C	29 D	30 B
31 D	32 C	33 C	34 D	35 C	36 A	37 B	38 A	39 C	40 C
41 D	42 C	43 B	44 B	45 B	46 C	47 C	48 B	49 D	50 D
51 A	52 B	53 A	54 B	55 D	56 D	57 C	58 B	59 C	60 B
61 C	62 C	63 C	64 A	65 B	66 C	67 B	68 A	69 C	70 A
71 B	72 C	73 C	74 D	75 C	76 A	77 A	78 B	79 C	80 D

CHAPTER

2

Drugs Acting on Peripheral Nervous System

1. **Which of the following is a neurotransmitter of sympathetic nervous system?**
   A. Acetyl choline
   B. Adrenaline
   C. Ephedrine
   D. Salbutamol

2. **Postganglionic fibres are nerve fibres that originate in the ganglia and terminate in fibre terminals around muscles or gland cells called ___________.**
   A. Post cells
   B. Kidney cells
   C. Neuronic cells
   D. Effector cells

3. **___________ phenomenon is produced by the actions of adrenaline and ergot.**
   A. Triple response
   B. Vasomotor reversal of Dale
   C. Myasthenia gravis
   D. Glaucoma

4. **The neurotransmitter __________ is a choline ester.**
   A. Acetylcholine
   B. Noradrenaline
   C. Dopamine
   D. None of the above

5. **Adrenergic antagonists are also known as___________.**
   A. Anticholinergic
   B. Sympatholytic
   C. Parasympatholytic
   D. Adrenergics

6. **_____________ receptors are found in the autonomic ganglia, skeletal muscles, and adrenal medulla.**
   A. Nicotinic receptors
   B. Alpha receptors
   C. Muscarinic receptors
   D. Gamma receptors

7. **The person fails to respond to bright light is known as ____________.**
   A. Glaucoma
   B. Photophobia
   C. Myopia
   D. Presbyopia

8. **The cholinergic drugs are also called __________.**
   A. Parasympathomimetics
   B. Sympathomimetics
   C. Parasympatholytics
   D. None of the above

9. **____________ is a drug of choice in myasthenia gravis.**
   A. D-tubocurarine
   B. Adrenaline
   C. Ephedrine
   D. Neostigmine

10. **The smooth muscles of the bronchial tubes are constricted, which can lead to ___________.**
    A. Contraction
    B. Apnoea
    C. Relaxation
    D. Antagonist action

11. **__________ receptors are present in skeletal muscles.**
    A. Muscarinic
    B. Nicotinic
    C. Alpha
    D. Beta

12. **Injection of Pralidoxime (1 g) is given by__________.**
    A. IV route
    B. Topical route
    C. Oral route
    D. Muscular route

13. **Cholinergic blocking drugs are also called ________.**
    A. Parasympatholytic
    B. Acetylcholinesterase
    C. Parasympathomimetics
    D. None of the above

14. **____________ means paralysis of accommodation of ciliary muscles of the eye.**
    A. Iritis
    B. Conjunctivitis
    C. Cycloplegia
    D. Myalgia

15. Atropine causes _________ by inhibiting the cholinergic nerve supply when injected locally.
A. Myosis B. Poisoning
C. Mydriasis D. Inhibition

16. The gastrointestinal tract's tone and motility are reduced by __________.
A. Belladonna B. Adrenaline
C. Hyoscine D. Atropine

17. __________ is an adrenergic neurone blocker.
A. Chlorpropamide B. Guanethidine
C. Quinine D. Cyclizine

18. Atropine has a higher affinity for ____________ than acetylcholine.
A. Muscarinic receptors
B. Efferent cells
C. Effector cells
D. None of the above

19. Which of the following drug is used in peptic ulcer?
A. Physostigmine
B. Atropine
C. Neostigmine
D. Pilocarpine

20. Noradrenaline acts on __________ receptor.
A. Gamma B. Beta
C. Alpha D. Muscarinic

21. __________ is always present as an emergency kit of the physician.
A. Ephedrine
B. Homatropine
C. Pilocarpine
D. Adrenaline

22. Isoprenaline acts on _________ receptor.
A. Gamma B. Beta
C. Alpha D. Muscarinic

23. __________ are the agents which reduce the appetite.
A. Anorexiant
B. Algesia
C. Analgesics
D. Dopaminergic agents

24. Which of the following drugs is used in Raynaud's disease?
A. Adrenaline B. Ephedrine
C. Amphetamine D. Phenoxybenzamine

25. ________________ depletes noradrenaline neurons, which means that nerve stimulation is not available for discharge.
A. Reserpine B. Acetylcholine
C. Noradrenaline D. None of the above

26. Xylocaine is popular brand name of __________.
A. Procaine B. Cinchocaine
C. Lignocaine D. Amethocaine

27. Sedation and direct peripheral vasodilation are other measures which can contribute to its total anti-hypertensive impact is __________.
A. Methyldopa
B. Dopamine
C. Alpha-methyldopa
D. None of the above

28. 5-hydroxy-tryptamine is also called __________.
A. Serotonin
B. Noradrenaline
C. Adrenaline
D. None of the above

29. ________ is added to injections of local anaesthetics.
A. Atropine B. Phenytoin
C. Adrenaline D. Physostigmine

30. Which of the following drugs can be used to reduce intraocular pressure in the treatment of glaucoma?
A. Pilocarpine B. Acetazolamide
C. Neostigmine D. All of the above

31. Metoprolol is __________.
A. Parasympatholytic
B. Sympatholytic and blocks alpha-1 receptors
C. Anticholinergic
D. Adrenergic agonist

32. In spinal anaesthesia the drug is injected through _____.
A. Thoracic puncture
B. Cervical puncture
C. Lumbar puncture
D. Sternal puncture

33. Antidote of atropine is __________.
A. Tubocurarine B. Neostigmine
C. Pralidoxime D. Physostigmine

34. Action of D-tubocurarine is __________.
A. Competitive blockade of muscarinic receptor
B. Competitive blockade of nicotinic receptor
C. Irreversible blockade of muscarinic receptor
D. None of the above

35. **NSAIDs stand for ___________.**
A. Non-steroidal anti-inflammatory dosage
B. Non-steroidal anti-inflammatory drugs
C. Non-steroidal aiding drugs
D. None of the above

36. **_______________ is agent which reduce elevated body temperature.**
A. Pyrexia B. Anti-inflammatory
C. Algesia D. Anti-pyretic

37. **The heat regulating centre (HRC) in the __________ is impacted by fever.**
A. Medulla oblongata B. Hypothalamus
C. Pons D. None of the above

38. **_____________ is a potent inhibitor of prostaglandin synthase that is derived from propionic acid.**
A. Mefenamic acid B. Ibuprofen
C. Salicylates D. None of the above

39. **__________ is an oxicam derivative that works similarly to aspirin and indomethacin in terms of analgesic, antipyretic, and anti-inflammatory properties.**
A. Piroxicam
B. Salicylates
C. Oxalic acid
D. None of the above

40. **Timolol reduces the intraocular pressure through ________.**
A. Carbonic anhydrase inhibitor
B. β-adrenoceptor antagonist
C. Muscarinic agonist
D. β-adrenoceptor antagonist

41. **_________ decreases skeletal muscle tone by CNS effect.**
A. D-Tubocurarine B. Diazepam
C. Methenamine D. Neomycin

42. **Acetylcholine is biosynthesized from __________.**
A. L-tryptophan B. L-choline
C. L-cysteine D. L-serine

43. **Mechanism of action of neostigmine is _________.**
A. Cholinomimetics
B. Muscarinic antagonist
C. Anticholinesterase
D. Nicotinic antagonist

44. **A common side effect associated with all NSAIDs drugs is __________.**
A. Drowsiness B. Gastric irritation
C. Xerostomia D. Constipation

45. **The two main divisions of the central nervous system are __________.**
A. Nerves and neurons
B. Cerebral cortex and cerebrospinal fluid
C. Brain and spinal cord
D. Spinal cord and nerves

46. **Which of the following chemical substances is NOT an example of a neurotransmitter?**
A. Acetylcholine B. Glucose
C. Dopamine D. Noradrenaline

47. **How many pairs of cranial nerves originate within the brain?**
A. Two B. Four
C. Eight D. Twelve

48. **The major postjunctional cholinergic receptor is of the muscarinic type at which of the following sites?**
A. Postganglionic parasympathetic
B. Adrenal medulla
C. Autonomic ganglia
D. Neuromuscular junction

49. **The cardiac muscarinic receptors __________.**
A. Are of the M1 subtype
B. Are of the M2 subtype
C. Are selectively blocked by pirenzepine
D. Function through the PIP2 IP3/DAG

50. **Pilocarpine is used for __________.**
A. Glaucoma B. Paralytic ileus
C. Urinary retention D. All of the above

51. **Which of the following mydriatic does not produce cycloplegia?**
A. Phenylephrine B. Tropicamide
C. Cyclopentolate D. Homatropine

52. **The most effective antidote for belladonna poisoning is ________.**
A. Neostigmine B. Physostigmine
C. Pilocarpine D. Methacholine

53. **Which of the following is a selective alpha-2-adrenoceptor antagonist?**
A. Prazosin B. Phentolamine
C. Yohimbine D. Clonidine

54. **Low doses of adrenaline dilate which of the following vascular bed?**
A. Cutaneous B. Mucosal
C. Renal D. Skeletal muscle

55. Anticholinergic used as a spasmolytic is __________.
A. Pyridostigmine
B. Intramuscular injection
C. Dicyclomine
D. Tropicamide

56. Amphetamine potentiates the actions of which of the following class of drugs?
A. Diuretics B. Analgesics
C. Neuroleptics D. Antihypertensives

57. Which of the following drugs is contraindicated in peptic ulcer?
A. Atropine B. Pilocarpine
C. Hyoscine D. Aspirin

58. Vasoconstrictors should not be used in __________.
A. Neurogenic shock
B. Haemorrhagic shock
C. Secondary shock
D. Hypotension due to spinal anaesthesia

59. Propranolol does not block the _______ action of adrenaline.
A. Bronchodilatation B. Lipolysis
C. Muscle tremor D. Mydriasis

60. Aspirin is generally taken after meals to __________.
A. Reduce gastric irritation
B. Increase gastric irritation
C. Both A and B
D. None of the above

61. Which hormone is a major contributor to the symptoms of inflammation?
A. Histamine B. Serotonin
C. Bradykinin D. Leukotrienes

62. __________ is used as anorexiant.
A. Acetaminophen B. Aceclofenac
C. Amphetamine D. Amphotericin

63. Which of the following promotes oedema?
A. Histamine B. Prostaglandins
C. Serotonin D. Bradykinin

64. Give the example of indole derivative.
A. Aspirin B. Ibuprofen
C. Phenylbutazone D. Indomethacin

65. Propranolol is used in __________.
A. Asthma
B. Ventricular tachycardia
C. Anaesthesia
D. Gout

66. Nicotinic receptor sites include all the following *except* __________.
A. Bronchial smooth muscle B. Adrenal medulla
C. Skeletal muscle D. Sympathetic ganglia

67. __________ is an antidote used in salicylate poisoning.
A. Sodium phosphate B. Sodium bicarbonate
C. Calcium carbonate D. Calcium phosphate

68. Which one of the following drugs does not induce mydriasis?
A. Phentolamine B. Ephedrine
C. Phenylephrine D. Cocaine

69. __________ is always given by oral route.
A. Diazepam B. Aspirin
C. Phenobarbitone D. Phenytoin

70. The antidote for nicotine poisoning is __________.
A. Neostigmine B. Atropine sulfate
C. Phentolamine D. Trimethorphan

Answer Key

1 B	2 D	3 B	4 A	5 B	6 C	7 B	8 A	9 D	10 B
11 B	12 A	13 A	14 C	15 C	16 D	17 B	18 A	19 B	20 C
21 D	22 B	23 A	24 D	25 A	26 C	27 C	28 A	29 C	30 D
31 B	32 C	33 D	34 B	35 B	36 D	37 B	38 B	39 A	40 B
41 A	42 D	43 C	44 B	45 C	46 B	47 D	48 A	49 B	50 A
51 A	52 B	53 C	54 D	55 C	56 B	57 D	58 C	59 D	60 A
61 A	62 C	63 B	64 D	65 B	66 B	67 B	68 A	69 B	70 D

CHAPTER 3

Drugs Acting on the Eye

1. **Dilation of pupils of the eye is known as __________**
   A. Miosis
   B. Mydriasis
   C. Synthesis
   D. Myopia

2. **Miosis is marked by __________**
   A. Increase in pupil size
   B. Stable pupil size
   C. Reduction in pupil size
   D. None of the above

3. **Which of the following drugs is commonly used topically and once a day in the treatment of open glaucoma?**
   A. Pilocarpine
   B. Tropicamide
   C. Latanoprost
   D. Carvedilol

4. **__________ is a miotic drug.**
   A. Pilocarpine
   B. Atropine
   C. Hyoscine
   D. Dicyclomine

5. **In human, intraocular pressure is about __________**
   A. 10 to 30 mmHg
   B. 20 to 50 mmHg
   C. 10 to 20 mmHg
   D. 10 to 60 mmHg

6. **The increased intraocular pressure in the eye is called __________**
   A. Glaucoma
   B. Miosis
   C. Mydriasis
   D. Iritis

7. **Timolol, Betaxolol and Levobunolol are __________ drugs effective in the treatment of glaucoma.**
   A. Alpha blockers
   B. Beta blockers
   C. Gamma blockers
   D. GABA blockers

8. **Homatropine is __________**
   A. Sympathomimetic mydriatic
   B. Parasympatholytic mydriatic
   C. Sympathomimetic miotic
   D. Osmotic miotic

9. **__________ is carbonic anhydrase inhibitor.**
   A. Acetazolamide
   B. Ephedrine
   C. Amphetamine
   D. Physostigmine

10. **Which of the following drugs produce cycloplegia?**
    A. Pilocarpine
    B. Physostigmine
    C. Atropine
    D. Pyridostigmine

11. **Which drug reduces IOP (intraocular pressure)?**
    A. Tropicamide
    B. Cyclopentolate
    C. Adrenaline
    D. Timolol

12. **Which of the following drugs is not used in open angle Glaucoma?**
    A. Latanoprost
    B. Phenylephrine
    C. Brimonidine
    D. Timolol

13. **All of the following drugs are miotics *except* __________**
    A. Acetylcholine
    B. Carbachol
    C. Pilocarpine
    D. Homatropine

14. **Which of the following drugs is used by IV route to treat eye disorder?**
    A. Adrenaline
    B. Mannitol
    C. Latanoprost
    D. Atropine

15. __________ means constriction of pupils of the eye.
    - A. Miosis
    - B. Mydriasis
    - C. Conjunctivitis
    - D. Iritis

16. Glaucoma is a disease characterized by __________
    - A. Medium intraocular pressure
    - B. Increased intraocular pressure
    - C. Decreased intraocular pressure
    - D. Stable intraocular pressure

17. Carbonic anhydrase inhibitor used in treatment of glaucoma is __________
    - A. Acetazolamide
    - B. Homatropine
    - C. Epinephrine
    - D. Mannitol

18. Atropine sulphate acts as __________
    - A. Miotic
    - B. Mydriatic
    - C. Anticonvulsant
    - D. Antihypertensive

19. ________ is a major cause of blindness in persons over 40 years of age.
    - A. Photophobia
    - B. Myopia
    - C. Glaucoma
    - D. Diplopia

20. __________ is a prostaglandin used to treat increase pressure inside the eye.
    - A. Latanoprost
    - B. Atrovastatin
    - C. Progestasert
    - D. Histoprat

Answer Key

1 B	2 C	3 B	4 A	5 C	6 A	7 B	8 B	9 A	10 C
11 D	12 B	13 D	14 B	15 A	16 B	17 A	18 B	19 C	20 A

CHAPTER 4

Drugs Acting on the Central Nervous System

1. **The drugs which produces calming and quietening effects on the individuals are called __________**
   A. Carminatives B. Tranquilizers
   C. Antiepileptics D. Anaesthetics

2. **__________ means the drugs used prior to anaesthetics agent.**
   A. Post-anaesthetics
   B. Post-labour anaesthetics
   C. Pre-anaesthetics
   D. Pre-labour anaesthetics

3. **Which drug induces a sleep resembling to natural sleep?**
   A. Sedative B. Hypnotic
   C. Analgesics D. NSAIDs

4. **Which of the following is a gaseous anaesthetic?**
   A. Cyclopropane
   B. Chloroform
   C. Ether
   D. Thiopentone

5. **__________ is used as an antidote in barbiturate poisoning.**
   A. Sodium phosphate
   B. Sodium bicarbonate
   C. Calcium carbonate
   D. Magnesium carbonate

6. **Minor surgical operations such as teeth extraction can be performed during the __________**
   A. Stage of delirium
   B. Stage of analgesia
   C. Stage of surgical anaesthesia
   D. None of the above

7. **__________ is ultra-short acting barbiturate.**
   A. Phenobarbitone B. Phenytoin
   C. Hexobarbitone D. Thiopentone

8. **__________ is a powerful anaesthetic that can induce all stages of anaesthesia without producing hypoxia.**
   A. Ethylene B. Ether
   C. Chloroform D. Ketamine

9. **Which of the following is a major inhibitory neurotransmitter?**
   A. GABA B. PABA
   C. ASA D. PAS

10. **__________ is a colourless gas with a slightly sweetish odour.**
    A. Cyclopropane B. Nitrous oxide
    C. Thiopentone D. Halothane

11. **NREM sleep stands for __________**
    A. Never rapid eye movement
    B. North rapid eye movement
    C. Non-rapid eye movement
    D. Negative rapid eye movement

12. **__________ is a sodium salt of phenobarbitone which can be used as an anaesthetic agent.**
    A. Ketamine B. Paraldehyde
    C. Thiopentone sodium D. Propanidid

13. **Nalorphine and naloxone are the antidotes used in __________**
    A. Salicylate poisoning
    B. Opium poisoning
    C. Barbiturate poisoning
    D. Iron poisoning

14. Daily dose of diazepam in an adult is _________
A. 5 to 40 mg B. 40 to 50 mg
C. 50 to 60 mg D. 80 to 100 mg

15. _________raises the pain threshold in the thalamus, impairing pain perception.
A. Morphine B. Opium
C. Narcotic D. None of the above

16. _________ is the most common neurological disorder characterized by paroxysmal cerebral dysrhythmia.
A. Neurosis B. Epilepsy
C. Psychosis D. Depression

17. CTZ stands for _________
A. Chemoreceptor Time Zone
B. Chemoreceptor Trigger Zone
C. Chemical Time Zone
D. Chemical Trigger Zone

18. _________ is the chemical name for codeine.
A. Methyl alcohol B. Ethyl alcohol
C. Methylmorphine D. None of the above

19. _________ is a drug of choice in the treatment of status epilepticus.
A. Clonazepam B. Diazepam
C. Nitrazepam D. Oxazepam

20. _________ is useful for washing away drugs that have been consumed and may be excreted in the stomach.
A. Gastric lavage B. Suffocation
C. Absorption D. All of the above

21. _________ is the medical term for a lack of sleep.
A. Appetite B. Insomnia
C. Pyrexia D. None of the above

22. Gardenal is a popular brand name of _________
A. Phenytoin B. Phenobarbitone
C. Carbamazepine D. Lithium carbonate

23. REM stands for _________.
A. Rise eye movement B. Rapid eye movement
C. Rapid ear movement D. None of the above

24. _________ is a drug of choice in grand mal epilepsy.
A. Phenobarbitone B. Phenformin
C. Phenytoin D. Phenoxybenzamine

25. _________ operate as an anti-convulsant by depressing both the motor and sensory parts of the brain.
A. Barbiturates B. Non-barbiturates
C. Sedatives D. None of the above

26. The main site of benzodiazepines acting is the _______
A. Brain B. Legs
C. Limbic system D. None of the above

27. MAOI stands for _________
A. More amino oxidase inhibitor
B. Monoamino oxidase inhibitor
C. Mono aryl oxidase inhibitor
D. Mono ally oxidase inhibitor

28. _________ is a neurological illness characterized by recurring, short-term occurrences of motor, sensory, or psychological dysfunction.
A. Anorexia B. Epilepsy
C. Insomnia D. Nausea

29. Imipramine and desipramine are _________
A. MAOI
B. Carbonic anhydrase inhibitors
C. Tricyclic antidepressants
D. ACE inhibitors

30. PTP stands for _________
A. Pressure tetanic potentiation
B. Post-tremor potentiation
C. Post-tetanic potentiation
D. None of the above

31. _________ prevents PTP by electrically stabilizing membranes.
A. Salicylates B. Barbiturates
C. Phenytoin D. None of these

32. _________ is a substitute of morphine.
A. Mephenesin B. Methadone
C. Metaxalone D. Methocarbamol

33. Eating of cheese is forbidden in patients with ________
A. MAOI
B. Carbonic anhydrase inhibitors
C. Tricyclic antidepressants
D. ACE inhibitors

34. _________ activates the cortex, spinal cord, and medulla, among other areas of the brain.
A. Amine group B. Barbiturates
C. Lobeline D. Amphetamine

35. _________ is a natural alkaloid found in the seeds of the *Strychnos nux-vomica*.
A. Strychnine B. Lobeline
C. Amphetamine D. Leptazole

36. _________ is called "Largactil".
A. Chlorpheniramine B. Chlorpromazine
C. Chloroquine D. Chlorpropamide

37. Which general anaesthetic selectively inhibits excitatory NMDA receptors?

A. Thiopentone B. Ketamine
C. Halothane D. Desflurane

38. Which of the following is a sign of deep anaesthesia?

A. Fall in blood pressure
B. Appearance of tears in eyes
C. Resistance to passive inflation of lungs
D. Patient makes swallowing movements.

39. _________ is a split mind condition characterized by disturbed thinking.

A. Epilepsy B. Depression
C. Schizophrenia D. Mania

40. Select the general anaesthetic having the most marked uterine relaxant action.

A. Ether B. Propofol
C. Halothane D. Nitrous oxide

41. Morphine stimulates _______ and produces vomiting.

A. Spinal cord
B. CTZ
C. Hypothalamus
D. Medulla oblongata

42. Dissociative anaesthesia is produced by _________

A. Ether B. Ketamine
C. Propofol D. None of the above

43. Barbiturates exert the following actions *except* ______

A. Antianxiety
B. Anticonvulsant
C. Analgesic
D. Respiratory depressant

44. ____________ are "smart drugs" that can boost brain performance.

A. Footropes B. Nootropics
C. Neuroleptic D. Psychotropics

45. Hypnotic dose of diazepam produces which of the following actions?

A. Decreased nocturnal gastric secretion
B. Tachycardia
C. Constipation
D. Hyperalgesia

46. Diazepam is indicated in the following conditions *except* _________

A. Tetanus
B. Febrile convulsions
C. Generalized tonic-colonic (grand mal) epilepsy
D. Cardiac catheterization

47. _________ are the examples of centrally acting muscle relaxants.

A. Mephenesin and chloroxazone
B. Paracetamol and aspirin
C. Aceclofenac and mefenamic acid
D. Phenybutazone and indomethacin

48. Which of the following are adverse effects of phenytoin related to high plasma drug concentration?

A. Hirsutism
B. Ataxia
C. Gum hyperplasia
D. All of the above

49. Which of the following drugs is used to produce basal anaesthesia?

A. Halothane B. Chloroform
C. Thiopentone sodium D. Althesin

50. Gabapentin acts _________

A. By enhancing GABA release
B. As GABAA agonist
C. As precursor of GABA
D. By GABA independent mechanism

51. _________ is also known as diacetylmorphine.

A. Cocaine B. Hyoscine
C. Heroin D. Indomethacin

52. The preferred drug for status epilepticus is _________

A. Intramuscular phenobarbitone
B. Intravenous diazepam
C. Intravenous phenytoin sodium
D. Rectal diazepam

53. Chlorpromazine therapy increases the secretion of which of the following hormones?

A. Gonadotropin
B. Corticotropin
C. Prolactin
D. Antidiuretic hormone

54. Hepatotoxicity and cardiotoxicity are the major toxic effects of _________

A. Ether B. Chloroform
C. Halothane D. Nitrous oxide

55. Euphoria is an adverse effect of _________

A. Atropine B. Paracetamol
C. Aspirin D. Heroin

56. Which of the following is an atypical neuroleptic drug?

A. Flupentixol B. Loxapine
C. Olanzapine D. Pimozide

57. **Which of the following is a non-sedative anxiolytic?**
 A. Hydroxyzine B. Chlorpromazine
 C. Buspirone D. Alprazolam

58. **Which of the following drugs produce constipation?**
 A. Ephedrine B. Morphine
 C. Carbachol D. Paracetamol

59. **Imipramine given to nondepressed individuals produces __________**
 A. Inappropriate behaviour
 B. Euphoria
 C. Insomnia
 D. Lethargy and light headedness

60. **All the following are barbiturates *except* __________**
 A. Phenobarbitone B. Chloral hydrate
 C. Pentobarbitone D. Hexobarbitone

61. **Nootropics are also known as __________**
 A. Cognitive enhancers
 B. Non-cognitive enhancers
 C. Medium cognitive enhancers
 D. Slow cognitive enhancers

62. **Baclofen is a __________**
 A. GABA derivative
 B. Mephenesin congener
 C. Benzodiazepine
 D. Centrally acting alpha-2 agonist

63. **Which of the following is called "laughing gas"?**
 A. Oxygen B. Carbon dioxide
 C. Nitrous oxide D. Sulphur dioxide

64. **Phenytoin consumed with which drug causes severe hypoglycaemia?**
 A. Morphine B. Phenobarbitone
 C. Chlorpropamide D. Benztropine

65. **Morphine is contraindicated in __________**
 A. Joint injury B. Muscle injury
 C. Tooth injury D. Head injury

66. **Benzodiazepines as anti-epileptic agents are used for treating following conditions *except* __________**
 A. Petit mal epilepsy
 B. Status epilepticus
 C. Grand mal epilepsy
 D. Infantile convulsions

67. **Class of drugs that cause cheese reaction is _______**
 A. Benzodiazepines
 B. MAO inhibitors
 C. Beta blockers
 D. Selective serotonin reuptake inhibitors

68. **Which of the following is an adverse effect of morphine?**
 A. Nausea B. Salivation
 C. Constipation D. Diarrhoea

69. **The benzodiazepine to be first used clinically is________**
 A. Diazepam B. Alprazolam
 C. Clonazepam D. Chlordiazepoxide

70. **__________ is given with atropine in the treatment of biliary colic.**
 A. Hyoscine B. Morphine
 C. Codeine D. Noscapine

Answer Key

1 B	2 C	3 B	4 A	5 B	6 B	7 D	8 C	9 A	10 B
11 C	12 C	13 B	14 A	15 A	16 B	17 B	18 C	19 B	20 A
21 B	22 A	23 B	24 C	25 A	26 C	27 B	28 B	29 C	30 C
31 C	32 B	33 A	34 D	35 A	36 B	37 B	38 A	39 C	40 C
41 B	42 B	43 C	44 B	45 A	46 C	47 A	48 B	49 C	50 A
51 C	52 B	53 C	54 B	55 D	56 C	57 C	58 B	59 D	60 B
61 A	62 A	63 C	64 C	65 D	66 C	67 B	68 C	69 D	70 B

CHAPTER

5

Drugs Acting on the Cardiovascular System

1. The drugs which increase the activity of heart are called __________

A. Haematinics
B. Cardiotonics
C. Nootropics
D. Analeptics

2. Digoxin is mainly used in the treatment of __________

A. Hypertension
B. Angina pectoris
C. Arrhythmia
D. Congestive heart failure

3. For fast action, nitro-glycerine should be given by __________.

A. Oral route
B. Sublingual route
C. Intramuscular route
D. Intrathecal route

4. Which of the following disorders is generally considered as "silent killer"?

A. Hypertension
B. Angina pectoris
C. Arrhythmia
D. Arthritis

5. Digitalis toxicity can be treated by __________

A. Sodium
B. Potassium
C. Calcium
D. Magnesium

6. Which of the following is calcium channel blocker?

A. Nicorandil
B. Captopril
C. Aspirin
D. Verapamil

7. Following are adverse effects of using digoxin *except* __________

A. Yellowish vision
B. Angioedema
C. Cardiac arrhythmia
D. Anorexia

8. Digitalis inhibits __________

A. Sodium–potassium pump
B. ACE pump
C. Calcium–potassium pump
D. MAOIs

9. __________ is a disease characterized by pains in the chest.

A. Arrhythmia
B. Angina pectoris
C. Epilepsy
D. Depression

10. Sodium nitroprusside works by __________

A. Suppressing angiotensin-11
B. Inhibiting Na^+/K^+-ATPase
C. Inhibiting HMG-CoA reductase
D. Activation vasodilation of guanylate cyclase causing vasodilation

11. Which of the following anti-anginal drugs also acts as a local anaesthetic?

A. Quinidine
B. Procainamide
C. Lidocaine
D. Timolol

12. Verapamil and nifedipine are __________

A. Calcium channel blockers
B. Alpha blockers
C. Beta blockers
D. Muscarinic blockers

13. All the following are adverse effects of amiodarone *except* __________

A. Pulmonary fibrosis
B. Hyperthyroidism
C. Hypothyroidism
D. Cinchonism

14. Following are examples of haematinics *except* __________

A. Iron
B. Folic acid
C. Vitamin B_{12}
D. Human serum albumin

15. Under physiological conditions the rate limiting enzyme in the generation of angiotensin II is _______

A. Renin
B. Angiotensin converting enzyme
C. Aminopeptidase
D. Angiotensinogen

16. Glyceryl trinitrate is used as _________

A. Diuretic B. Antianginal
C. Antihistaminic D. Analgesic

17. The plasma half-life of digoxin is _________

A. 10 hours B. 15 hours
C. 25 hours D. 36 hours

18. The principal action common to all class I antiarrhythmic drugs is _________

A. Na^+ channel blockade
B. K^+ channel opening
C. Depression of impulse conduction
D. Prolongation of effective refractory period

19. Calciguard is a popular brand name of _________

A. Verapamil B. Meprobamate
C. Methyldopa D. Nifedipine

20. Which of the following drugs is used to reduce the frequency of angina pectoris as well as to terminate an acute attack?

A. Isosorbide dinitrate
B. Pentaerythritol tetranitrate
C. Diltiazem
D. Dipyridamole

21. _________ is a drug used in atherosclerosis.

A. Methyldopa B. Clofibrate
C. Quinine D. Verapamil

22. CVD stands for _________

A. Cardio vessel digoxin B. Cardiovascular drugs
C. Cardio vessel drugs D. None of the above

23. The abnormal increase in blood pressure is called _________

A. Hypotension B. Hypertension
C. Hyperglycaemia D. Hypoglycaemia

24. Amyl nitrate is used in _________

A. Barbiturate poisoning B. Iron poisoning
C. Cyanide poisoning D. Opium poisoning

25. The patient on digitalis therapy is given a _________ supplement.

A. Calcium B. Potassium
C. Sodium D. Magnesium

26. Which of the following drugs is contraindicated in patients with asthma?

A. Propranolol B. Prazosin
C. Amlodipine D. Chlorthalidone

27. _________ is called cardiotonic.

A. Senna B. Aloe
C. Datura D. Digitalis

28. _________ is contraindicated in atrial fibrillation.

A. Digitalis B. Quinidine
C. Propranolol D. Atenolol

29. Which antihypertensive drug is recommended for use in pregnancy?

A. Verapamil B. Furosemide
C. Clonidine D. Methyldopa

30. Lanoxin is a popular brand name of _________

A. Quinine B. Atropine
C. Loperamide D. Digoxin

Answer Key

1 B	2 D	3 B	4 A	5 B	6 D	7 B	8 A	9 B	10 C
11 C	12 A	13 D	14 D	15 A	16 B	17 B	18 A	19 D	20 A
21 B	22 B	23 B	24 C	25 B	26 A	27 D	28 B	29 D	30 D

CHAPTER 6

Drugs Acting on Blood and Blood Forming Organs

1. _________ are the drugs which raise the number of red blood cells and the haemoglobin to normal level and above when they are below normal.

A. Anti-tuberculosis B. Analgesics
C. Anti-anginal D. Haematinics

2. Antiplatelet agents are also known as _________

A. Haematinics B. Haemostatics
C. Blood thinners D. Plasma expanders

3. _________ are the drug which promotes clotting.

A. Coagulants B. Anticoagulants
C. Plasma expanders D. Haemostatics

4. All the following drugs used for iron deficiency anaemia, *except* _________

A. Ferrous gluconate B. Ferrous sulphate
C. Folic acid D. Ferrous fumarate

5. _________ is arachidonic acid pathway inhibitor.

A. Aspirin B. Abciximab
C. Ticlopidine D. Dipyridamole

6. A decrease in oxygen carrying capacity of blood is known as _________

A. Anaemia B. Polycythemia
C. Leukaemia D. Leukopenia

7. The vitamin essential for blood clotting is _________

A. Vitamin K B. Vitamin A
C. Vitamin B D. Vitamin C

8. The following are thrombolytics (fibrinolytic) *except* _________

A. Streptokinase B. Urokinase
C. Altepase D. Diastase

9. _________ is the process of formation of RBCs in the red bone marrow.

A. Erythrocytes B. Erythropoiesis
C. Thrombosis D. Atherosclerosis

10. Which of the following prevents clotting of blood in blood vessels?

A. Fibrinogen B. Heparin
C. Fibrin D. Serotonin

11. Megaloblastic anaemia is caused due to deficiency of _________

A. Vitamin C B. Vitamin B_{12}
C. Vitamin D D. Vitamin A

12. _________ is an antiplatelet agent/blood thinner.

A. Aspirin B. Paracetamol
C. Aceclofenac D. Mefenamic acid

13. The term _________ refers to a decrease in blood's oxygen carrying capacity.

A. Algesia B. Pyrexia
C. Anaemia D. Necrosis

14. Oral anticoagulants take about _________ hours for anticoagulant effect.

A. 10 to 12 hours B. 15 to 20 hours
C. 36 to 48 hours D. 20 to 25 hours

15. Desferrioxamine is an antidote used in the treatment _________ poisoning.

A. Opium B. Barbiturate
C. Salicylate D. Iron

16. Cyanocobalamin is the other name for _________

A. Vitamin A B. Vitamin B_{12}
C. Vitamin D D. Vitamin K

17. _________ is an adverse effect of heparin.
A. Alopecia B. Myopia
C. Diplopia D. Presbyopia

18. _________ medicines are used to prevent intra-vascular coagulation from spreading and to reduce the risk of embolism.
A. Anti-ulcer B. Anti-arrhythmia
C. Anticoagulant D. Anti-parkinsonism

19. Oral anticoagulants act by competitively antagonising the actions of _________
A. Vitamin C B. Vitamin K
C. Vitamin E D. Vitamin D

20. _________ is also known as anti-pernicious anaemia agent.
A. Thiamine B. Niacin
C. Cyanocobalamin D. Riboflavin

21. The daily requirement of folic acid in pregnant women is _________
A. 0.2 mg/day B. 0.57 mg/day
C. 1 mg/day D. 0.5 mg/day

22. Heparin is _________ anticoagulant.
A. Oral B. Parenteral
C. Topical D. None of the above

23. Dicoumarol is an _________ drug.
A. Diuretic B. Cardiotonic
C. Anticoagulant D. Haematinic

24. Iron is stored in human body as _________
A. Haemoglobin B. Parenchymal iron
C. Tubulin D. Ferritin

25. _________ is called coagulation vitamin.
A. Vitamin C B. Vitamin K
C. Vitamin E D. Vitamin D

26. _________ injection is given in pernicious anaemia.
A. Vitamin B_1 B. Vitamin B_3
C. Vitamin B_6 D. Vitamin B_{12}

27. Iron toxicity/poisoning can be treated by _________
A. Cyanocobalamin
B. Desferrioxamine
C. Hydroxocobalamin
D. Sindarin

28. Which of the following is a source of vitamin B_{12}?
A. Banana B. Carrots
C. Legumes D. Apples

29. _________ drug inhibits platelet aggregation by inhibiting the enzyme cycloxygenase and formation of thromboxane A2.
A. Warfarin B. Aspirin
C. Aceclofenac D. Clopidogrel

30. The site of action of heparin is _________
A. Prostacyclin B. Anti-thrombin III
C. Fibrinogen D. None of the above

Answer Key

1 D	2 C	3 A	4 C	5 A	6 A	7 A	8 D	9 B	10 B
11 B	12 A	13 C	14 C	15 D	16 B	17 A	18 C	19 B	20 C
21 C	22 B	23 C	24 D	25 B	26 D	27 B	28 C	29 B	30 B

CHAPTER 7

Drugs Acting on Respiratory System

1. **The drugs which dilate the bronchi and improves the rate of breathing are known as _________**
   A. Expectorant B. Bronchodilator
   C. Antitussives D. Nasal decongestants

2. **Drug that removes sputum from the respiratory tract are known as _________**
   A. Emetics B. Expectorants
   C. Antidotes D. None of the above

3. **The central cough suppressants inhibit cough reflex by depressing the cough centre in the _________**
   A. Cerebrum B. Cerebellum
   C. Medulla oblongata D. Pons Varolii

4. **_________ is a drug used to relieve nasal congestion in the upper respiratory tract.**
   A. Urinary decongestant
   B. Antitussives
   C. Nasal decongestants
   D. Expectorant

5. **All are the clinical forms of bronchial asthma *except* _________**
   A. Episodic form B. Status asthmaticus
   C. Unique form D. Chronic form

6. **Which of the following is selective beta-2 agonist?**
   A. Salbutamol B. Theophylline
   C. Guaifenesin D. Codeine

7. **Which of the following is the drug of choice in the treatment of productive cough?**
   A. Noscapine
   B. Ammonium chloride
   C. Bromhexine
   D. Dextromethorphan

8. **All are examples of expectorants *except* _________**
   A. Potassium iodide B. Sodium phosphate
   C. Guaifenesin D. Ipecac

9. **Which drug depolymerises mucopolysaccharides of mucus?**
   A. Theophylline B. Noscapine
   C. Guaifenesin D. Diphenhydramine

10. **Codeine is used clinically as _________**
    A. Antidiarrheal B. Analgesic
    C. Antitussive D. All of the above

11. **_________ is a mucolytic agent.**
    A. Bromhexine B. Guaifenesin
    C. Ipecac D. Potassium iodide

12. **_________ is a paroxysmal dyspnoea and wheeze described as a result of an increase in respiratory resistance in narrower bronchus.**
    A. Glaucoma
    B. Bronchial asthma
    C. Loss of appetite
    D. Respiration loss

13. **Which of the following drugs used in treatment of bronchial asthma?**
    A. Antitussives B. Expectorants
    C. Bronchodilators D. Nasal decongestants

14. **In _________ an acute attack is severe, persistent and does not respond to adrenaline and aminophylline.**
    A. Status asthmaticus
    B. Episodic form
    C. Chronic form
    D. None of the above

15. __________ is a drug of choice in the treatment of status asthmaticus.

A. Prednisolone B. Hydrocortisone
C. Methohexitone D. Aldosterone

16. _____________ is beneficial for the termination of nocturnal asthma attack in oral doses of 30 mg at bed time.

A. Aminophylline
B. Salbutamol
C. Ephedrine hydrochloride
D. Orciprenaline

17. Which of the following expectorant acts both directly on the airway mucosa as well as reflexly?

A. Guaifenesin
B. Potassium iodide
C. Terpene hydrate
D. Bromhexine

18. The central cough suppressant is __________

A. Noscapine B. Ipecac
C. Potassium iodide D. Guaifenesin

19. What is the synonym of ammonium chloride?

A. Baker's ammonia
B. Ammonium muriate
C. Tartare antimony
D. Preston salt

20. __________ is a response that helps to remove irritants from the airway.

A. Redness B. Allergy
C. Cough D. Irritation

21. Which of the following inhibits acetylcholine-mediated bronchospasm?

A. Salmeterol B. Theophylline
C. Ephedrine D. Ipratropium

22. Adrenaline and salbutamol are ___________ used in bronchial asthma.

A. Bronchoconstrictors
B. Bronchodilators
C. Bronchospasm
D. Expectorants

23. Which of the following drugs is contraindicated in bronchial asthma?

A. Ipratropium bromide
B. Theophylline
C. Propranolol
D. Ketotifen

24. Which drug depolymerises mucopolysaccharides of mucus?

A. Guaifenesin B. Noscapine
C. Bromhexine D. Diphenhydramine

25. Which of the following expectorant acts both directly on the airway mucosa as well as reflex?

A. Bromhexine B. Potassium iodide
C. Guaifenesin D. Terpin hydrate

26. Which of the following inhibits acetylcholine-mediated bronchospasm?

A. Theophylline B. Ephedrine
C. Ipratropium D. Salmeterol

27. Mucokinetic is a drug which __________

A. Reduce airway mucus secretion
B. Increase airway mucus secretion
C. Makes respiratory secretions more watery
D. None of the above

28. Which of the following is the drug of choice in the treatment of productive cough?

A. Dextromethorphan B. Bromhexine
C. Noscapine D. Pholcodine

29. Dextromorphan is used as __________

A. Analgesic B. Antitussive
C. Expectorants D. Antihistaminic

30. Which of the following pharmacological agents that antagonizes adenosine?

A. Theophylline B. Terbutaline
C. Glucocorticoids D. Cromolyn sodium

31. Which one of the following is sedative type of expectorant?

A. Lemon oil
B. Ammonium chloride
C. Potassium iodide
D. Both B and C

32. Ammonium chloride is used as __________

A. A diuretic
B. An acidifying agent
C. An expectorant
D. All of the above

33. Sodium cromoglycate has a role in the treatment of the following conditions *except* __________

A. Chronic bronchial asthma
B. Chronic allergic rhinitis
C. Chronic allergic conjunctivitis
D. Chronic urticaria

34. _________ is a mucolytic agent that breaks up thick and sticky mucus.

A. Potassium iodide B. Noscapine
C. Bromhexine D. Ipecac

35. The drugs which increase bronchial secretion and protects irritated mucosa are called _________

A. Antitussive
B. Expectorant
C. Bronchoconstrictors
D. Mucolytics

36. _________ is an anticholinergic bronchodilator drug.

A. Potassium iodide
B. Ipratropium bromide
C. Hyoscine
D. Phencyclidine

37. Bromhexine acts by _________

A. Inhibiting cough centre
B. Irritating gastric mucosa and reflexly increasing bronchial secretion
C. Deploymerizing mucopolysaccharides present in sputum.
D. Desensitizing stretch receptors in the lungs

38. Which of the following antiasthmatic drug is not a bronchodilator?

A. Sodium chromoglycate
B. Theophylline
C. Ipratropium bromide
D. Formoterol

39. The antitussive present in opium but has no analgesic or addicting properties is _________

A. Codeine B. Pholcodine
C. Noscapine D. Ethyl morphine

40. _________ is an antihistamine used to relieve allergy symptoms such as watery eyes, runny nose, sneezing, itching of eyes.

A. Aceclofenac B. Cetrizine
C. Noscapine D. Cimetidine

Answer Key

1 B	2 B	3 C	4 C	5 C	6 A	7 C	8 B	9 C	10 D
11 A	12 B	13 C	14 A	15 B	16 C	17 B	18 A	19 B	20 C
21 D	22 B	23 C	24 C	25 A	26 B	27 C	28 C	29 B	30 A
31 D	32 C	33 D	34 C	35 B	36 B	37 C	38 A	39 C	40 B

CHAPTER 8

Drugs Acting on Gastrointestinal Tract

1. _______ are drugs that neutralize acid in the stomach.
   A. Anti-basic
   B. Antacids
   C. Anti-ulcer
   D. None of the above

2. The drugs which prevent vomiting are called __________
   A. Analeptics
   B. Emetics
   C. Antiemetics
   D. Neuroleptic

3. ______________ is a condition where defaecation is delayed.
   A. Diarrhoea
   B. Purgation
   C. Constipation
   D. Gastritis

4. The process of vomiting is called __________
   A. Kinesis
   B. Emesis
   C. Synthesis
   D. Autolysis

5. PPIs means__________
   A. Protein pump inhibitors
   B. Proton pump inhibitors
   C. Proline pump inhibitors
   D. Proguanil pump inhibitors

6. GERD stands for __________
   A. Gastric Oesophageal Role Disease
   B. Gastric Oesophageal Reflux Drug
   C. Gastric Oesophageal Reflux Disorder
   D. Gas Oesophageal Reflux Disease

7. __________ is a 5-HT3 receptor antagonist.
   A. Ondansetron
   B. Metoclopramide
   C. Promethazine
   D. Meclizine

8. Avomine is a popular brand name of __________
   A. Omeprazole
   B. Promethazine
   C. Rabiprazole
   D. Pentaprazole

9. __________ is defined as the frequent passage of liquid faeces with or without blood mucous.
   A. Vomiting
   B. Dysentery
   C. Nausea
   D. Diarrhoea

10. The percentage of elemental iron in hydrated ferrous sulfate is __________
    A. 20%
    B. 5%
    C. 10%
    D. 33%

11. __________ are used in the treatment of constipation.
    A. Carminatives
    B. Purgatives
    C. Antihypertensives
    D. Haematinics

12. The side effect which primarily limits acceptability of oral iron therapy is __________
    A. Metallic taste
    B. Epigastric pain and bowel upset
    C. Black stools
    D. Staining of teeth

13. Dulcolax is a popular brand name of __________
    A. Calcium carbonate
    B. Bisacodyl
    C. Promethazine
    D. Podophyllum

14. Which of the following factors is required for the absorption of dietary vitamin B_{12}?
    A. Gastric intrinsic factor
    B. Gastric acid
    C. Transcobalamin
    D. Both A and B

15. **Which salt causes diarrhoea?**
   A. Calcium carbonate
   B. Sodium bicarbonate
   C. Magnesium trisilicate
   D. Aluminium hydroxide

16. **__________ is an example of emollient purgative.**
   A. Cellulose B. Liquid paraffin
   C. Senna D. Castor oil

17. **Which of the following is H2 antihistamine?**
   A. Sucralfate B. Omeprazole
   C. Misoprostol D. Cimetidine

18. **GERD treatment option is __________**
   A. Ondansetron B. Misoprostol
   C. Omeprazole D. Metronidazole

19. **Which of the following antiemetic act by blocking D2-receptor in the CTZ?**
   A. Cisapride B. Chlorpromazine
   C. Metoclopramide D. Domperidone

20. **Castro oil is an example of __________ purgative.**
   A. Stimulant/irritant B. Bulk
   C. Saline D. Emollient

21. **Motion sickness can be treated by __________**
   A. Diazepam B. Hyoscine
   C. Grinston D. Dronabinol

22. **Which drug is safe for use during pregnancy?**
   A. Promethazine
   B. Apomorphine
   C. Droperidol
   D. Metoclopramide

23. **All of the following are examples of stimulant purgatives *except* __________**
   A. Bisacodyl B. Lactulose
   C. Senna D. Castor oil

24. **Which of the following drugs acts by reducing gastric acid secretion *except* __________**
   A. Omeprazole B. Famotidine
   C. Sucralfate D. Cimetidine

25. **Increase in prolactin release is seen administration of __________**
   A. Diazepam B. Promethazine
   C. Metoclopramide D. Dihydroazepine

26. **Following are examples of bulk laxatives *except* ______**
   A. Tannic acid B. Psyllium
   C. Agar D. Setulose

27. **Phenolphthalein use has side effects like ________**
   A. Rectal bleeding B. Amenorrhoea
   C. Pink coloured urine D. Vomiting

28. **Which of the following drugs is a histamine blocker and reduces levels of gastric acid?**
   A. Omeprazole B. Metoclopramide
   C. Cimetidine D. Magnesium hydroxide

29. **Amongst the following all are adsorbents *except* ______**
   A. Croton oil B. Light kaolin
   C. Activated charcoal D. Pectin

30. **Which of the following drugs is a dopamine antagonist? __________**
   A. Cimetidine B. Metoclopramide
   C. Cetrizine D. Promethazine

Answer Key

1 B	2 C	3 C	4 B	5 B	6 C	7 A	8 B	9 D	10 A
11 B	12 C	13 B	14 D	15 C	16 B	17 D	18 C	19 C	20 A
21 B	22 A	23 B	24 C	25 C	26 A	27 C	28 C	29 A	30 B

CHAPTER

9

Drugs Acting on the Kidney

1. __________ are substances that speed up and increase the volume of urine produced.
   A. Anti-ulcer drugs B. Anti-anginal drugs
   C. Haematinics D. Diuretics

2. Which of the following is called natural/physiological diuretic?
   A. Urea B. Mannitol
   C. Water D. Alcohol

3. __________ is a carbonic anhydrase inhibitor
   A. Benzothiadiazine
   B. Acetazolamide
   C. Aminophylline
   D. Mannitol

4. Parenteral furosemide is an alternative diuretic to mannitol in the following condition __________
   A. Pulmonary oedema
   B. Cirrhotic oedema
   C. Cerebral oedema
   D. Cardiac oedema

5. The primary site of action of thiazide diuretic in the nephron is __________
   A. Distal tubule
   B. Collecting duct
   C. Proximal tubule
   D. Loop of Henle

6. Spironolactone, triamterene and amiloride are examples of __________
   A. Weak diuretics
   B. Potassium sparing diuretics
   C. Thiazide diuretics
   D. Osmotic diuretic

7. All of the following are diuretics *except* __________
   A. Frusemide B. Ethacrynic acid
   C. Mannitol D. Cimetidine

8. Which one among the following is not an osmotic diuretic?
   A. Urea nitrate B. Glycerol
   C. Mannitol D. Isosorbide

9. The following are the indications of diuretic therapy *except* __________
   A. In oedema B. In hypertension
   C. In hepatic coma D. In glaucoma

10. Ethacrynic acid is used primarily as __________
    A. Antiemetic B. Diuretic
    C. Laxative D. Sedative

11. ADH stands for __________
    A. Anti-diuretic histidine
    B. Anti-diuretic hormone
    C. Anti-drug hormone
    D. None of the above

12. The major side effect of spironolactone is __________
    A. Hypokalemia B. Hyponatremia
    C. Hyperkalemia D. Hypernatremia

13. Daily dose of frusemide is __________
    A. 20 to 80 mg orally
    B. 100 to 200 mg daily
    C. 250 to 300 mg daily
    D. 300 to 400 mg daily orally

14. The side effect of loop diuretic is __________
    A. Hypokalemia B. Hyperkalemia
    C. Hypocalcemia D. Hypercalcemia

15. The risk of digitalis toxicity is significantly increased by concomitant administration of __________

A. Triamterene B. Lidocaine
C. Captopril D. Hydrochlorthiazide

16. Which of the following actions is related to thiazide diuretics?

A. Hyperuricemia
B. Hyperkalaemia
C. Hypoglycaemia in diabetes
D. Hypercalcemia

17. Which of the following drugs interacts with vasopressin (ADH)?

A. Chloroquine B. Chloramphenicol
C. Chlorpropamide D. Chlorpheniramine

18. __________ is an aldosterone antagonist.

A. Testosterone B. Spironolactone
C. Chlorthiazide D. Mannitol

19. A short acting diuretic that has side effects that include hypokalaemia metabolic alkalosis and reversible ototoxicity.

A. Acetazolamide B. Chlorothiazide
C. Furosemide D. Triamterene ceiling

20. Loop diuretics are also known as __________

A. Low ceiling B. High ceiling
C. Medium ceiling D. None of the above

21. The symptoms related to the toxicity of loop diuretics is __________

A. Allergic reaction B. Deafness
C. Hypomagnesemia D. Hyperuricemia

22. The following are the examples of anti-diuretics *except* __________

A. Oxytocin B. Aldosterone
C. Desmopressin D. Lypressin

23. Long-term use of loop diuretics causes __________

A. Cirrhosis of liver
B. Deafness
C. Distal nephron hypertrophy
D. Renal insufficiency

24. Which one of the following diuretics is effective in severe renal failure?

A. Loop diuretics
B. K^+ sparing diuretics
C. Thiazides
D. Carbonic anhydrase inhibitors

25. Lasix is a popular brand name of __________

A. Acetazolamide B. Frusemide
C. Spironolactone D. Chlorthiazide

26. Identify the correct drug with alpha and beta effects of sympathomimetics amines __________

A. Isoprenaline B. Ephedrine
C. Orciprenaline D. Atropine

27. __________ is a self-limiting diuretic.

A. Frusemide B. Chlorthiazide
C. Mannitol D. Acetazolamide

28. Osmotic diuretics are contraindicated in ________

A. Increased intracranial tension
B. Increased intraocular tension
C. Established acute renal failure
D. Poisonings

29. ________ salts are given along with thiazide diuretics.

A. Sodium B. Potassium
C. Calcium D. Magnesium

30. Example of weak diuretic includes __________

A. Propranolol B. Spironolactone
C. Mannitol D. Furosemide

31. ADH is released by __________ of the pituitary gland.

A. Middle lobe B. Posterior lobe
C. Anterier lobe D. None of the above

32. Spironolactone belongs to the class of drug ________

A. Potassium sparing diuretics
B. Weak diuretics
C. Other electrolytes
D. Potent diuretics

33. Which diuretic competes with aldosterone and is used for the treatment of hyperaldosteronism?

A. Hydrochlorthiazide
B. Isosorbide
C. Frusemide
D. Spironolactone

34. Furosemide increases the excretion of all of the following *except* __________

A. Sodium
B. Potassium
C. Uric acid
D. Calcium and magnesium

35. ________ is used in the treatment of patient suffering from diabetes insipidus.

A. ADH B. ACTH
C. TSH D. FSH

36. **Which one of the following diuretics acts on loop of Henle?**
   A. Spironolactone
   B. Ethacrynic acid
   C. Dichlorphenamide
   D. Cortexolone

37. **Lithium toxicity is increased by __________**
   A. Beta blockers
   B. Clonidine
   C. Calcium channel blockers
   D. Diuretics

38. **Which one of the following diuretics acts on the loop of Henle?**
   A. Spironolactone
   B. Ethacrynic acid
   C. Clorexolone
   D. Dichlorphenamide

39. **The drugs which reduce the urine volume are called __________**
   A. Diuretics
   B. Antidiuretics
   C. Carminative
   D. Purgatives

40. **Action of ADH causes __________**
   A. More reabsorption of water
   B. Less reabsorption of water
   C. Medium reabsorption of water
   D. None of the above

Answer Key

1 D	2 C	3 B	4 C	5 A	6 B	7 D	8 A	9 C	10 B
11 B	12 C	13 A	14 A	15 D	16 C	17 C	18 B	19 C	20 B
21 B	22 B	23 C	24 A	25 B	26 B	27 D	28 C	29 B	30 C
31 B	32 A	33 D	34 C	35 A	36 B	37 D	38 B	39 B	40 A

CHAPTER 10

Hormones and Hormone Antagonists

1. **The primary route of administration of insulin is __________**
   - **A.** Subcutaneous
   - **B.** Intradermal
   - **C.** Intramuscular
   - **D.** Intravenous

2. **__________ are the drugs which lower excessive sugar level to normal level.**
   - **A.** Hyperglycaemic agents
   - **B.** Hypoglycaemic agents
   - **C.** Hypotensive agents
   - **D.** Hypertensive agents

3. **__________ controls serum calcium level.**
   - **A.** Growth hormone
   - **B.** Aldosterone
   - **C.** Parathormone
   - **D.** Oxytocin

4. **__________ is used in the treatment of rickets.**
   - **A.** Vitamin D
   - **B.** Vitamin C
   - **C.** Iron
   - **D.** Magnesium

5. **Which of the following glands is not activated by products of the anterior pituitary?**
   - **A.** The mammary gland
   - **B.** The adrenal cortex
   - **C.** The pancreas
   - **D.** The thyroid gland

6. **Deficiency of insulin leads to __________**
   - **A.** Dysphagia
   - **B.** Diabetes mellitus
   - **C.** Diabetes insipidus
   - **D.** Depression

7. **__________ are chemical messengers that convey information from one cell to the next.**
   - **A.** Neurons
   - **B.** Hormones
   - **C.** Agonist
   - **D.** None of the above

8. **Diabetes insipidus is caused due to deficiency of __________**
   - **A.** TSH
   - **B.** ACTH
   - **C.** FSH
   - **D.** ADH

9. **__________ is a polypeptide hormone produced by beta cells in the pancreatic islets of Langerhans.**
   - **A.** Insulin
   - **B.** Glucagon
   - **C.** Glucose
   - **D.** Adrenaline

10. **Which of the following is an example of sulphonyl urea?**
    - **A.** Metformin
    - **B.** Propranolol
    - **C.** Tolbutamide
    - **D.** Methotrexate

11. **Insulin is a polypeptide hormone produced by __________ in the pancreatic islets of Langerhans.**
    - **A.** Alpha cells
    - **B.** Beta cells
    - **C.** Gamma cells
    - **D.** Delta cells

12. **__________ is a natural androgen produced by the testes' interstitial cells in response to the luteinizing hormone.**
    - **A.** Progesterone
    - **B.** Testosterone
    - **C.** FSH
    - **D.** None of the above

13. **__________ is used to control postpartum haemorrhage.**
    - **A.** Insulin
    - **B.** Oxytocin
    - **C.** Aldosterone
    - **D.** Hydrocortisone

14. **Which of the following is a hypoglycaemic agent obtained from the plant source?**
    - **A.** Phenformin
    - **B.** Chlorpropamide
    - **C.** Guar gum
    - **D.** Metformin

15. ___________ is the main mineralocorticoid.
A. Calcitrol
B. Insulin
C. Aldosterone
D. Hydrocortisone

16. Protamine zinc insulin is a ___________
A. Long acting insulin
B. Short acting insulin
C. Intermediate acting insulin
D. None of the above

17. The main hormone secreted by the thyroid gland is ___________
A. T3
B. T4
C. Both A and B
D. TSH

18. Which of the following activities occurs following the stimulation of H2 receptors?
A. Bronchial smooth muscle contraction
B. Vasodilation
C. Uterine contraction
D. Enhanced secretion of hydrochloric acid in the stomach

19. Iodine deficiency can cause ___________
A. Goitre
B. Thyroid cancer
C. Thyroiditis
D. Solitary thyroid nodules

20. The thyroid symptoms are mistaken for ___________ condition.
A. Pregnancy
B. Menopause
C. Crohn's disease
D. Post-traumatic stress

21. What is the first-line drug for patients with type 2 diabetes and obesity?
A. Acarbose
B. Insulin
C. Metformin
D. Sulphonyl ureas

22. Propyl thiouracil and methyl thiouracil are ________
A. Antihypertensive drugs
B. Antithyroid drugs
C. Antidiabetic drugs
D. Antidiuretic drugs

23. ___________ hormone acts at cell membrane receptor.
A. Thyroid
B. Oxytocin
C. Calcitriol
D. Steroidal

24. Deficiency of vitamin D causes ___________ in adults.
A. Rickets
B. Paget's disease
C. Osteomalacia
D. Malabsorption syndrome

25. All of the following are oral hypoglycaemic drugs *except* ___________
A. Metformin
B. Chlorpropamide
C. Glibenclamide
D. Insulin

26. Which one is short acting insulin?
A. Insulin zinc suspension
B. Insulin lispro
C. Insulin glargine
D. Insulin detemir

27. Calcitonin is a hormone secreted by ___________
A. Parathyroid gland
B. Adrenal gland
C. Thyroid gland
D. Pituitary gland

28. ___________ is the sulfonyl urea derivative.
A. Metformin
B. Repaglinide
C. Tolbutamide
D. Acarbose

29. Estrogen is used in the following conditions, *except* _____
A. To treat menopausal syndrome
B. Hypertension
C. Functional uterine bleeding
D. As a oral contraceptive

30. ___________ is also called "sunshine" vitamin.
A. Vitamin D
B. Vitamin C
C. Vitamin K
D. Vitamin E

31. ___________ is the anti-progestin drug.
A. Allyl mestranol
B. Megestrol acetate
C. Mifepristone
D. Hydroxy progesterone caproate

32. Phenformin and metformin are the examples of _______
A. Hypnotics
B. Hypoglycaemic agents
C. Hypotensives
D. Hypertensives

33. Actions of growth hormone include the __________
A. Increased protein synthesis
B. Increased carbohydrate utilization
C. Increased fat utilization
D. Glucose intolerance

34. **Somatostatin inhibits the release of __________**

A. Insulin
B. Growth hormone
C. Thyrotropin
D. All of the above

35. **The most reliable guide to adjustment of thyroxine dose in a patient of hypothyroidism is __________**

A. Serum TSH level
B. Pulse rate
C. Body weight
D. Serum thyroxine level

36. **Over treatment with the following thyroid inhibitor results in enlargement of the thyroid __________**

A. Lugol's iodine
B. Carbimazole
C. Radioactive iodine
D. All of the above

37. **The thyroid inhibitor which produces the fastest response is __________**

A. Radioactive iodine
B. Propylthiouracil
C. Lugol's iodine
D. Lithium carbonate

38. **The insulin receptor is a __________**

A. G-protein coupled receptor
B. Ion channel regulating receptor
C. Tyrosine protein kinase receptor
D. None of the above

39. **The hypoglycaemic action of sulfonylureas is likely to be attenuated by the concurrent use of __________**

A. Aspirin
B. Hydrochlorothiazide
C. Propranolol
D. Theophylline

40. **__________ stimulate uterus and produce contraction uterus to expel the baby (parturition)**

A. Insulin
B. Oxytocin
C. Renin
D. Aldosterone

Answer Key

1 A	2 B	3 C	4 A	5 C	6 B	7 B	8 D	9 A	10 C
11 B	12 B	13 B	14 C	15 C	16 A	17 C	18 D	19 A	20 B
21 C	22 B	23 B	24 C	25 D	26 B	27 C	28 C	29 B	30 A
31 C	32 B	33 B	34 D	35 A	36 B	37 C	38 C	39 B	40 B

CHAPTER

11

Autocoids

1. ___________ are self-regulating substances.
   A. Lipids B. Autocoids
   C. Proteins D. Carbohydrates

2. 5-hydroxytryptamine is also known as ___________
   A. Oxytocin B. Calcitonin
   C. Thyrocalcitonin D. Serotonin

3. ___________ is produced by histamine.
   A. Dale's vasomotor reversal
   B. Double response
   C. Triple response
   D. Single response

4. Which of the following actions of 5-hydroxytryptamine is mediated by the 5-HT3 receptor.
   A. EDRF release B. Vasoconstriction
   C. Bradycardia D. Platelet aggregation

5. Which histamine H2 blocker has most marked inhibitory effect on microsomal cytochrome P-450 enzyme.
   A. Famotidine B. Cimetidine
   C. Ranitidine D. Roxatidine

6. Which one of the following is an appetite suppressant?
   A. Cyproheptadine B. Morphine
   C. Diphenhydramine D. Promethazine

7. The most efficacious drug for inhibiting round the clock gastric acid output is ___________
   A. Pirenzepine B. Omeprazole
   C. Cimetidine D. Misoprostol

8. Which of the following histamine receptors increases the release of gastric acid?
   A. H1 receptor B. H2 receptor
   C. H3 receptor D. H4 receptor

9. ___________ is example of 5-HT receptor antagonist.
   A. Cyproheptadine
   B. Histidine
   C. Histones
   D. Cytosine

10. Ondansetron blocks emetogenic impulses at which of the following sites?
    A. Chemoreceptor trigger zone
    B. Vagal afferents in intestines
    C. Nucleus tractus solitarius
    D. All of the above

11. Triple response does not include ___________
    A. Flare B. Flush
    C. Floar D. Wheal

12. Which of the following drugs belongs to ethylene diamine class of antihistamines?
    A. Mepyramine
    B. Diphenhydramine
    C. Cyclizine
    D. Buclizine

13. Following are H2-receptor antagonists *except* ______
    A. Famotidine
    B. Ranitidine
    C. Clonidine
    D. Cimetidine

14. Which prostaglandin is used in abortion of pregnancy?
    A. Prostacyclin (PGI2)
    B. Prostaglandin E1
    C. Prostaglandin D2 (PGD2)
    D. Prostaglandin F20 (PGF2a)

15. **Methysergide is used in the treatment of __________**
A. Migraine B. Epilepsy
C. Depression D. Mania

16. **Triple response of histamine is described by scientist __________**
A. Dale B. Lewis
C. Fleming D. Edward

17. **Histamine is released in many allergic states due to __________**
A. Antigen–antibody reactions
B. Chemical reactions
C. Irritation
D. Hormonal secretions

18. **Which drug is used in migraine prophylactically?**
A. Methysergide B. Ondansetron
C. Prostaglandins D. Cyproheptadine

19. **__________ are present in cardiac muscles, mast cells and gastric parietal cells.**
A. H1 receptors B. H2 receptors
C. Alpha receptors D. Beta receptors

20. **Which one of the following are not autocoid drug?**
A. 5-HT B. Serotonin
C. Tryptophan D. Prostaglandin E1

21. **Benadryl is a popular brand name of __________**
A. Chlorpheniramine B. Diphenhydramine
C. Promethazine D. Chlorpromazine

22. **__________ is a potent biogenic amine.**
A. Noradrenaline B. Histamine
C. Acetylcholine D. None of the above

23. **__________ is 5-HT3 antagonist.**
A. Ondansetron B. Chlorpromazine
C. Promethazine D. Metoclopramide

24. **COX stands for __________**
A. Cyclic oxygen
B. Cyclooxygenase
C. Cyclo oxygen
D. Cyclic oxygen compound

25. **Avomine is brand name of __________**
A. Emetine B. Cyclizine
C. Promethazine D. Buclizine

26. **__________ are carboxylic acids that are unsaturated and consist of a skeleton of 20 carbon and a five-member ring.**
A. Dopaminergic compounds
B. Prostaglandins
C. Noradrenaline
D. None of the above

27. **Which class of antibody is associated with allergic reactions?**
A. IgE B. IgA
C. IgM D. IgG

28. **Which of the following is H1-antihistaminic?**
A. Metiamide B. Burimamide
C. Meclizine D. Cimetidine

29. **__________ are synthesized by oxidation of essential fatty acids.**
A. Histamines B. Enzymes
C. Hormones D. Prostaglandins

30. **GPCR stands for __________**
A. G-protein complex receptor
B. G-protein coupled receptor
C. G-protein complex role
D. None of the above

Answer Key

1 B	2 D	3 C	4 C	5 B	6 A	7 B	8 B	9 A	10 D
11 C	12 A	13 C	14 B	15 A	16 B	17 A	18 A	19 B	20 C
21 B	22 B	23 A	24 B	25 C	26 B	27 A	28 C	29 D	30 B

CHAPTER 12

Chemotherapeutic Agents

1. **The use of chemical compounds in the treatment of infectious diseases so as to destroy the microorganisms without damaging the host tissues is called _______**
   A. Antagonist B. Chemotherapy
   C. Agonist D. None of the above

2. **__________ is a disease which causes characteristic lesion in the peripheral neurons.**
   A. Cancer B. Tuberculosis
   C. Parkinsonism D. Leprosy

3. **__________ are the agents that prevent the growth of bacteria.**
   A. Fungistatics B. Bactericidal
   C. Fungicidal D. Bacteriostatics

4. **Anaphylactic shock is a major toxic effect of ________**
   A. Streptomycin B. Penicillin
   C. Metronidazole D. Erythromycin

5. **__________ is a macrolide antibiotic.**
   A. Streptomycin B. Ciprofloxacin
   C. Erythromycin D. Amoxicillin

6. **Anthelmintics are administered along with ________**
   A. Carminatives B. Purgatives
   C. Cardiotonic D. Appetizers

7. **__________ should be avoided with milk or antacid.**
   A. Sulphonamides B. Chloramphenicol
   C. Tetracycline D. Ciprofloxacin

8. **Which of the following antibiotics has a beta-lactam ring?**
   A. Streptomycin B. Cephalosporin
   C. Penicillin D. Tetracycline

9. **Amoebiasis causes __________**
   A. Dysentery B. Headache and cold
   C. Fever D. Severe cold

10. **Peripheral neuritis is a toxicity of __________**
    A. PAS B. INH
    C. DEC D. CPM

11. **Which of the following drugs is not an aminoglycoside?**
    A. Neomycin B. Amikacin
    C. Streptomycin D. Azithromycin

12. **Penicillin was discovered in 1929 by __________ in England.**
    A. Griffin B. Alexander Fleming
    C. Dale D. Edward

13. **The causative agent of tuberculosis is __________**
    A. Protozoan B. Virus
    C. Bacterium D. Malnutrition

14. **Penicillin acts by interfering with __________**
    A. Synthesis of proteins
    B. Synthesis of cell wall
    C. Synthesis of enzymes
    D. Synthesis of hormones

15. **Which of the following is the most common adverse effect of Amphotericin-B?**
    A. Bone marrow suppression
    B. Nephrotoxicity
    C. Hypokalaemia
    D. Hypomagnesemia

16. **Resochin is a popular brand name of __________**
    A. Metronidazole B. Chloroquine
    C. Mefloquine D. Mebendazole

17. The agents which kill the bacteria are called ________

A. Fungicidal B. Virucidal
C. Bactericidal D. Amoebicidal

18. The daily dose of ciprofloxacin is __________

A. 250 to 750 mg twice daily
B. 100 to 150 mg twice daily
C. 150 to 200 mg twice daily
D. 50 to 100 mg twice daily

19. Which one of the following is urinary antiseptic?

A. Oxalic acid B. Acetic acid
C. Nalidixic acid D. Boric acid

20. The following are used as anticancer agents *except* __________

A. Azithromycin
B. Cyclophosphamide
C. Chlorambucil
D. Busulphan

21. Which one of the following drugs inhibits herpes viruses?

A. Amantadine B. Oseltamivir
C. Azidothymidine D. Acyclovir

22. Macrolides are derived from __________

A. *Saccharopolyspora erythraea*
B. *Streptomyces griseus*
C. *Streptomyces racemosus*
D. *Penicillium notatum*

23. Metronidazole is a drug of choice in the treatment of __________

A. Helminthiasis
B. Amoebiasis
C. Candidiasis
D. Blastomycosis

24. The drug used for Malaria chemoprophylaxis and treatment is __________

A. Quinine B. Chloroquine
C. Quinidine D. Sulphonamides

25. Quinine is __________

A. Viricidal B. Fungicidal
C. Schizoonticidal D. Bacteriocidal

26. Althrocin is a popular brand name of __________

A. Azithromycin
B. Streptomycin
C. Erythromycin
D. Actinomycin

27. __________ is a major toxic effect of chloroquine.

A. Allergy
B. Black water fever
C. Peripheral neuritis
D. Retinopathy

28. Which of the following drugs is used for Trichomoniasis treatment?

A. Tetracycline B. Metronidazole
C. Suramin D. Pyrimethamine

29. __________ is an antibiotic used in the treatment of cancer.

A. Kanamycin B. Neomycin
C. Actinomycin-D D. Bleomycin

30. DEC stands for __________

A. Diethyl carbamazine
B. Diethelene carboxamide
C. Diethyl chloride
D. Diethyl chromium

31. Defective formation of bone and teeth is a major toxicity of __________

A. Penicillins
B. Chloramphenicol
C. Tetracycline
D. Erythromycin

32. ____________ is indicated for the treatment of eye infection.

A. Sulphacetamide
B. Sulphaguanidine
C. Sulphamethoxazole
D. Sulphadimidine

33. The cancer-causing agents are called __________

A. Parkinsonism agents
B. Carcinogenic agents
C. Diabetic agents
D. None of the above

34. __________ is a major toxic effect of streptomycin.

A. Nephrotoxicity
B. Cardiotoxicity
C. Ototoxicity
D. Liver toxicity

35. In tuberculosis treatment the drugs are given _______

A. Frequently
B. Synergistically
C. Antagonistically
D. None of the above

36. Metallic taste in mouth is an adverse effect of ________

A. Mebendazole B. Albenzole
C. Metronidazole D. Thibendazole

37. Busulfan is anticancer drug belongs to the class of __________

A. Alkyl sulfonates B. Antibiotics
C. Hormones D. Antimetabolites

38. Methamoglobinemia is an adverse effect of ________

A. Insulin B. Dapsone
C. Warfarin D. Phenindione

39. Which of the following sulphonamide is used in GIT infections?

A. Sulphacetamide
B. Sulphadiazine
C. Sulphaguanidine
D. Sulphadimidine

40. Undecylenic acid is __________

A. Antiviral agent
B. Anticancer agent
C. Antifungal agent
D. Antiamoebic agent

41. Which of the following is folic acid antagonist?

A. Busulfan
B. Methotrexate
C. Rubidomycin
D. None of the above

42. Tetracyclines acts by inhibiting __________ of bacterial cells.

A. Enzyme system B. Cell wall
C. Nucleus D. Cytoplasm

43. Vincristine and vinblastine are the alkaloids used in the treatment of __________

A. Leprosy B. Cancer
C. Tuberculosis D. Amoebiasis

44. PABA stands for ___________

A. Para-amino benzene
B. Para-aldehyde benzene
C. Para-aminobenzoic acid
D. None of the above

45. ___________ is used in "travellers diarrhoea"

A. Penicillin
B. Ciprofloxacin
C. Tetracycline
D. Neomycin

46. ___________ is a folic acid antagonist.

A. Methotrexate
B. Fluorouracil
C. 6-mercaptomerine
D. Chlorambucil

47. Tuberculosis is an infectious disease caused by _______

A. *Mycobacterium tuberculosis*
B. *E. coli*
C. *Shigella*
D. None of the above

48. INH stands for ___________

A. Isonicotinic acetyl hydrazide
B. Isonicotinic acid hydrazide
C. Isonicotinic acidic hydrazide
D. None of the above

49. Gray baby syndrome is an adverse effect of _________

A. Chloroquine
B. Chlorpropamide
C. Chloramphenicol
D. Chlorpheniramine

50. Which of the following drugs is called life saving as well as life threatening?

A. Penicillin B. Streptomycin
C. Actinomycin D. Neomycin

51. PAS stands for ___________

A. Para-amino salicylic aldehyde
B. Para-aminosalicylic acid
C. Para-amino salicylic anhydride
D. None of the above

52. Pigmentation of teeth is a major toxic effect of _______

A. Amphotericin B
B. Neomycin
C. Tetracycline
D. Streptomycin

53. Bone marrow depression is an adverse effect of ______

A. Chloramphenicol
B. Streptomycin
C. Neomycin
D. Clotrimazole

54. ___________ means the drugs which expels the worms.

A. Vermicide B. Vermifuge
C. Bacteriostatic D. Bactericidal

55. Hypoplasia of gums is an adverse effect of ___________

A. Atenolol B. Penicillin
C. Tetracycline D. Ciprofloxacin

56. **Micro-organism causing leprosy is __________**
A. *Mycobacterium leprae*
B. *Mycobacterium tuberculosis*
C. Mycobacterium Lepromatous
D. None of the above

57. **Sulphonamides compete with __________ in bacterial metabolism.**
A. GABA B. PABA
C. ACTH D. INH

58. **Which of the following is a drug of choice in the treatment of plague?**
A. Metronidazole B. Kanamycin
C. Tetracycline D. Erythromycin

59. **__________ is a drug of choice in leprosy.**
A. Levodopa B. Dapsone
C. Bromocriptine D. Methyldopa

60. **Crystalluria is a toxicity of __________**
A. Penicillins B. Tetracyclines
C. Sulphonamides D. Thiazides

61. **__________ is selectively effective for skin, nail, and hair dermatophyte infections.**
A. Methyldopa
B. Lignocaine
C. Griseofulvin
D. None of the above

62. **RNA stands for __________**
A. Ribonucleic acid
B. Riboxy nucleic acetic acid
C. Riboxy nucleic aldehyde
D. None of the above

63. **Co-trimoxazole is a combination of __________**
A. 2 parts of sulphamethoxazole + 2 parts of trimethoprim
B. 5 parts of sulphamethoxazole + 1 part of trimethoprim
C. 3 parts of sulphamethoxazole + 3 parts of trimethoprim
D. 1 part of sulphamethoxazole + 3 parts of trimethoprim

64. **__________ is a globe distributive infectious disease produced by *Plasmodium* protozoa, which are spread by the anopheles mosquito from man to man.**
A. Gonorrhoea
B. Diarrhoea
C. Malaria
D. None of the above

65. **__________ have structural similarity to that of PABA.**
A. Tetracyclines B. Sulphonamides
C. Chloramphenicol D. Macrolides

66. **There are __________ plasmodium species that have a similar life cycle and are harmful to man.**
A. Four B. Five
C. Three D. Two

67. **__________ is useful in the treatment of candidiasis.**
A. Metronidazole B. Fluconazole
C. Ornidazole D. Cloxacillin

68. **Idoxuridine is __________**
A. Antianginal drug
B. Antiemetic drug
C. Antiviral drug
D. Anticancer drug

69. **__________ is an acute or chronic *Entamoeba histolytica* protozoan infection.**
A. Diarrhoea B. Amoebic dysentery
C. Tuberculosis D. None of the above

70. **The drugs used to treat worms are called ________**
A. Antimalarials B. Anthelmintics
C. Antivirals D. Antihypertensives

71. **__________ is characterized by local itching, redness, swelling, and pain at the site of injection.**
A. Insulin resistance
B. Insulin lipodystrophy
C. Insulin allergy
D. Insulin neuropathy

72. **All the following are ß-lactam antibiotics *except* ______**
A. Penicillin B. Chloramphenicol
C. Penicillin G D. Cephalosporins

73. **__________ is used in the treatment of Covid-19.**
A. Penicillin B. Remedesivir
C. Tetracyclines D. Rifamycin

74. **The major toxicity of isoniazid is __________**
A. Gray baby syndrome
B. Pruritis
C. Neurotoxicity
D. Rashes

75. **Which antifungal agent can be used systemically as well as topically?**
A. Benzoic acid B. Ketoconazole
C. Griseofulvin D. Nystatin

76. Cinchonism and black water fever are the adverse effects of ___________

A. Chloroquine
B. Quinine
C. Amodiaquine
D. Mefloquine

77. Diloxanide furoate is a ___________

A. Tissue amoebicide
B. Hepatic amoebicide
C. Luminal amoebicide
D. Extra-intestinal amoebicide

78. Broad spectrum anthelmintics include ___________.

A. Mebendazole
B. Albendazole
C. Thiabendazole
D. All of the above

79. Which is a contraindication in the use of chloroquine?

A. Pregnancy
B. Lactation
C. Vision abnormalities
D. No contraindication

80. Zidovudine and lamivudine are the antiviral drugs used in the treatment of ___________

A. Fungal infections
B. HIV infections
C. Amoebic infections
D. GIT infections

Answer Key

1 B	2 D	3 D	4 B	5 C	6 B	7 C	8 C	9 A	10 B
11 D	12 B	13 C	14 B	15 B	16 B	17 C	18 A	19 C	20 A
21 D	22 A	23 B	24 B	25 C	26 C	27 D	28 B	29 C	30 A
31 C	32 A	33 B	34 C	35 B	36 C	37 A	38 B	39 C	40 C
41 B	42 A	43 B	44 C	45 B	46 A	47 A	48 B	49 C	50 A
51 B	52 C	53 A	54 B	55 C	56 A	57 B	58 C	59 B	60 C
61 C	62 A	63 B	64 C	65 B	66 A	67 B	68 C	69 B	70 B
71 C	72 B	73 B	74 C	75 B	76 B	77 C	78 D	79 C	80 B

Section VII

Community Pharmacy and Management

Syllabus (As Per ER 2020) Community Pharmacy and Management

Chapter	Topics
1	**Community Pharmacy Practice** Definition, history and development of community pharmacy: International and Indian scenarios
2	Professional responsibilities of community pharmacists Introduction to the concept of Good Pharmacy Practice and SOPs
3	**Prescription and Prescription Handling** ■ Definition, parts of prescriptions, legality of prescriptions, prescription handling, labelling of dispensed medications (Main label, ancillary label, pictograms), brief instructions on medication usage ■ Dispensing process, Good Dispensing Practices, dispensing errors and strategies to minimize them
4	**Communication Skills** ■ Definition, types of communication skills ■ Interactions with professionals and patients ■ Verbal communicationskills (one-to-one, over the telephone) ■ Written communication skills ■ Body language ■ Patient interview techniques
5	**Patient Counselling** ■ Definition and benefits of patient counselling ■ Stages of patient counselling: Introduction, counselling content, counselling process, and closing the counselling session ■ Barriers to effective counselling: Types and strategies to overcome the barriers ■ Patient counselling points for chronic diseases/disorders: Hypertension, Diabetes, Asthma, Tuberculosis, Chronic obstructive pulmonary disease, and AIDS ■ Patient Package Inserts: Definition, importance and benefits, scenarios of PPI use in India and other countries ■ Patient information leaflets: Definition and uses
6	**Medication Adherence** Definition, factors influencing non-adherence, strategies to overcome non-adherence
7	**Health Screening Services in Community Pharmacy** Introduction, scope, and importance of various health screening services—for routine monitoring of patients, early detection, and referral of undiagnosed cases
8	**Over The Counter (OTC) Medications** ■ Definition, need and role of Pharmacists in OTC medication dispensing ■ OTC medications in India, counselling for OTC products ■ Self-medication and role of pharmacists in promoting the safe practices during self-medication ■ Responding to symptoms, minor ailments, and advice for self-care in conditions such as—Pain management, Cough, Cold, Diarrhea, Constipation, Vomiting, Fever, Sore throat, Skin disorders, Oral health (mouth ulcers, dental pain, gum swelling)
9	**Community Pharmacy Management** Definition, classification, pharmacological actions, dose, indications, and contraindications of: ■ Legal requirements to set up a community pharmacy ■ Site selection requirements ■ Pharmacy designs and interiors ■ Vendor selection and ordering ■ Procurement, inventory control methods, and inventory management ■ Financial planning and management ■ Accountancy in community pharmacy—Day book, Cash book ■ Introduction to pharmacy operation softwares—usefulness and availability ■ Customer Relation Management (CRM) ■ Audits in Pharmacies ■ SOP of Pharmacy Management ■ Introduction to Digital Health, mHealth and Online pharmacies

CHAPTER 1

Community Pharmacy Practice

1. **Pharmacists are registered under the Pharmacy Act __________**
   A. 1968 B. 1938
   C. 1948 D. 1958

2. **Which of the following is role of community pharmacist?**
   A. Dispensing of medicines
   B. Patient counselling
   C. Processing of prescription
   D. All of the above

3. **The minimum area required for a medical store is ______**
   A. 20 sq m B. 30 sq m
   C. 10 sq m D. 40 sq m

4. **CHC stands for __________**
   A. Community Health Centre
   B. Common Health Centre
   C. Collective Health centre
   D. Causal Health Centre

5. **Which of the following is known as retail pharmacy?**
   A. Hospital pharmacy
   B. Clinical pharmacy
   C. Community pharmacy
   D. None of the above

6. **Community pharmacy is a link between __________**
   A. Community and drug
   B. Community and health
   C. Community and disease
   D. Community and social pharmacy

7. **As per Drugs and Cosmetics Rules 1945, which one of the following rules indicate the presence of pharmacist is legally required during the dispensing and selling of medicines?**
   A. Rule 65 (15) B. Rule 45 (15)
   C. Rule 65 (25) D. Rule 75 (15)

8. **The first Pharmacopoeia of World is published in __________**
   A. Italy
   B. Greece
   C. Nuremberg Germany
   D. Pennsylvania

9. **The history of community pharmacy in India starts with opening of chemist shop in __________**
   A. 1831 B. 1801
   C. 1811 D. 1821

10. **The community pharmacists who actually manage __________**
    A. Retail drug outlets or medical store
    B. Retail pharmacy
    C. Place where medicines are stored, dispensed and sold
    D. All of the above

11. **WHO published the First International Pharmacopoeia in __________ 1951.**
    A. Geneva, Switzerland
    B. Nuremberg Germany
    C. Italy
    D. Russia

12. **All India Organization of Chemists and Druggists (AIOCD) was formed in ________**
    A. 1979 B. 1977
    C. 1978 D. 1980

13. Community Pharmacy received the official recognition in India through ___________

A. Drugs and Cosmetics Act
B. Pharmaceutical Education Regulations
C. Pharmacy Practice Regulations
D. AICTE's intervention

14. In which year the first degree program in pharmacy was started in Banaras Hindu University?

A. 1940 **B.** 1932
C. 1937 **D.** 1955

15. The "first qualified person" to get recognition as chemist and druggist in India in 1866 was ___________

A. ML Schroff
B. HW Honey
C. PC Ray
D. Jonathan Roberts

16. The most accessible healthcare professional is ______

A. Practising nurse
B. Community pharmacist
C. Hospital pharmacist
D. Practising doctor

17. First regular two years course for "Chemists and Druggists Diploma" was started at ___________

A. Kolkata
B. Delhi
C. Chennai
D. Mumbai

18. "Chemists and Druggist Diploma" course of MMC, Chennai made equivalent to diploma issued by Royal Pharmaceutical Society of Great Britain, in ___________

A. 1895 **B.** 1893
C. 1897 **D.** 1899

19. Which type of pharmacy offers maximum opportunity of career growth for an employed community pharmacist?

A. Pharmacy owned by a businessman
B. Chain pharmacies
C. Pharmacy owned by other pharmacists
D. E-pharmacies

20. Bengal Dispensary and Pharmacopoeia-Vol 1 was published in ___________

A. 1861
B. 1831
C. 1841
D. 1851

21. Which of the following retail pharmacy types is illegal in India?

A. On-line pharmacy
B. Independent community pharmacy
C. Chain store pharmacy
D. Community pharmacy in a hospital

22. Which of the following is not an alternative (or synonym) of community pharmacy in India?

A. Internet pharmacy
B. Retail pharmacy
C. Pharmacy
D. Chemist and druggist

23. Who is the licensing authority for establishing a community pharmacy?

A. State Pharmacy Council
B. Central Drugs Control Authority
C. State Drugs Control Authority
D. Pharmacy Council of India

24. Community pharmacy requires ___________

A. Retail sale license
B. Manufacturing license
C. Export license
D. Wholesale license

25. The minimum qualification for registration as a registered pharmacist is ___________

A. Bachelor of Pharmacy
B. Master of Pharmacy
C. Diploma in Pharmacy
D. Doctor of Pharmacy

26. In 1729, the first community pharmacy was founded in ___________

A. Philadelphia
B. Italy
C. Germany
D. Sweden

27. The first community pharmacy in India was started by ___________

A. Smith Stan Street & Co
B. Bathgate & Co
C. Kemp & Co
D. Thomson & Co

28. While processing a prescription for dispensing, the community pharmacist needs to look into ___________

A. Safety of medications
B. The legality of the prescription
C. Appropriateness of the prescription
D. All of the above

29. Pharmacists working in India must have a pharmacist registration certificate issued by the state it comes under which Act __________.

A. Drugs and Cosmetics Act 1940

B. Provisions of the Pharmacy Act 1948

C. Medicinal and Toilet Preparation Act

D. Drugs Price Control Order 1995

30. To obtain a registration certificate, the pharmacist must acquire the minimum qualification of

A. Diploma in Pharmacy (DPharm)

B. Pharm D

C. Bachelor of Pharmacy (BPharm)

D. All of the above

Answer Key

1 C	2 D	3 C	4 A	5 C	6 B	7 A	8 C	9 C	10 D
11 A	12 A	13 C	14 B	15 B	16 B	17 C	18 B	19 B	20 C
21 A	22 A	23 C	24 A	25 C	26 A	27 B	28 D	29 B	30 D

CHAPTER 2

Professional Responsibilities of Community Pharmacists

1. **Good Pharmacy Practice for community pharmacy setting is developed by __________.**
   A. WHO and UNICEF
   B. WHO and FIP
   C. FIP and UNICEF
   D. WHO

2. **What is GPP?**
   A. Good Pharmacy Practices
   B. Good Physician Practices
   C. Good Practical Practices
   D. All of the above

3. **Standard operating procedures (SOPs) are __________.**
   A. The rules of conduct of manufacturing
   B. The set of written instructions
   C. Laws of sale
   D. None of the above

4. **GPP is practice of pharmacy that responds to _______.**
   A. The needs of the people
   B. The needs of the pharmacists
   C. The needs of the nurses
   D. The needs of the doctors

5. **What is FIP?**
   A. International Federation of Police
   B. Federation of Indian Police
   C. International Pharmaceutical Federation
   D. None of the above

6. **GPP guidelines are based on the __________.**
   A. Hospital care
   B. Nursing care
   C. Pharmaceutical care
   D. None of the above

7. **FIP Congress held in Tokyo adopted the FIP/GPP in year __________.**
   A. 1993 B. 1994
   C. 1992 D. None of the above

8. **The FIP Congress held in __________ adopted the FIP/GPP text under the Tokyo declaration on standards for quality of pharmacy services.**
   A. Beijing in 1992
   B. Tokyo in 1994
   C. Tokyo in 1993
   D. None of the above

9. **PMR stands for __________.**
   A. Postmedication record
   B. Patients medication record
   C. Preanesthetic medication record
   D. Preoperative medication record

10. **SOP is recognized abbreviation for __________.**
   A. Standards of parameter
   B. Staff of pharmacy
   C. Student of pharmacy
   D. Standard operating procedure

11. **Model Pharmacy is a requirement of Diploma in Pharmacy conducting institution under __________.**
   A. Education Regulations 2020
   B. Education Regulations 1991
   C. Pharmacy Practice Regulations 2015
   D. Pharmacy Practice (Amendment) Regulations 2021

12. **The year in which the Indian Pharmaceutical Association developed GPP Guidelines was __________.**
   A. 2004 B. 2007
   C. 2003 D. 2001

13. **The Seven Star Pharmacist concept is given by ______**
    - A. WHO
    - B. FIP and IPA
    - C. FIP
    - D. FIP and WHO

14. **Roles for community pharmacists were suggested by WHO in 1988 at a meeting held in __________.**
    - A. New Delhi
    - B. Geneva
    - C. Alma Ata
    - D. Tokyo

15. **The counselling area should be equipped with _______.**
    - A. Weight and height scale
    - B. Refrigerator
    - C. Computer
    - D. All of the above

16. **Upon receiving the prescription, first responsibility of Pharmacist is __________.**
    - A. Counselling of client
    - B. To dispense medicine
    - C. To confirm identity of client
    - D. To explain the price of medicine

17. **Preparation of SOPs in pharmacy is responsibility of __________.**
    - A. Drug inspector
    - B. Pharmacist
    - C. Pharmacy assistant
    - D. None of these

18. **Which one of the following things is not necessary in counselling area?**
    - A. Sound system
    - B. Chair for the pharmacist and a couple of patients
    - C. Cabinet for storing patient medication records
    - D. Television

19. **A necessary document needs to start the community pharmacy is __________.**
    - A. NOC from local government organization
    - B. FDA license
    - C. Pharmacist registrations
    - D. All of the above

20. **Which of the following is a professional responsibility of community pharmacists?**
    - A. Dealing with general health of the patients
    - B. Drug information source
    - C. Patient safety
    - D. All of the above

Answer Key

1 B	2 A	3 B	4 A	5 C	6 C	7 A	8 C	9 B	10 D
11 A	12 C	13 D	14 A	15 D	16 C	17 B	18 A	19 D	20 D

CHAPTER 3

Prescription and Prescription Handling

1. **The prescription must be received and checked by the ________.**
   A. Physician B. Pharmacist
   C. Patient D. Nurse

2. **The following are the parts of prescription *except* ________.**
   A. Signatura B. Subscription
   C. Date D. Disease state

3. **Drug labelling is also known as ________.**
   A. Analytical labelling
   B. Compounding labelling
   C. Prescription labelling
   D. All of the above

4. **The superscription is represented by a symbol _____.**
   A. Tx B. Rx
   C. Mx D. Phx

5. **________ is responsible for proper handling of the prescription.**
   A. Nurses B. Science graduates
   C. Pharmacists D. Physicians

6. **In which language, the abbreviations in the prescription writing is very common especially in dosage instruction?**
   A. Italian B. Latin
   C. Greek D. French

7. **The drug labelling requirements in India are provided in Drugs and Cosmetics Act Rules 1945, under ________.**
   A. Sections 40 and 45 B. Sections 35 and 37
   C. Sections 45 and 50 D. Sections 96 and 97

8. **The prescription is an order written by a registered medical practitioner to ________.**
   A. Nurse
   B. Patient
   C. Pharmacist
   D. Compounder

9. **The prescriber indicates the ________ for the use of the medication in the portion of the prescription called signatura.**
   A. Directions for the doctor
   B. Directions for the patients
   C. Directions for the pharmacist
   D. Directions for the nurse

10. **The main label is also known as ________.**
    A. Manufacturers label
    B. Dispensing label
    C. Store label
    D. None of the above

11. **In the day of mythology, the symbol Rx was considered as a prayer to ________.**
    A. Dhanvantari B. Jupiter
    C. Jesus D. Neptune

12. **Auxiliary label is also known as ________.**
    A. Manufacturer's label
    B. Warehouse label
    C. Cautionary advisory label
    D. Transport label

13. **The abbreviation of Latin word Rx is ________.**
    A. To sold B. You take
    C. To make D. To use

14. Pictogram is also known as __________.

A. Pictorange B. Pictograph
C. Pictodrum D. Pictocard

15. The part of the prescription called inscription contains __________.

A. Name, Age
B. Signature, Address
C. Registration number and patient information
D. Name and quantity of ingredients

16. Rx is denoted for __________.

A. Inscription
B. Superscription
C. Subscription
D. Transcription

17. The last item written in the inscription is __________.

A. Medicament
B. Vehicle, diluent
C. Active ingredients
D. Quantity

18. __________ is a simple drawing, a chart or graph that uses pictures to represent data in simple way.

A. Histogram B. Cardiogram
C. Pictogram D. Hectogram

19. The part of prescription called subscription contains __________.

A. Direction to the patient's relatives
B. Direction to the pharmacist
C. Direction to the patient
D. All of the above

20. BID means __________.

A. Every other day B. Twice a day
C. Once a day D. Three times a day

21. Which of the following is a type of medication error?

A. Transcription error
B. Prescription error
C. Dispensing error
D. All of the above

22. "Prescription" is derived from the Latin term

A. Prescribe B. Precriptus
C. Praescriptus D. None of the above

23. When drug is placed under the tongue, then it is called __________.

A. Subcutaneous B. Transdermal
C. Buccal D. Sublingual

24. Pictogram is available for __________.

A. "Dilute with water" B. "Take by mouth"
C. "Take at bed time" D. All of the above

25. "Keep in a refrigerator" is __________.

A. Instruction
B. Indication
C. Precaution
D. None of the above

26. Which of the following is a reason of dispensing error?

A. Poor handwriting of the prescriber
B. Wrong prescription
C. Dispensing wrong medication
D. All of the above

27. "PIL" stands for __________.

A. Pathology information leaflet
B. Pharmacist information leaflet
C. Patient information leaflet
D. Physician information leaflet

28. Which of the following professional is not usually a prescriber?

A. Dentist B. Doctor
C. Pharmacist D. Veterinary doctor

29. Post-cibos means __________.

A. After a drink B. After food
C. Before food D. Before a drink

30. Dispensing is governed by __________.

A. Patent Rules
B. Pharmacy Rules
C. Drugs and Cosmetics Rules
D. All of the above

31. The instruction to the patient in a prescription is called __________.

A. Signatura
B. Inscription
C. Superscription
D. None of the above

32. "Store in a cool dry place" is __________.

A. Precaution B. Instruction
C. Indication D. None of the above

33. The dispenser is duty bound to keep a copy of the prescription while __________.

A. Dispensing veterinary drug
B. Dispensing of schedule 'X' drug
C. Dispensing any drug
D. None of the above

34. Shake well before use is a labelling requirement for _________.

A. Emulsion B. Suspension
C. Both A and B D. All of the above

35. Pictograms are helpful for persons who have _______.

A. Difficulty in reading/hearing
B. Difficulty in reading
C. Difficulty in hearing
D. All of the above

36. Subscription means _________.

A. Direction for patient
B. It lists the names and dosages of the medications prescribed
C. The prescriber gives the instructions to the pharmacist
D. None of the above

37. Inscription contains _________.

A. Direction for patient
B. The names and dosages of the medications prescribed
C. The prescriber gives the pharmacist instructions
D. None of the above

38. Signatura means _________.

A. The prescriber gives the pharmacist instructions
B. The names and dosages of the medications prescribed
C. Direction for patient
D. None of the above

39. Pictogram is an _________.

A. Instruction on label as image
B. Main label
C. Ancillary label
D. None of the above

40. "Shake well before use" is _________.

A. Indication
B. Precaution
C. Instruction
D. None of the above

Answer Key

1 B	2 D	3 C	4 B	5 C	6 B	7 D	8 C	9 B	10 B
11 B	12 C	13 B	14 B	15 D	16 B	17 B	18 C	19 B	20 B
21 D	22 C	23 D	24 D	25 A	26 D	27 C	28 C	29 B	30 C
31 A	32 A	33 B	34 C	35 B	36 C	37 B	38 C	39 A	40 C

CHAPTER 4

Communication Skills

1. **Communication is a part of __________.**
   A. Hard skills
   B. Soft skills
   C. Medium skills
   D. None of the above

2. **__________ is an act of giving, receiving and sharing intended information.**
   A. Observation
   B. Communication
   C. Cooperation
   D. Distribution

3. **Normally, communication is __________ in which the information or message is transferred from one person to another.**
   A. Alternative B. Interpersonal
   C. Personal D. Impersonal

4. **Oral communication ensures __________.**
   A. Speedy interaction and immediate response
   B. Fluency speed and attention
   C. Adequate attention and immediate response
   D. None of the above

5. **The healthiest way of greeting clients/patients in community pharmacy practice is __________.**
   A. Smiling B. Shaking hands
   C. Namaste D. Patting on the back

6. **Which of the following is an advantage of written communication?**
   A. Easy to preserve
   B. Accurate presentation
   C. Effective communication
   D. All of the above

7. **Sharing a patient information leaflet with the patient is a type of __________.**
   A. Not considered as communication
   B. Verbal communication
   C. Non-verbal communication
   D. All of the above

8. **__________ aims at making the people to work together for the common goal of the organization.**
   A. Combination
   B. Communication
   C. Coincidence
   D. Confirmation

9. **__________ is an example of positive body language.**
   A. Tense facial expression
   B. Maintaining good eye contact
   C. Arms folded
   D. Keeping hands on the hips

10. **E-mails and websites are the types of __________ communication.**
    A. Non-verbal B. Oral
    C. Written D. Informal

11. **Face to face communication falls under __________.**
    A. Telephonic communication
    B. Verbal communication
    C. Non-verbal communication
    D. None of the above

12. **Which of the following is considered as a requirement for a good communicator?**
    A. Caring B. Politeness
    C. Positiveness D. All of the above

13. The primary goal of communication is __________.

A. To create noises
B. To create barrier
C. To effect a change
D. None of the above

14. Response to senders message is __________.

A. Transport B. Hearing
C. Visualizing D. Feedback

15. Which of the following are communication skills?

A. Effective listening
B. Non-verbal communication
C. Conflict resolution
D. All of the above

16. The word 'communication' comes from the Latin word __________

A. Communicareon B. Communicare
C. Communicate D. Communica

17. Communication by ________________ is called verbal communication.

A. Written material and gestures
B. Spoken words and written material
C. Body language and spoken words
D. None of the above

18. Effective communication with the patient is essential for __________.

A. Improving therapeutic outcomes
B. Improving interpersonal relationship
C. Promoting medication adherence
D. All of the above

19. At each stage in the process of communication, there is a possibility of interference which may hinder the process. Such interference is known as __________.

A. Receiver B. Barrier
C. Sender D. None of the above

20. Our dress code is an example of __________ communication.

A. Verbal B. Non-verbal
C. Written D. Spoken

21. __________ communications are pre-planned.

A. Informal B. Formal
C. Uniformal D. Unformal

22. The person who transmits the message is called __________.

A. Receiver B. Channel
C. Sender D. Response

23. __________ is the primary way of obtaining comprehensive information about the patient.

A. Nurse interview
B. Pharmacist interview
C. Patient interview
D. Physician interview

24. Which of the following improves verbal communication?

A. Familiar language
B. Smiling facial expression
C. Modulating the tone of the voice
D. All of the above

25. Communication through __________ is called verbal communication.

A. Body language and gestures
B. Written material and gestures
C. Gestures and spoken words
D. Spoken words and written material

26. Communication is an interaction between sender and receiver involving a transfer of __________.

A. Pronunciation
B. Information
C. Verbal elements
D. Power

27. Which of the following is a type of body language?

A. Manner of walking
B. Head tilts
C. Hand gestures
D. All of the above

28. __________ is an exchange of facts, ideas, opinions, or emotions by two or more persons.

A. Connection
B. Communication
C. Combination
D. Conversation

29. Using a metered dose inhaler can best be communicated/explained to the patient through __________.

A. Verbal communication
B. Visual communication
C. Non-verbal communication
D. Written communication

30. ____________ is the study of touches as non-verbal communication.

A. Haptics B. Body language
C. Gestures D. Prosody

31. __________ is example of negative body language.
A. Keeping hands on the hips
B. Arms folded
C. Tense facial expression
D. All of the above

32. ____________ includes sounds, words, language, and speech.
A. Non-verbal communication
B. Verbal communication
C. Both of the above
D. None of the above

33. ____________ refers to the factors that disrupts the communication.
A. Nonsense
B. Noise
C. No body
D. Silence

34. Which of the following skills are important to communicate properly?
A. Speaking
B. Reading
C. Writing
D. All of the above

35. In body language, implication of frequent throat clearing is __________.
A. Receptiveness
B. Hopelessness
C. Disagreement
D. Confidence

36. Which of the following is a type of communication?
A. Visual communication
B. Written communication
C. Electronic communication
D. All of the above

37. __________ means communication without words.
A. Object communication
B. Written communication
C. Oral communication
D. Non-verbal communication

38. Prescription is the example of __________.
A. Non-verbal communication
B. Verbal communication
C. Written communication
D. Visual communication

39. Identify the example of body language__________.
A. Coughing
B. Breathing rate
C. Facial expression
D. All of the above

40. Message is any signal that triggers the response of a __________.
A. Driver
B. Receiver
C. Sender
D. Cleaner

Answer Key

1 B	2 B	3 B	4 C	5 C	6 D	7 C	8 B	9 B	10 C
11 B	12 D	13 C	14 D	15 D	16 B	17 C	18 D	19 B	20 B
21 B	22 C	23 C	24 D	25 C	26 B	27 D	28 B	29 B	30 A
31 D	32 B	33 B	34 D	35 C	36 D	37 D	38 C	39 D	40 B

CHAPTER 5

Patient Counselling

1. **The __________ is the heart of the patient counselling session.**
   A. Counselling content
   B. Preparing for the session
   C. Opening the session
   D. Closing the session

2. **__________ is beneficial in understanding the patient and their illness.**
   A. Dispensing
   B. Compounding
   C. Counselling
   D. Prescribing

3. **The objective of patient counselling is __________**
   A. To know him the importance of medication
   B. To improve active participation of the patient in drug usage
   C. To avoid drug interaction
   D. All of the above

4. **Patient counselling helps to__________**
   A. Develop business relationship
   B. Pass time at old age
   C. Know chemical structure of the drug
   D. Motivate the patient to take medicine for improvement if his/her health status

5. **Barriers to effective communication cited by pharmacists include**
   A. Economic considerations
   B. Poor communication skills
   C. Lack of time
   D. All of the above

6. **GATHER principle may be used for __________**
   A. Dispensing
   B. Counselling
   C. Preparing an SOP
   D. Complying with regulatory requirements

7. **The success of the patient counselling depends on the __________**
   A. Language
   B. Tone
   C. Facial expressions
   D. Knowledge and skill

8. **The step to be followed during patient counselling is __________**
   A. Counselling content
   B. Preparing for the session
   C. Opening of the session
   D. All of the above

9. **Counselling is a __________**
   A. Mass communication
   B. One way communication
   C. Two ways communication
   D. None of the above

10. **PPI stands for __________**
    A. Patient package insert
    B. Patient promotional insert
    C. Pre-package insert
    D. Post-package insert

11. **The quality of good counsellor in patient counselling is __________**
    A. Be good listener
    B. Be empathetic
    C. Be flexible
    D. All of the above

12. **Ibuprofen is to be taken ________**
    A. After food
    B. Before food
    C. In between meals
    D. Any time

13. **COPD stands for ________**
    A. Chronic obese pulmonary disease
    B. Chronic obstructive pulmonary disorder
    C. Chronic open pulmonary disease
    D. Chronic obstructive pulse disorder

14. **Which of the following bodies determines the requirement of patient package inserts?**
    A. FIP
    B. FDA
    C. DCC
    D. DEC

15. **When food interferes with absorption, ideally the medicine is to be taken ________**
    A. Any time before food
    B. At least an hour before food
    C. Two hours after food
    D. At least an hour before food or two hours after food

16. **Restricted salt intake is recommended in ________**
    A. Diabetes
    B. High blood pressure
    C. Low blood pressure
    D. Asthma

17. **Which of the following country issued the 'Guidelines on the readability of the label and package leaflet and medicinal products for human use'?**
    A. Japanese
    B. European
    C. Chinese
    D. Indian

18. **Advice must be given to patient while using MAO inhibitors is ________**
    A. Do not drive vehicle
    B. Avoid cheese, alcoholic beverages and liver yeast extract
    C. Use of purgatives
    D. Do not work on dangerous machineries

19. **PIL stands for ________**
    A. Product inbuilt leaflet
    B. Process information leaflet
    C. Patient information leaflet
    D. Public information leaflet

20. **The normal BMI for Indian adults is ________**
    A. <18.5 kg/m²
    B. 23–24.9 kg/m²
    C. 25 kg/m²
    D. 18.5–22.9 kg/m²

21. **Medication history should be taken of at least last ________**
    A. 6 months
    B. 8 months
    C. 3 months
    D. 7 months

22. **Which of the following is third stage of counselling?**
    A. Counselling content
    B. Closing session
    C. Preparing counselling session
    D. Open the counselling session

23. **In USA, the concept of a patient package insert is in practice since ________**
    A. 1955
    B. 1968
    C. 1978
    D. 1988

24. **OTC stands for ________**
    A. Over-the-counselling
    B. Over-the-counter
    C. Over-the-cabin
    D. Over-the-concept

25. **Which of the following is the most effective technique to address patient's emotional issues?**
    A. Empathic reactions
    B. Consultations
    C. By assuring
    D. By maintaining privacy

26. **Increased concentration of glucose in blood is a sign of ________**
    A. COPD
    B. Diabetes
    C. AIDS
    D. High blood pressure

27. **Non-pharmacological measure for diabetes is ________**
    A. Stress management
    B. Nutrition, exercise and activity
    C. Maintenance of blood sugar level
    D. All of the above

28. **The major role of clinical pharmacist is ________**
    A. Pre-marketing surveillance
    B. Pre-clinical study
    C. Post-clinical study
    D. Patient counselling

29. **Insulin-dependent diabetes is also known as ________**
    A. Drug-induced diabetes
    B. Type 1 diabetes
    C. Type 2 diabetes
    D. Gestational diabetes

30. ________ or a medication guide is a document provided along with prescription medication to provide additional information about that drug.
A. Prescription
B. Label
C. Patient package insert
D. None of the above

31. CMI stands for ________.
A. Community medication information
B. Consumer medication information
C. Counter medication information
D. Care medication information

32. Which of the following is an example of patient information leaflet?
A. Electronic message
B. Loose leaflet
C. Package insert
D. All of the above

33. Patient package insert (PPI) is a part of ________ requirement of prescription medicine.
A. Analytical
B. Regulatory
C. Advisory
D. Subsidiary

34. The following is a barrier to effective counselling____.
A. Emotional factor
B. Pharmacy environment
C. Patient-related barrier
D. All of the above

35. Insulin is to be stored at home in ________.
A. Freezer of the refrigerator
B. In the coolest place in the house
C. A refrigerator but not in the freezer
D. Any place as temperature has no influence on potency

36. The phase one of the counselling session is used for ________.
A. Talking with relatives
B. Information gathering
C. Gathering other pharmacists
D. Gathering other nurses

37. Patient package insert (PPI) is also known as ________.
A. Packaging drug label
B. Prescription drug label
C. Carton drug label
D. Unit drug label

38. Which is not a component of patient education?
A. Relevance
B. Individualization
C. Feedback
D. Composition

39. Which is used as written information material?
A. Package inserts
B. Labels on drug cartons
C. Booklets
D. All of the above

40. Patient package insert is a ________ approved document provided along with prescription medication to provide additional information about that drug.
A. FDA
B. FIP
C. PCI
D. DIC

Answer Key

1 A	2 C	3 D	4 D	5 D	6 B	7 D	8 D	9 C	10 A
11 D	12 A	13 B	14 B	15 D	16 B	17 B	18 B	19 C	20 D
21 C	22 A	23 B	24 B	25 A	26 B	27 D	28 D	29 B	30 C
31 B	32 D	33 B	34 D	35 C	36 B	37 B	38 D	39 D	40 A

CHAPTER 6

Medication Adherence

1. **A faithful adherence by the patient to the prescriber's instruction is called __________.**
   A. Non-compliance
   B. Non-adherence
   C. Patient compliance
   D. Patient information

2. **Taking prescription medication correctly is called**
   A. Medication adverseness
   B. Medication adherence
   C. Medication avoidance
   D. Medication attentiveness

3. **"A patient is considered adherent if they take _____. of their medication as prescribed".**
   A. 80% B. 60%
   C. 70% D. 90%

4. **The term __________ is used in place of compliance/ adherence.**
   A. Concordance
   B. Co-operation
   C. Co-ordination
   D. Counter action

5. **The prescription related factor for medication adherence is __________.**
   A. Illegible and inaccurate prescription
   B. Failure to refill prescription
   C. Polypharmacy
   D. All of the above

6. **Which of the following best defines adherence drug treatment?**
   A. Understanding possible side effects of taking drug
   B. Filling a prescription
   C. Taking a drug as directed
   D. Writing down the doctor's instructions for taking the drugs.

7. **Nonadherent patients are those who do not take at least __________ of their prescribed medication.**
   A. 90% B. 60%
   C. 70% D. 80%

8. **Social and economic factors for non-adherence are __________.**
   A. Cultural beliefs
   B. The cost of medications and poverty
   C. Financial stress with transportation problem
   D. All of the above

9. **What should people do if they are adhering to their drug treatment and they experience unpleasant side effects?**
   A. Stop taking the drug immediately
   B. Skip a few doses until the unpleasant effects stops
   C. Adjust the drug dose to lower dose
   D. Report the side effect to their healthcare practitioners

10. **Factors influencing non-adherence are __________.**
    A. Lack of understanding of the disease
    B. Social and economic factors
    C. Patient-related factors
    D. All of the above

11. **Which one of the following is not a reason for intentional non-adherence?**
    A. Reducing doses to avoid side effects
    B. Forgetfulness
    C. Concern about addiction
    D. Unable to afford the prescription drugs

12. Patient-related factors for non-adherence is ______

A. Physical impairments
B. Forgetfulness
C. Medication beliefs
D. All of the above

13. Which of the pairs have similar meaning?

A. Concordance/Dosing
B. Adherence /Compliance
C. Adherence/Dosing
D. Compliance/Dosing

14. Non-adherence to medication may lead to _______.

A. Development of resistance
B. Treatment failure
C. Increasingly difficult to treat the illness
D. All of the above

15. 'Pill count' is a method of measurement of_________.

A. Number of units given free
B. Medication adherence
C. Number of units sold
D. Number of units consumed

16. Which of the following factors are responsible for medication non-adherence?

A. Low level of education
B. Tight work schedules
C. Poor health literacy
D. All of the above

17. _________ can lead to hospital readmissions and expensive treatments that drive higher healthcare costs.

A. Medication non-adherence
B. Medication adherence
C. Effective treatment
D. All of the above

18. Which of the following factors is not related to medication adherence?

A. Health system factors
B. Environmental factors
C. Social and economic factors
D. Condition factors

19. Which of the following strategies can overcome medication non-adherence?

A. Reduce complexity
B. Nurture relationships with patients
C. Follow-up with patients
D. All of the above

20. EHR stands for _________.

A. Elective Health Record
B. Electronic Health Room
C. Electronic Health Record
D. None of the above

Answer Key

1 C	2 B	3 A	4 A	5 D	6 C	7 D	8 D	9 D	10 D
11 B	12 D	13 B	14 D	15 B	16 D	17 A	18 B	19 D	20 C

CHAPTER 7

Health Screening Services in Community Pharmacy

1. **Health screening services are the services provided by the healthcare professionals including __________.**
   A. Nurses
   B. Medical practitioners
   C. Pharmacists
   D. All of the above

2. **__________ is the screening test for diabetes mellitus.**
   A. Renal clearance test
   B. Glucose tolerance test
   C. Lipid profile test
   D. Pulmonary function test

3. **LDL cholesterol is called "bad cholesterol" because __________.**
   A. It causes low blood counts
   B. It can cause blockage in the arteries
   C. It changes heart rhythm
   D. None of the above

4. **Body Mass Indexing (BMI) is the most common screening test for __________.**
   A. Hypertension
   B. Obesity
   C. Asthma
   D. Cancer

5. **The normal level of glucose during fasting is ________.**
   A. 40–60 mg/dl
   B. 70–110 mg/dl
   C. 120–140 mg/dl
   D. 140–160 mg/dl

6. **Sphygmomanometer is used to measure__________.**
   A. Blood sugar
   B. Blood pressure
   C. Blood cholesterol
   D. All of the above

7. **Which of the following is used for the assessment of lung function in COPD and asthma?**
   A. Glucometer
   B. Speedometer
   C. Peak flow meter
   D. Manometer

8. **Referral of patient from primary healthcare facility or community pharmacy to a specialized medical practitioner or hospital is called __________.**
   A. Social referral
   B. Down-referral
   C. Up-referral
   D. None of the above

9. **The normal value of blood pressure is _________.**
   A. 120/80 mmHg
   B. 140/100 mmHg
   C. 160/120 mmHg
   D. 90/100 mmHg

10. **Defects in the secretion or action of insulin observed in patient suffering from __________.**
    A. Eye diseases
    B. Diabetes
    C. Skin disorders
    D. Lung cancer

11. **HDL is called 'good cholesterol" because ________.**
    A. It keeps cholesterol from building up in the lining of the arteries
    B. Your body makes more of it as you get older
    C. It helps to keep your blood from clotting
    D. None of the above

12. **Mammogram is look for early signs of __________.**
    A. Anaemia
    B. Bone disorder
    C. Breast cancer
    D. None of the above

13. **The normal level of glucose after meal is about ______.**
    A. 140–180 mg/dl
    B. 70–100 mg/dl
    C. 120–150 mg/dl
    D. 200–300 mg/dl

14. **Lipid profile check-up is suggested for individual suffering from __________.**
    A. Obesity
    B. Fever
    C. Anaemia
    D. Sore throat

15. The risk factors for type 2-diabetes mellitus includes __________.

A. Family history
B. Being overweight
C. High intake of dietary fat
D. All of the above

16. Which of the following health screening services is non-invasive?

A. Blood haemoglobin levels
B. Blood glucose levels
C. Blood pressure levels
D. Blood lipid levels

17. _____________ is a condition in which the kidneys are unable to conserve water.

A. Diabetes mellitus
B. Diabetes insipidus
C. Gestational diabetes
D. Diabetic coma

18. Which of the following is not a beneficial effect of exercise in people with diabetes?

A. Reduction of triglycerides
B. Increase of insulin sensitivity
C. Hypoglycaemia
D. Helps in controlling hypertension

19. Which of the following is not an advantage of health screening services in community pharmacies?

A. Costly
B. Easy to access
C. Saves on time
D. Helps in early detection

20. Glucometers used in community pharmacy measure glucose levels in the __________

A. Plasma
B. Blood
C. Capillaries
D. Veins

21. Type 2 diabetes can cause long-term damage in the __________

A. Kidneys
B. Eyes
C. Nerves
D. All of the above

22. Which of the following is a complication of uncontrolled hypertension?

A. Liver failure
B. Dizziness
C. Stroke
D. Bleeding

23. A peak flow meter is useful to monitor __________.

A. Whether the asthma is in control
B. The progression of COPD
C. If asthma has reached its peak
D. None of the above

24. Pap smear test is used for the screening of __________.

A. Cervical cancer
B. Lung cancer
C. Skin cancer
D. Blood cancer

25. When the body does not respond to the insulin it makes, this is called __________.

A. Type-1 diabetes
B. Type-2 diabetes
C. Both A and B
D. None of the above

26. Screening test of women's breast cancer __________.

A. HPV test
B. Cervical cancer screening
C. Pap smear test
D. All of the above

27. Diabetes screening test are __________.

A. Glucose-fasting blood test
B. Glycosylated haemoglobin test
C. Both A and B
D. None of the above

28. The tapping sounds used while measuring blood pressure by using a sphygmomanometer are called __________.

A. Carotid sounds
B. Karaoke sounds
C. Korotkoff sounds
D. Carotenoid sounds

29. Which of these can increase the risk of high BP?

A. Obesity
B. Family history
C. Smoking
D. All of the above

30. Which test is used to determine the cholesterol levels?

A. HDL cholesterol
B. Total cholesterol
C. LDL cholesterol
D. All of the above

Answer Key

1 D	2 B	3 B	4 B	5 B	6 B	7 C	8 C	9 A	10 B
11 B	12 C	13 A	14 A	15 B	16 C	17 B	18 C	19 A	20 B
21 D	22 C	23 A	24 A	25 B	26 C	27 C	28 C	29 D	30 D

CHAPTER 8

Over-the-Counter (OTC) Medications

1. **Over-the-counter (OTC) medicines are available for the treatment of __________.**

   A. Hepatitis B. Diarrhoea
   C. Cancer D. Tuberculosis

2. **Full form of OTC is __________.**

   A. Over the count
   B. Over-the-counter
   C. Over the countable
   D. All of the above

3. **__________ can be defined as the self-consuming and medication without getting advice from a physician for either diagnosis or treatment.**

   A. Self-attention
   B. Self-medication
   C. Self-withdrawal
   D. Self-achievement

4. **What is the role of pharmacist in promoting the safe practices during self medication?**

   A. As a trainer
   B. As a health promoter
   C. As a quality drug supplier
   D. All of the above

5. **__________ drugs are purchased without prescription of RMP.**

   A. Schedule C & C1 B. OTC drugs
   C. Schedule H D. Schedule X

6. **__________ are known as non-prescription drugs.**

   A. Schedule C & C1 drugs
   B. OTC drugs
   C. Schedule X drugs
   D. Schedule H drugs

7. **Which of the following is a reason of self-medication practice?**

   A. Perception and simplicity
   B. Healthcare costs
   C. Social lifestyle
   D. All of the above

8. **Cold is a viral infection of __________ .**

   A. Upper respiratory tract
   B. Lower respiratory tract
   C. Urinary tract
   D. Gastrointestinal tract

9. **OTC analgesic options include __________ .**

   A. Aspirin B. Paracetamol
   C. Ibuprofen D. All of the above

10. **Questions for OTC counselling will be __________ .**

    A. Closed ended questions
    B. Open ended questions
    C. Both A and B
    D. None of the above

11. **__________ of Drugs and Cosmetics Rules 1945, contains the list of substances described as household remedies.**

    A. Schedule K B. Schedule Y
    C. Schedule U D. Schedule V

12. **Laxatives are used in the treatment of __________ .**

    A. Sore throat B. Cough
    C. Constipation D. Vomiting

13. **__________ is the study of cause of disease.**

    A. Myology B. Etiology
    C. Arthrology D. Angiology

14. Pharmacist can carry out the counselling of ______
A. Drug–alcohol interactions
B. Food–drug interactions
C. Drug–drug interactions
D. All of the above

15.__________ has a significant responsibility to assist and educate patient about a variety of effective self-medication options.
A. Nurses B. Pharmacists
C. Physicians D. All of the above

16. Loperamide is used in the treatment of __________.
A. Vomiting B. Constipation
C. Diarrhoea D. Sore throat

17. __________ is a symptom of fever.
A. Pigmentation of teeth
B. Hypoplasia of gums
C. Chattering of teeth
D. Loosening of teeth

18. Low grade temperature means temperature increases to __________ .
A. 100.4°F (38°C) B. 80°F
C. 103°F D. 92°F

19. __________ are used in the treatment of constipation.
A. Laxatives
B. Carminatives
C. Antacids
D. Antidiarrhoeals

20. Which types of drugs are to be sold by pharmacist only on prescription of a registered medical practitioner?
A. Schedules H B. Schedules X
C. Schedules H1 D. All of the above

21. __________ is the cause of vomiting.
A. Motion sickness
B. Travellers diarrhoea
C. Placebo
D. Euphoria

22. High grade temperature means temperature increases to __________.
A. 103°F (39.4°C) B. 70°F
C. 100°F D. 90°F

23. Guaifenesin is used as __________.
A. Expectorant B. Decongestant
C. Demulcent D. Antitussive

24. __________ is a complex protective mechanism that protects the body from danger or harm.
A. Epilepsy B. Pain
C. Diarrhoea D. Dysentery

25. Identify the anti-itching agent.
A. Calamine B. Mupirocin
C. Salicylic acid D. Permethrin

26. Sore throat is an infection of __________.
A. Upper respiratory tract
B. Lower respiratory tract
C. Urinary tract
D. Gastrointestinal tract

27. __________ means swelling of gums.
A. Conjunctivitis B. Otitis
C. Meningitis D. Gingivitis

28. Wet cough is also called __________.
A. Productive cough
B. Unproductive cough
C. Dry cough
D. All of the above

29. __________ is the disorder in which stools become hard and dry which further difficult to pass from the bowel.
A. Purgative B. Constipation
C. Diarrhoea D. Dysentery

30. Calamine is __________.
A. Antiepileptic
B. Anti-itching agent
C. Anti-cough agent
D. Antidepressant

31. Which of the following types of drugs can be given as OTC medication?
A. Antacids
B. Antidepressants
C. Antianxiety drugs
D. Antipsychotics

32. Which of the following drugs is used in diarrhoea?
A. Acetazolamide B. Metoclopramide
C. Loperamide D. Chlorpropamide

33. Medicines like Ibuprofen, naproxen is __________.
A. Schedule X drugs in India
B. OTC in India
C. Schedule H drugs in India
D. None of the above

34. The process of vomiting is known as __________.

A. Helminthiasis
B. Emesis
C. Candidiasis
D. Amoebiasis

35. __________ means study of causes and development of diseases.

A. Etiopathogenesis
B. Pathogenesis
C. Pre-pathogenesis
D. Organogenesis

36. Psoriasis and warts are __________.

A. GIT disorders
B. Skin disorders
C. Urinary disorders
D. CNS disorders

37. One of the medicines used in Dandruff is __________.

A. Sulphur
B. Ketoconazole
C. Salicylic acid
D. All of the above

38. IBS stands for __________.

A. Intestinal bowel syndrome
B. Irritable bowel syndrome
C. Intact bowel syndrome
D. Inter bowel syndrome

39. Pruritus means __________.

A. Itchy sensation requiring scratching of the area
B. Swelling
C. Redness
D. White patches

40. Which type of medications is commonly abbreviated as OTC?

A. Generic medication
B. Children's medication
C. Prescription medication
D. Over-the-counter medication

Answer Key

1 B	2 B	3 B	4 D	5 B	6 B	7 D	8 A	9 D	10 C
11 A	12 C	13 B	14 D	15 B	16 C	17 C	18 A	19 A	20 D
21 A	22 A	23 A	24 B	25 B	26 A	27 D	28 A	29 B	30 B
31 A	32 C	33 C	34 B	35 A	36 B	37 D	38 B	39 A	40 D

CHAPTER

9

Community Pharmacy Management

1. **Community pharmacists is also known as _________.**
   A. Drug researcher
   B. Drug specialist
   C. Drug inventor
   D. Clinical pharmacist

2. **The minimum space required for retail drug store is _________.**
   A. 50 m^2 B. 20 m^2
   C. 30 m^2 D. 10 m^2

3. **Economic order quantity used for _________.**
   A. Purchase B. Inventory
   C. Finance D. None of the above

4. **______ means retail pharmacy owned by corporation.**
   A. Medical shop
   B. Chain shop
   C. Bulk pharmacy
   D. Isolated pharmacy

5. **Frequent purchasing in quantities to meet the demand until the next ordering time is called _________.**
   A. Instant demand B. Just-in-time
   C. Out-of time D. Excess-in time

6. **A stock of physical commodity is referred to as _____.**
   A. Inventory B. Budget
   C. Loan D. Cash

7. **_________ is a plan explaining proper and maximum utilization of space inside the four walls of business.**
   A. Drug design
   B. Patent design
   C. Layout design
   D. Dosage design

8. **Which is not a part of accountancy?**
   A. Cash book B. Work book
   C. Day book D. Petty cash book

9. **Purchase invoice is an important document to be retained by community pharmacy for at least ______.**
   A. 05 years B. 02 years
   C. 10 years D. 03 years

10. **The cool storage condition means temperature range between __________.**
    A. 2°C and 8°C B. 8°C and 25°C
    C. 0°C and 8°C D. 30°C and 40°C

11. **CPMM stands for ___________.**
    A. Common Pharmacy Medicine Management
    B. Co-ordinated Pharmacy Medicine Management
    C. Community Pharmacy Medicine Management
    D. Community Performance Medicine Management

12. **Based on the business potential the choice of site for a community pharmacy would be ___________.**
    A. Near a shopping mall B. Near a hospital
    C. Near a clinic D. All of the above

13. **Who is the licensing authority for issuing retail sale license?**
    A. District Collector
    B. Central Drugs Control Authority
    C. State Drugs Control Authority
    D. Chief Medical Officer of the District

14. **____________ is rightly referred to as company's life blood.**
    A. Audit B. Finance
    C. Staff D. Managers

15. When a quantity of stock falls below safety stock or minimum level, it is known as ___________.

A. Reorder level B. Danger level
C. Buffer level D. Minimum level

16. ABC analysis is based on ___________.

A. Ordering B. Value of items
C. Consumption D. All of the above

17. Inventory turnover ratio (ITR) is the index of______.

A. Efficiency of peoples
B. Efficiency of marketing management
C. Efficiency of material management
D. Efficient equipments conditions

18. Petty cash book is a book of account which records the transactions of ___________.

A. Big amounts B. Medium amounts
C. Minor amounts D. None of the above

19. Lead time refers to ___________.

A. Time to order economic order quantity
B. Time to get the supply after ordering
C. Ideal time to order supply
D. None of the above

20. ___________ is a person who supplies goods or services to another business.

A. Vendor B. Auditor
C. Financer D. Cashier

21. VED stands for ___________.

A. Vital emergency desirable
B. Valid essential desirable
C. Vital essential desirable
D. Vital essential detail

22. The process of assessing the capital required and choosing its competition is known as ___________.

A. Sourcing
B. Finance
C. Financial planning
D. Financial management

23. ___________ is a process of checking examination and observation of supplier's premises and transport facility.

A. Pre-audit B. Post-audit
C. Vendor audit D. Sales audit

24. ___________ is the level between maximum and minimum stock levels.

A. Reorder level B. Safety level
C. Danger level D. Buffer level

25. The following are the methods of inventory control *except* ___________.

A. Setting of stock levels B. EOQ
C. VED D. CRM

26. Cash memo is the testimony of ___________.

A. Counselling record
B. Purchase record
C. Sales record
D. None of the above

27. PMS stands for ___________.

A. Potential management system
B. Pharmacy management system
C. Pharmacy major system
D. Pharmacy monopoly system

28. Storage at cold condition indicates

A. Keeping at below 0°C
B. Keeping at 2°C to 8°C
C. Keeping at 0°C
D. Keeping at –0°C to –18°C

29. CRM stands for ___________.

A. Core relationship management
B. Care relationship management
C. Customer relationship management
D. Customer real management

30. Patient counselling area in pharmacy should have_____.

A. Sphygmomanometer
B. Peak flow meter
C. Weighing scale
D. All of the above

31. EOQ is the balance between ___________.

A. Sales cost and purchase cost
B. Ordering cost and carrying cost
C. Ordering cost and sales cost
D. Carrying cost and purchase cost

32. SOP stands for ___________.

A. Sequence operating procedure
B. Some operating procedure
C. Standard operating procedure
D. Standard organization procedure

33. From following features, what is applicable to petty cash?

A. The easy and quick way for payment
B. Small amount of cash
C. Used for minor expenses
D. All of the above

34. **Effective purchase procedure is a method of ________.**
A. Sales control
B. Inventory control
C. Budget control
D. Staff control

35. **Minimum practical training required for registration of pharmacist ___________.**
A. NLT 100 hrs
B. NLT 500 hrs
C. NLT 600 hrs
D. NLT 200 hrs

36. **___________ is an unbiased examination and evaluation of the financial statement of the organization.**
A. Cash B. Loan
C. Cash book D. Audit

37. **Cash memo must have the signature of ___________.**
A. Any employee of pharmacy
B. Owner
C. Registered pharmacist
D. Any one of the above

38. **___________ is a book of original entries.**
A. Day book B. Ledger
C. Audit D. Balance sheet

39. **A stock of a physical commodity is referred to as _______.**
A. Management
B. Purchase
C. Inventory
D. None of the above

40. **________ refers to the use of information and communication technologies in medicine and other health profession to manage illness and health risks and to promote wellness.**
A. Physical health
B. Digital health
C. Mental health
D. Spiritual health

41. **___________ is the amount contributed by proprietor of the business.**
A. Liability B. Asset
C. Cash credit D. Debenture

42. **Following sites are good for pharmacy ___________.**
A. Residential areas
B. Nearby Hospital
C. Business Locality
D. All of the above

43. **The following are some of the variables to consider while choosing a vendor *except* ___________.**
A. Slow delivery
B. Quality
C. Price
D. Assurance of supply

44. **___________ is an event in which there is an exchange of goods or services, in cash or on credit.**
A. Capital B. Loan
C. Transaction D. Solvency

45. **___________ is a perfect example of mhealth (mobile health)**
A. Youchart B. Uschart
C. Mychart D. Dochart

46. **Long-term finance means duration is for ___________.**
A. More than 2 years
B. More than 3 years
C. More than 1 years
D. More than 5 years

47. **Form 19-C is used for seeking sale license for drugs listed in ___________.**
A. Schedule X
B. Schedule C and C1
C. Schedule G
D. Schedule H1

48. **___________ is launched by Government of India during the fight against Covid-19.**
A. Ayurvedic Setu app
B. Aromatic Setu app
C. Aarogya Setu app
D. Agriculture Setu app

49. **When capital is divided into small units, each unit is described as ___________.**
A. Cash B. Share
C. Loan D. debt

50. **The efficiency of a procurement system depends on the capability of the purchasing agency to ensure ___________.**
A. Right source
B. Right quality
C. Right quantity
D. All of the above

51. **___________ refers to the stock of products held to meet future demand.**
A. Goods B. Inventory
C. Procurement D. None of the above

52. **Telehealth and telemedicine are the examples of______.**
   A. Mental health
   B. Spiritual health
   C. Digital health
   D. Social health

53. **ABC analysis __________.**
   A. Almost Better Control
   B. Always Best Control
   C. Always Better Control
   D. None of the above

54. **Use of pharmacy operation software __________.**
   A. Maintain Separate Registers/Folders
   B. Recognizes Obsolete Products
   C. Systematic Marketing
   D. All of the above

55. **______________ refers to the use of information and communications technologies in medicine and other health professions to manage illnesses and health risks and to promote wellness.**
   A. Digital health
   B. Health literacy
   C. Medical health
   D. None of the above

56. **Following are the pharmacy operation software, *except* __________.**
   A. PrimeRx
   B. Pharmaserv
   C. Practo
   D. Liberty Software

57. **mhealth refers to __________.**
   A. Mental health
   B. Mobile health
   C. Mono health
   D. Manipulated health

58. **Following are the examples of online pharmacies, *except* __________.**
   A. Netmeds
   B. Pharmaserv
   C. Medlife
   D. Healthcart

59. **Online pharmacy (e-Pharmacy) is also known as______.**
   A. General drug store
   B. Medicine store
   C. Wholesale drug store
   D. Web drug Store

60. **The following is an objective of inventory control____.**
   A. Low cost plant operation
   B. Maximum customer satisfaction
   C. Minimum inventory investment
   D. All of the above

Answer Key

1 B	2 D	3 A	4 B	5 B	6 A	7 C	8 B	9 D	10 B
11 C	12 B	13 C	14 B	15 B	16 B	17 C	18 C	19 B	20 A
21 C	22 C	23 C	24 A	25 D	26 C	27 B	28 B	29 C	30 D
31 B	32 C	33 D	34 B	35 B	36 D	37 C	38 A	39 C	40 B
41 B	42 D	43 A	44 C	45 C	46 D	47 A	48 C	49 B	50 D
51 B	52 C	53 C	54 D	55 A	56 C	57 B	58 B	59 D	60 D

Section VIII

Biochemistry and Clinical Pathology

1. Introduction to Biochemistry (The Cell)
2. Carbohydrates
3. Proteins
4. Lipids
5. Nucleic Acids
6. Enzymes
7. Vitamins
8. Metabolism
9. Minerals
10. Water and Electrolytes
11. Introduction to Biotechnology
12. Organ Function Tests
13. Pathology of Blood and Urine

Syllabus (As Per ER 2020) Biochemistry and Clinical Pathology

Chapter	Topics
1	**Introduction to biochemistry:** Scope of biochemistry in pharmacy; Cell and its biochemical organization.
2	**Carbohydrates** ■ Definition, classification with examples, chemical properties ■ Monosaccharides: Structure of glucose, fructose, and galactose ■ Disaccharides: Structure of maltose, lactose, and sucrose ■ Polysaccharides: Chemical nature of starch and glycogen ■ Qualitative tests and biological role of carbohydrates
3	**Proteins** ■ Definition, classification of proteins based on composition and solubility with examples ■ Definition, classification of amino acids based on chemical nature and nutritional requirements with examples ■ Structure of proteins (four levels of organization of protein structure) ■ Qualitative tests and biological role of proteins and amino acids ■ Diseases related to malnutrition of proteins.
4	**Lipids** ■ Definition, classification with examples ■ Structure and properties of triglycerides (oils and fats) ■ Fatty acid classification: Based on chemical and nutritional requirements with examples ■ Structure and functions of cholesterol in the body ■ Lipoproteins: Types, composition and functions in the body ■ Qualitative tests and functions of lipids
5	**Nucleic acids** ■ Definition, purine and pyrimidine bases ■ Components of nucleosides and nucleotides with examples ■ Structure of DNA (Watson and Crick model), RNA and their functions
6	**Enzymes** ■ Definition, properties and IUB and MB classification ■ Factors affecting enzyme activity ■ Mechanism of action of enzymes, enzyme inhibitors ■ Therapeutic and pharmaceutical importance of enzymes
7	**Vitamins** ■ Definition and classification with examples ■ Sources, chemical nature, functions, coenzyme form, recommended dietary requirements, deficiency diseases of fat- and water-soluble vitamins
8	**Metabolism (study of cycle/pathways without chemical structures)** ■ Metabolism of carbohydrates: Glycolysis, TCA cycle and glycogen metabolism, regulation of blood glucose level. Diseases related to abnormal metabolism of carbohydrates ■ Metabolism of lipids: Lipolysis, β-oxidation of fatty acid (palmitic acid) ketogenesis and ketolysis. Diseases related to abnormal metabolism of lipids such as ketoacidosis, fatty liver, hypercholesterolemia ■ Metabolism of amino acids (proteins): General reactions of amino acids and its significance– Transamination, deamination, urea cycle and decarboxylation. Diseases related to abnormal metabolism of amino acids, disorders of ammonia metabolism, phenylketonuria, alkaptonuria and jaundice. ■ Biological oxidation: Electron transport chain and oxidative phosphorylation
9	■ **Minerals:** Types, functions, deficiency diseases, recommended dietary requirements

Contd...

10	**Water and Electrolytes** ■ Distribution, functions of water in the body ■ Water turnover and balance ■ Electrolyte composition of the body fluids, dietary intake of electrolyte and electrolyte balance ■ Dehydration, causes of dehydration and oral rehydration therapy
11	**Introduction to Biotechnology**
12	**Organ function tests** ■ Functions of kidney and routinely performed tests to assess the functions of kidney and their clinical significances ■ Functions of liver and routinely performed tests to assess the functions of liver and their clinical significances ■ Lipid profile tests and its clinical significances
13	**Introduction to Pathology of Blood and Urine** ■ Lymphocytes and platelets, their role in health and disease ■ Erythrocytes—abnormal cells and their significance ■ Normal and abnormal constituents of urine and their significance

CHAPTER 1

Introduction to Biochemistry
The Cell

1. __________ is the basic structural and functional unit of organism.

A. Enzyme
B. Protein
C. Carbohydrate
D. Cell

2. The term biochemistry has originated from the word __________.

A. 'Trios'
B. 'Bios'
C. 'Pentose'
D. 'Hexose'

3. _________ of the cell controls all the cellular activities.

A. Mitochondria
B. Lysosomes
C. Microsomes
D. Nucleus

4. ___________ known as powerhouse/energy coin of the cells.

A. Nucleolus
B. Mitochondria
C. Nucleus
D. Endoplasmic reticulum

5. __________ surrounds the cytoplasm of a cell.

A. Cell membrane
B. Chromosome
C. Chromatin
D. Nucleolus

6. _____________ are the main site for the synthesis and storage of ATP.

A. Golgi complex
B. Ribosomes
C. Lysosomes
D. Mitochondria

7. The enzymes which involve in glycolytic pathway are present in __________.

A. Cytoplasm
B. Cell membrane
C. Nucleus
D. Mitochondria

8. Mitochondrial DNA is __________.

A. Circular single stranded
B. Linear double helix
C. Circular double stranded
D. None of the above

9. The spherical and largest part of the cell is __________.

A. Mitochondria
B. Nucleus
C. Lysosomes
D. Microsomes

10. ______________ represents the genetic material of the prokaryotes.

A. Nucleoplasm
B. Proto-nucleus
C. Nucleus
D. Nucleoid

11. ATP means __________.

A. Adenine triphosphate
B. Adenosine triphosphate
C. Aldol triphosphate
D. Acetyl triphosphate

12. In prokaryotic cells, ribosomes are __________.

A. 80S
B. 60S + 40S
C. 70S
D. 50S + 40S

13. The tiny granules present on the surface of endoplasmic reticulum are called __________.

A. Microsomes
B. Ribosomes
C. Lysosomes
D. Centrosomes

14. Who discovered the cell?

A. De Bary B. Schwann
C. Tatum D. Robert Hooke

15. The function of Golgi complex is to __________.

A. Provide a pathway for transporting chemicals
B. Synthesize proteins
C. Produce ATP
D. Form glycoproteins

16. The substances pass through semipermeable membrane which depends upon their __________.

A. Particle size
B. Lipid solubility
C. Concentration
D. All of the above

17. __________ have well-defined nucleus.

A. Bacteria cells
B. Prokaryotic cells
C. Eukaryotic cells
D. Animal cells

18. The "maintain cell integrity" is a function of _______.

A. Nucleus B. Golgi body
C. Cell membrane D. Mitochondria

19. __________ is the main site for citric acid cycle, beta-oxidation, urea cycle and ETS.

A. Ribosomes B. Mitochondria
C. Lysosomes D. Golgi complex

20. Which of the following is example of prokaryotic cells?

A. Bacterial cell B. Animal cell
C. Human cell D. All of the above

21. Which one is the heaviest particulate component of cell?

A. Golgi apparatus B. Microsomes
C. Nucleus D. Cytoplasm

22. Inner surface of the mitochondria has many cristae and are covered with __________ particles.

A. F2 B. F1
C. F3 D. F4

23. Golgi complex __________ .

A. Forms glycoproteins B. Synthesize protein
C. Produces ATP D. All of the above

24. The digestive enzymes of cellular compounds are confirmed to __________ .

A. Polysomes B. Lysosomes
C. Ribosomes D. Centrioles

25. Which of the following is located in the mitochondria?

A. Dihydrolipoyl dehydrogenase
B. Cytochrome oxidase
C. Succinate dehydrogenase
D. All of the above

26. Organisms which do not posses well-formed nucleus is called __________.

A. Unicellular B. Prokaryotes
C. Eukaryotes D. Multicellular

27. ____________ plays major role in countless biological process.

A. Potassium B. Sulphur
C. Calcium D. Copper

28. Protein biosynthesis has major function of _______.

A. Lipid B. DNA
C. RNA D. Polysaccharides

29. The cell nucleus is surrounded by __________.

A. Nuclear membrane
B. Nucleolemma
C. Karyotheca
D. All of the above

30. _________ responsible for the production of hormones and other secretory products.

A. Endoplasmic reticulum
B. Mitochondria
C. Nucleus
D. Nucleolus

31. The most important component of the nucleus is ______.

A. Centrioles B. Chromatin
C. Chromosome D. Nucleolus

32. The degradative processes are categorized under the heading of __________.

A. Metabolism B. Anabolism
C. Catabolism D. None of the above

33. The exchange of material takes place __________.

A. Only by pinocytosis
B. Only by diffusion
C. Only by active transport
D. All of the above

34. Fatty acids can be transported into and out of cell membrane by __________.

A. Osmosis B. Active transport
C. Facilitated transport D. Diffusion

35. The following are various stages of cell reproduction or cell division *except* __________.

A. Anaphase
B. Prophase
C. Telophase
D. Gamma phase

36. Lysosomes are known as "suicidal bags" because of __________.

A. Parasitic activity
B. Hydrolytic activity
C. Catalytic activity
D. Presence of food vacuole

37. The oxygen and carbon dioxide cross the plasma membrane by the process of __________.

A. Passive diffusion
B. Active diffusion
C. Random diffusion
D. Facilitated diffusion

38. Cell membrane/cell wall performs following function __________.

A. Give shape to the cell
B. Covers and protects the cell
C. Acts as a physiological sieve
D. All of the above

39. Which cell organelle is involved in apoptosis?

A. Lysosome
B. Mitochondria
C. Golgi bodies
D. Endoplasmic reticulum

40. Which of the following cell organelles is absent in animal cells and present in a plant cell?

A. Vacuoles
B. Mitochondria
C. Cell wall
D. Cytoplasm

Answer Key

1 D	2 B	3 D	4 B	5 A	6 D	7 A	8 C	9 B	10 D
11 B	12 C	13 B	14 D	15 A	16 D	17 C	18 C	19 B	20 A
21 C	22 B	23 A	24 B	25 D	26 B	27 C	28 C	29 D	30 A
31 B	32 C	33 D	34 C	35 D	36 B	37 A	38 D	39 B	40 C

CHAPTER 2

Carbohydrates

1. **The general formula of monosaccharides is ________.**
   A. $C_{2n}H_2O_n$ B. $C_nH_{2n}O_n$
   C. $C_nH_2O_{2n}$ D. $C_nH_{2n}O_{2n}$

2. **Two sugars which differ from one another only in configuration around a single carbon atom are termed ________.**
   A. Anomers
   B. Stereoisomers
   C. Epimers
   D. Optical isomers

3. **____________ is a polysaccharide used as an anti-coagulant.**
   A. Starch B. Heparin
   C. Cellulose D. Glycogen

4. **Isomers differing as a result of variations in the configuration of –OH and –H on carbon atoms 2, 3 and 4 of glucose are known as ________.**
   A. Anomers
   B. Optical isomers
   C. Stereoisomers
   D. Epimers

5. **________ is an important food reserve for the plant and foodstuff for men and the animals.**
   A. Starch B. Cellulose
   C. Gelatin D. Glycogen

6. **Alpha-D-glucose and beta-D-glucose are ________.**
   A. Anomers
   B. Stereoisomers
   C. Epimers
   D. Keto-aldo pairs

7. **The chemical test used to differentiate reducing sugar is ________.**
   A. Osazone test
   B. Iodine test
   C. Mucic acid test
   D. Seliwanoff's test

8. **Sugar alcohol is ________.**
   A. Trehalose B. Xylulose
   C. Arabinose D. Mannitol

9. **The sugar found in DNA is ________**
   A. Deoxyribose B. Xylose
   C. Ribose D. Ribulose

10. **Sucrose consists of ________.**
    A. Glucose + mannose
    B. Glucose + glucose
    C. Glucose + fructose
    D. Glucose + galactose

11. **________ are special carbohydrates being provided to the nervous tissue.**
    A. Polysaccharides
    B. Cerebrosides
    C. Polysaccharides
    D. Monosaccharides

12. **Which of the following is a reducing sugar?**
    A. Agar B. Sucrose
    C. Trehalose D. Fructose

13. **Osazones are not formed with the ________.**
    A. Sucrose B. Glucose
    C. Fructose D. Lactose

14. **The general test for detection of carbohydrates is ________.**
   A. Osazone test
   B. Iodine test
   C. Molisch test
   D. Barfoed test

15. **Which of the following is not a polymer of glucose?**
   A. Dextrin B. Amylose
   C. Cellulose D. Inulin

16. **Amylose is a constituent of ________.**
   A. Glycogen B. Starch
   C. Cellulose D. None of the above

17. **Invert sugar is ________.**
   A. Hydrolytic products of sucrose
   B. Lactose
   C. Sucrose
   D. Fructose

18. **Carbohydrates are also called ________.**
   A. Glycolipids
   B. Saccharides
   C. Glycoproteins
   D. All of the above

19. **Glycogen in animals are stored in ________.**
   A. Liver and adipose tissue
   B. Liver and biles
   C. Liver and muscles
   D. Liver and spleen

20. **The number of isomers of glucose is ________.**
   A. 16 B. 2
   C. 4 D. 8

21. **Which is non-reducing sugar?**
   A. Maltose B. Glucose
   C. Fructose D. Sucrose

22. **The inner portion of starch is formed by ________.**
   A. Sucrose B. Cellulose
   C. Amylose D. Amylopectin

23. **Lactose composed of ________.**
   A. Glucose and fructose
   B. Glucose and galactose
   C. Glucose and pentose
   D. Glucose and glucose

24. **The most important epimer of glucose is ________.**
   A. Fructose B. Arabinose
   C. Galactose D. Xylose

25. **The storage form of carbohydrate in the animal is known as ________.**
   A. Glucose B. Glycogen
   C. Starch D. Mannose

26. **The possible number of isomers for glucose due to presence of asymmetric carbon atom is ________.**
   A. 18 B. 14
   C. 16 D. 20

27. **The sugar found in RNA is ________.**
   A. Erythrose B. Ribose
   C. Deoxyribose D. Ribulose

28. **Optically active molecules which rotate plane-polarized light in a counterclockwise direction are said to be ________.**
   A. S configuration
   B. R configuration
   C. Levorotary
   D. Dextrorotary

29. **Which of the following sugar are tetrose?**
   A. Erythrose B. Galactose
   C. Fructose D. Idose

30. **Mutarotation refers to change in ________.**
   A. Conductance
   B. pH
   C. Optical rotation
   D. Chemical properties

31. **The sugar found in milk is ________.**
   A. Galactose B. Glucose
   C. Lactose D. Fructose

32. **Iodine solution produces no colour with ________.**
   A. Glycogen
   B. Cellulose
   C. Starch
   D. Dextrin

33. **Which of the following biomolecules simply refers to as "Staff of life"?**
   A. Lipids
   B. Proteins
   C. Carbohydrates
   D. Vitamins

34. **______ is a polysaccharide used as an anticoagulant.**
   A. Heparin
   B. Cellulose
   C. Hexose
   D. Lactose

35. **Fructose and glucose can be distinguished by _______.**
    A. Barfoed's reagent
    B. Fehling's reagent
    C. Seliwanoff's reagent
    D. Benedict's reagent

36. **Other name for osazone test is _________.**
    A. Sodium acetate test
    B. Glacial acetic test
    C. Fehling's test
    D. Kowarsky test

37. **Which class of carbohydrates is considered as non-sugar?**
    A. Polysaccharides
    B. Monosaccharides
    C. Disaccharides
    D. Oligosaccharides

38. **Minimum number of carbon required for mono-saccharides _________.**
    A. 8 B. 2
    C. 3 D. 4

39. **Class of carbohydrates which cannot be hydrolysed further, is known as _________.**
    A. Monosaccharides
    B. Disaccharides
    C. Polysaccharides
    D. Proteoglycan

40. **The red precipitate formed when glucose is heated with "Benedict's reagent" is _________.**
    A. Cuprous oxide
    B. Cuprous hydroxide
    C. Cupric oxide
    D. Cupric hydroxide

Answer Key

1 B	2 C	3 B	4 D	5 A	6 B	7 A	8 D	9 A	10 C
11 B	12 D	13 A	14 C	15 D	16 B	17 A	18 B	19 C	20 A
21 D	22 C	23 B	24 C	25 B	26 C	27 B	28 C	29 A	30 C
31 C	32 B	33 C	34 A	35 C	36 D	37 A	38 C	39 A	40 D

CHAPTER

3

Proteins

1. **The building blocks of proteins are __________.**
   A. Nucleotides B. Amino acids
   C. DNA D. RNA

2. **How many amino acids make up a protein?**
   A. 50 B. 10
   C. 20 D. 30

3. **__________ is a complete protein containing all essential amino acids.**
   A. Tyrosine B. Glycine
   C. Casein D. Leucine

4. **The bond between amino acids is called __________.**
   A. Hydrogen bond
   B. Ionic bond
   C. Acidic bond
   D. Peptide bond

5. **The naturally occurring proteins consist of __________.**
   A. L-amino acids
   B. D-amino acids
   C. Both A and B
   D. None of the above

6. **Secondary structure is defined by __________.**
   A. Ionic bonding
   B. Hydrogen bonding
   C. van der Waals force
   D. Covalent bonding

7. **The reaction between protein and conc. HNO_3 is ____.**
   A. Xanthoproteic test
   B. Biuret test
   C. Millon's test
   D. Ninhydrin test

8. **The breakdown of primary, secondary and tertiary structure of protein is called __________.**
   A. Mutarotation
   B. Zwitterion
   C. Denaturation of proteins
   D. Diazotisation

9. **All alpha amino acids are optically active *except* ____.**
   A. Tryptophan B. Glycine
   C. Alanine D. Serine

10. **Amino acid exists as a __________.**
    A. Lipid B. Cations
    C. Anions D. Zwitterions

11. **__________ is a genetic disorder related to the phenylalanine metabolism.**
    A. Phenyl albuminuria
    B. Phenyl ketonuria
    C. Alkaptonuria
    D. Proteinuria

12. **__________ water-soluble proteins.**
    A. Prolamin's
    B. Globulins
    C. Albumin
    D. Glutelin's

13. **Which among the following is a neutral amino acid __________.**
    A. Serine B. Histidine
    C. Arginine D. Lysine

14. **Millon's test is used for the identification of __________.**
    A. Lysine B. Tyrosine
    C. Serine D. Tryptophan

15. **Which of the following diseases is caused by protein deficiency?**
A. Hypothyroidism
B. Anaemia
C. Kwashiorkor
D. All of the above

16. **Peptide bond is a _________.**
A. Hydrogen bond
B. Covalent bond
C. Ionic bond
D. Metallic bond

17. **An aromatic amino acid is _________.**
A. Arginine
B. Phenylalanine
C. Cysteine
D. Methionine

18. **Which linkage is present in proteins?**
A. Amide B. Ester
C. Peptide D. Aliphatic

19. **____________ is a hair protein which is made up of alpha-helix only.**
A. Gelatin B. Keratin
C. Maize D. Soya

20. **The process of protein synthesis takes place in which of the following cell organelles?**
A. Mitochondria B. Nucleus
C. Vacuoles D. Ribosomes

21. **Protein deficiency disease is known as _________.**
A. Cushing's disease
B. Kwashiorkor and marasmus
C. Fabry's disease
D. Parkinson's disease

22. **___________ are involved in the formation of stable tertiary structure of protein.**
A. Hydrogen bond B. van der Waals bond
C. Peptide bond D. Sulphur bond

23. **An essential amino acid in man is _________.**
A. Methionine B. Aspartate
C. Tyrosine D. Serine

24. **Primary structure of a protein is formed by ________.**
A. Disulphide bonds
B. Hydrogen bonds
C. Peptide bonds
D. All of the above

25. **Kwashiorkor occurs when the diet is severely deficient in _________.**
A. Essential fatty acids B. Iron
C. Calories D. Proteins

26. **The optically inactive amino acid is _________.**
A. Valine B. Glycine
C. Serine D. Threonine

27. **Which of the following factors is not responsible for the denaturation of proteins?**
A. Organic solvent B. Heat
C. Charge D. pH change

28. **Sulphur containing amino acid is _________.**
A. Asparagine B. Methionine
C. Leucine D. Valine

29. **Which of the following diseases is caused by protein deficiency?**
A. Hypothyroidism B. Anaemia
C. Kwashiorkor D. All of the above

30. **A coiled peptide chain held in place by hydrogen bonding between peptide bonds in the same chain is _________.**
A. Tertiary structure
B. Primary structure
C. Alpha-helix
D. Beta-pleated sheets

31. **Name the product obtained by the reaction of proteins with NaOH and 1% $CuSO_4$.**
A. Aspartic acid B. Tyrosine
C. Biuret D. Xanthoproteic acid

32. **Casein, the milk protein, is _________.**
A. Glycoprotein
B. Nucleoprotein
C. Chromoprotein
D. Phosphoprotein

33. **All of the following are sulphur containing amino acids found in proteins *except* _________.**
A. Threonine B. Cysteine
C. Cystine D. Methionine

34. **Amino acids are mostly synthesized from __________.**
A. Volatile acids
B. Fatty acids
C. Mineral salts
D. Alpha-ketoglutaric acid

35. Which of the following are positively charged basic amino acids?

A. Lysine and glutamine
B. Lysine and arginine
C. Lysine and asparagine
D. Glutamine and arginine

36. __________ amino acid has highest isoelectric point.

A. Arginine **B.** Lysine
C. Alanine **D.** Proline

37. __________ is a metabolic disorder associated with abnormal metabolism of tyrosine

A. Marasmus
B. Phenylketonuria
C. Alkaptonuria
D. Kwashiorkor

38. An example of chromoprotein is __________.

A. Nucleon
B. Haemoglobin
C. Casein
D. Gliadin

39. Sakaguchi's reaction is specific for __________.

A. Arginine
B. Tyrosine
C. Proline
D. Cysteine

40. __________ is an example of incomplete protein.

A. Soya proteins
B. Gclatin
C. Milk proteins
D. Egg proteins

Answer Key

1 B	2 C	3 C	4 D	5 A	6 B	7 A	8 C	9 B	10 D
11 B	12 C	13 A	14 B	15 C	16 B	17 B	18 C	19 B	20 D
21 B	22 B	23 A	24 C	25 D	26 B	27 C	28 B	29 C	30 C
31 C	32 D	33 A	34 D	35 B	36 A	37 C	38 B	39 A	40 B

CHAPTER 4

Lipids

1. **The importance of phospholipids as a constituent of cell membrane is because they possess __________**
   A. Phosphoric acid
   B. Fatty acids
   C. Both polar and non-polar groups
   D. Glycerol

2. **Cholesterol is the precursor for the synthesis of ______**
   A. Estrogen
   B. Glucocorticoids
   C. Progestins
   D. All of the above

3. **Deterioration of food (rancidity) is due to presence of __________**
   A. Peroxidation of lipids
   B. Cholesterol
   C. Vitamin E
   D. Phenolic compounds

4. **Rancid oil shows higher __________**
   A. Acetyl values
   B. Iodine values
   C. Acid values
   D. Sap values

5. **Lipids are stored in the body mainly in the form of __________**
   A. Fatty acids B. Phospholipids
   C. Glycolipids D. Triglycerides

6. **Biological functions of lipids include __________**
   A. Maintenance of cellular integrity
   B. Source of energy
   C. Insulating material
   D. All of the above

7. **_______ forms a structural part of the biomembranes.**
   A. Proteins
   B. Cholesterol
   C. Carbohydrates
   D. Waxes

8. **Lipid stored in the form of energy in the body adipose tissue is __________**
   A. Sphingolipid
   B. Steroid
   C. Fatty acid
   D. None of the above

9. **Higher alcohol present in waxes is __________**
   A. Cetyl alcohol
   B. Benzyl alcohol
   C. Methyl alcohol
   D. Ethyl alcohol

10. **An oil which contains cyclic fatty acids and once used in the treatment of leprosy is __________**
    A. Elaidic oil
    B. Chaulmoogric oil
    C. Rapeseed oil
    D. Lanoline

11. **__________ indicates/expresses the unsaturation in fat or oil.**
    A. Acetyl value B. Iodine value
    C. Sap value D. Acid value

12. **Unpleasant odours and taste in a fat (rancidity) can be delayed or prevented by the addition of __________**
    A. Ergosterol B. Lead
    C. Copper D. Tocopherol

13. __________ is an essential fatty acid.
A. Arachdonic acid
B. Palmitic acid
C. Stearic acid
D. Oleic acid

14. The number of ml of N/10 KOH required to neutralize fatty acids in the distillate from 5 gm of fat is called __________
A. Acetyl number
B. Reichert-Meissl number
C. Polenske number
D. Non-volatile fatty acid number

15. Salkowski test is performed for the detection of _____
A. Vitamin D B. Glycerol
C. Cholesterol D. Fatty acids

16. Long chain fatty acids are first activated to acetyl-CoA in __________
A. Nucleus B. Cytosol
C. Microsomes D. Mitochondria

17. The enzymes of beta-oxidation are found in ________
A. Nucleus
B. Mitochondria
C. Cytosol
D. Golgi apparatus

18. Gaucher's disease is due to the deficiency of the enzyme ____________
A. B-Galactosidase
B. Sphingomyelinase
C. Glucocerebrosidase
D. Galactocerebrosidase

19. __________ gives an idea about rancidity of fats or oil
A. Acetyl values B. Iodine values
C. Acid values D. Sap values

20. Which of the following molecules serve as fuel reserve of the body?
A. Triglycerides B. Glycogen
C. Glucose D. Proteins

21. The lipids are transported throughout the body as _____
A. Triacylglycerols
B. Lipoproteins
C. Phospholipids
D. Glycolipids

22. In humans, a dietary essential fatty acid is __________
A. Linoleic acid B. Palmitic acid
C. Stearic acid D. Oleic acid

23. The cholesterol molecule is __________
A. Straight chain acid B. Benzene derivative
C. Quinoline derivative D. Steroid

24. Lipid stores are mainly present in __________
A. Adipose tissue B. Liver
C. Brain D. Muscles

25. The cyclic ring present in all the steroids is __________
A. Cycloheptadiene
B. Cyclopentano-phenanthrene
C. Nitro pentane
D. Quinoline

26. Liebermann-Burchard reaction is performed to detect __________
A. Glycerol B. Fatty acid
C. Cholesterol D. Vitamin D

27. Acrolein test is used to detect __________
A. Proteins B. Glycerol
C. Prostaglandins D. Carbohydrates

28. Which one of the following is an example of a saturated fatty acid?
A. Oleic acid B. Linoleic acid
C. Palmitic acid D. Erucic acid

29. Drying oil, oxidized spontaneously by atmospheric oxygen at ordinary temperature and forms a hard waterproof material is __________
A. Linseed oil B. Coconut oil
C. Peanut oil D. Rapeseed oil

30. Excessive deposition of fats in the body with decreased mobility causes __________
A. Pellagra B. Obesity
C. Beriberi D. Goitre

31. Sphingomyelins are __________
A. Alcohols B. Phospholipids
C. Nitro lipids D. None of the above

32. A fatty acid which is not synthesized in the body and must be supplied in the diet is __________
A. Palmitoleic acid B. Palmitic acid
C. Lauric acid D. Linolenic acid

33. Number of carbon atoms in cholesterol is __________
A. 27 B. 17
C. 19 D. 30

34. Phospholipid acting as a surfactant is __________
A. Phosphatidyl serine B. Cephalin
C. Lecithin D. Phosphatidylinositol

35. The enzyme acyl-CoA synthase catalyses the conversion of a fatty acid of an active fatty acid in the presence of __________

A. GTP B. AMP
C. ADP D. ATP

36. The molecular formula of cholesterol is __________

A. $C_{25}H_{42}OH$ B. $C_{27}H_{45}OH$
C. $C_{24}H_{41}OH$ D. $C_{26}H_{43}OH$

37. Acid number gives __________

A. Idea about molecular weight
B. Idea about rancidity
C. Solubility of fats and oils
D. Hydroxyl group present in fats and oils

38. A triglyceride is called a fat if it is a solid at __________

A. 25°C B. 27°C
C. 28°C D. 29°C

39. The important manifestation of Niemann-Pick disease is __________

A. Corneal opacity
B. Leukopenia
C. Hepatosplenomegaly
D. Cardiac enlargement

40. The linoleic, linolenic and arachidonic acids are examples of __________

A. Non-essential fatty acids
B. Carcinogens
C. Mutagens
D. Essential fatty acids

41. The highest phospholipids content is found in ______

A. Chylomicrons B. HDL
C. VLDL D. LDL

42. __________ is an example of fat.

A. Glyceryl trioleate
B. Groundnut oil
C. Coconut oil
D. Vegetable ghee

43. Which of the following is a symptom of Fabry's disease?

A. Mental retardation
B. Skin rash
C. Exophthalmos
D. Haemolytic anaemia

44. Hydrolysis of fats by alkali is called __________

A. Saponification
B. Acidification
C. Both A and B
D. None of the above

45. Sphingomyelins are __________

A. Alcohols B. Phospholipids
C. Nitro lipids D. None of the above

46. Rancidity is prevented by addition of __________

A. Vit K
B. Lead
C. Copper
D. Vit. E. (tocopherol)

47. Saturated fats are a type of fat wherein the fatty acids possess __________

A. Coordinate covalent bonds
B. Triple bonds
C. Single bond
D. Double bonds

48. Oleic acid is an example of __________

A. Saturated fat
B. Inert fatty acids
C. Neutral fatty acids
D. Unsaturated fat

49. Which of the following is a polyunsaturated fatty acid?

A. Linoleic acid
B. Palmitic acid
C. Palmitoleic acid
D. Oleic acid

50. Gallstone is a chief source of __________

A. Carbohydrates B. Proteins
C. Cholesterol D. Waxes

51. Fatty liver is caused due to accumulation of ________

A. Triacylglycerol B. Fatty acids
C. Cholesterol D. Phospholipids

52. Hypocholesterolaemia is found in __________

A. Nephrotic syndrome
B. Thyrotoxicosis
C. Diabetes mellitus
D. Obstructive jaundice

53. A lipotropic factor is __________

A. Vitamin C B. Choline
C. Palmitic acid D. Calcium

54. All enzymes involved in the synthesis of cholesterol are found in __________

A. Endoplasmic reticulum and cytosol
B. Mitochondria
C. Golgi apparatus
D. Nucleus

55. Cholesterol by a feedback mechanism inhibits the activity of __________

A. Mevalonate kinase
B. HMG-CoA synthetase
C. HMG-CoA reductase
D. Thiolate

56. The principal sterol excreted in faeces is __________

A. Coprostanol B. Desmosterol
C. Zymosterol D. Lanosterol

57. The major source of extracellular cholesterol for human tissue is __________

A. Very low-density lipoprotein
B. High density lipoprotein
C. Low density lipoprotein
D. Albumin

58. The source of all carbon atoms in cholesterol is ________

A. Succinyl-CoA
B. Acetyl-CoA
C. Bicarbonate
D. Propionyl-CoA

59. Fatty liver is also caused by __________

A. Riboflavin
B. CH_3CI
C. CCl_4
D. Na_2SO_4

60. Hypercholesterolemia is found in __________

A. Malabsorption syndrome
B. Xanthomatosis
C. Thyrotoxicosis
D. Hemolytic jaundice

Answer Key

1 C	2 D	3 A	4 C	5 D	6 D	7 B	8 C	9 A	10 B
11 B	12 D	13 A	14 B	15 C	16 B	17 B	18 C	19 C	20 A
21 B	22 A	23 D	24 A	25 B	26 C	27 B	28 C	29 A	30 B
31 B	32 D	33 A	34 C	35 D	36 B	37 B	38 A	39 C	40 D
41 B	42 D	43 B	44 A	45 B	46 D	47 C	48 D	49 A	50 C
51 A	52 B	53 B	54 A	55 C	56 B	57 C	58 B	59 C	60 B

CHAPTER 5

Nucleic Acids

1. __________ is regarded as a reserve bank of genetic information.
   A. RNA B. DNA
   C. m-RNA D. t-RNA

2. The double helix structure of DNA was proposed by __________
   A. Miescher
   B. Paul Erich
   C. Watson and Crick
   D. Louise pasture

3. RNA contains uridine, it is a __________
   A. Nucleotide
   B. Pyrimidine
   C. Nucleoside
   D. Purine

4. The complementary base pairing in DNA helix proves __________
   A. Chargaff's rule
   B. Grignard's rule
   C. Hensons rule D. Hirarcheal rule

5. The type of coiling in DNA is __________
   A. Left-handed B. Right-handed
   C. Zigzag D. Opposite

6. RNA transcript that is produced during DNA transcription is __________
   A. mRNA B. rRNA
   C. tRNA D. None of the above

7. DNA strands are separated by __________
   A. DNA polymerase B. DNA ligase
   C. DNA helicase D. Both A and B

8. Transferring the genetic information from one cell to its daughter is __________
   A. Replication process
   B. Mutation
   C. Development
   D. Transcription

9. __________ helps in transporting chemical signals and metabolic regulation.
   A. ADP B. cAMP
   C. ATP D. Both A and B

10. RNA is __________
    A. Tetra stranded
    B. Double stranded
    C. Single stranded
    D. None of the above

11. RNA does not consist of __________
    A. Aliphatic B. Adenine
    C. Guanine D. Thymine

12. The combination of a base and sugar is called ______
    A. Nucleoside B. Adenine
    C. Ribosomes D. Nucleotides

13. ______________ is a site of chromosomes and DNA synthesis.
    A. Mitochondria
    B. Cytoplasm
    C. Nucleus
    D. Endoplasmic reticulum

14. Nucleotide does not compose of __________
    A. Phosphate B. Nitrogenous base
    C. Triose sugar D. Pentose sugar

15. **Pyrimidine dihydrouracil is used in treatment of __________**
    A. Fever B. Tuberculosis
    C. Malaria D. Cancer

16. **The main function of RNA is __________**
    A. Cell protection
    B. Protein synthesis
    C. Transfer of offsprings
    D. None of the above

17. **Nucleotides are phosphoric acid __________ of nucleosides.**
    A. Ester B. Ether
    C. Methyl D. None of the above

18. **DNA is the master blueprint for life and constitutes the __________ in all free-living organisms and most viruses.**
    A. Acidic material
    B. Genetic material
    C. Chemicals
    D. None of the above

19. **The 3'-5' phosphodiester linkage joins __________**
    A. Two nucleosides
    B. Two DNA strands
    C. Two nucleotides
    D. A nitrogenous base with pentose sugar

20. **A form of DNA possesses right-handed helix with a diameter of __________**
    A. 18 A° B. 20 A°
    C. 22 A° D. 26 A°

21. **The __________ functions by transferring the genetic material into ribosomes.**
    A. r-RNA B. m-RNA
    C. t-RNA D. All of the above

22. **DNA is __________**
    A. Tetra strand
    B. Double strand
    C. Single strand
    D. None of the above

23. **A pyrimidine nucleotide is __________**
    A. GMP B. AMP
    C. CMP D. IMP

24. **The sugar moiety present in RNA is __________**
    A. Deoxyribose B. Ribulose
    C. Arabinose D. Ribose

25. **__________ serves as repository and transmitters of genetic information.**
    A. Fatty acids
    B. Nucleic acids
    C. Essential fatty acids
    D. Non-essential fatty acids

26. **DNA does not contain __________**
    A. Deoxyribose B. Thymine
    C. Adenine D. Uracil

27. **A nucleotide consists of __________**
    A. A sugar, a base and three phosphates
    B. A sugar, a base and a phosphate
    C. A sugar and a phosphate
    D. Paired bases

28. **Which of the following is not a base of RNA?**
    A. Adenine (A)
    B. Cytosine (C)
    C. Thymine (T)
    D. Guanine (G)

29. **The sugar moiety present in DNA is __________**
    A. Ribulose B. Deoxyribose
    C. Ribose D. Xylose

30. **Uracil is found only in __________**
    A. DNA B. RNA
    C. Both A and B D. Cytoplasm

31. **In DNA, three hydrogen bonds are formed between __________**
    A. Thymine and cytosine
    B. Adenine and guanine
    C. Adenine and thymine
    D. Guanine and cytosine

32. **The attachment between the base and sugar in a nucleotide is through which bond.**
    A. Hydrogen
    B. Glycosidic
    C. Peptide
    D. Phosphodiester

33. **The first true pyrimidine ribonucleotide synthesized is __________**
    A. UDP B. TMP
    C. UMP D. CTP

34. **Adenine always pairs with __________**
    A. Guanine B. Cytosine
    C. Thymine D. Adenine

35. Nucleotides are formed by pyrimidine and purine bases which are __________

A. Hydrogen bonded to a sugar
B. Covalently bonded to a sugar
C. Conically bonded to a sugar
D. None of the above

36. UDP and UTP are formed by phosphorylation from __________

A. GTP B. AMP
C. ADP D. ATP

37. Conversion of deoxy-uridine monophosphate to thymidine monophosphate is catalysed by the enzyme __________

A. Uridylic acid decarboxylase
B. Ribonucleotide reductase
C. Thymidylate synthetase
D. CTP synthetase

38. A purine nucleotide is __________

A. TMP B. AMP
C. UMP D. CMP

39. Ribosomal RNA accounts for about __________ of total weight of ribosomes.

A. 40–60% B. 20%
C. 10% D. 50–60%

40. A substrate for enzymes of pyrimidine nucleotide biosynthesis is __________

A. Puromycin B. Allopurinol
C. Tetracycline D. Chloramphenicol

Answer Key

1 B	2 C	3 C	4 A	5 B	6 A	7 C	8 A	9 B	10 C
11 D	12 A	13 C	14 C	15 D	16 B	17 A	18 B	19 C	20 B
21 B	22 B	23 C	24 D	25 B	26 D	27 B	28 C	29 B	30 B
31 D	32 B	33 C	34 C	35 B	36 D	37 C	38 B	39 A	40 B

CHAPTER 6.

Enzymes

1. ___________ is a biocatalyst that increases the rate of the reaction without being changed.
   A. Hydrogen peroxide
   B. Aluminium oxide
   C. Enzyme
   D. Silicon dioxide

2. The protein part of holoenzyme is known as _________
   A. Coenzyme B. Active site
   C. Allosteric site D. Apoenzyme

3. The term enzymes are coined by ___________
   A. Kuhne B. Pasteur
   C. Buchhner D. Urey miller

4. Hexokinase belongs to the class of enzyme ___________
   A. Hydrolase B. Isomerase
   C. Transferase D. Ligase

5. Amylases is an ___________
   A. Co-factor
   B. Exoenzyme
   C. Endoenzymes
   D. Prosthetic factor

6. IUB stands for ___________
   A. International unit of biology
   B. International union of biochemistry
   C. International unique biochemistry
   D. International unity of biomolecules

7. Which of the following enzyme is produced with the combination of apoenzyme and coenzyme?
   A. Prosthetic group
   B. Enzyme product complex
   C. Holoenzyme
   D. Enzyme substrate complex

8. The temperature at which an enzyme shows maximum activity is called ___________
   A. High temperature
   B. Optimum temperature
   C. Low temperature
   D. Moderate temperature

9. Blocking of enzyme action by blocking its active site is called ___________
   A. Uncompetitive inhibition
   B. Allosteric inhibition
   C. Competitive inhibition
   D. Non-competitive inhibition

10. Enzymes are made up of ___________
    A. Fats B. Vitamins
    C. Nucleic acid D. Proteins

11. Multiple forms of the same enzymes is called ______
    A. Apoenzyme B. Holoenzyme
    C. Isoenzyme D. Proenzyme

12. Which model was proposed by Koshland?
    A. Fluid mosaic model
    B. Lock and key model
    C. Induced fit model
    D. Refractive index model

13. The increase in concentration of enzyme ___________
    A. Decreases the rate of reaction
    B. Increases the rate of reaction
    C. Neutralize the rate of reaction
    D. None of the above

14. The ion which activates salivary amylase activity is __________

A. Potassium
B. Chloride
C. Bicarbonate
D. Sodium

15. The increase in temperature above the optimum temperature may result into inactivation of enzymes, is known as __________

A. Protein synthesis
B. Thermal denaturation
C. Rancidification
D. Tautomerization

16. The unit of enzyme activity measurement is _______

A. Katal
B. Curie
C. Mg
D. Base pair

17. In Henri-Michaelis-Menten equation Km stands for _____________

A. Substrate concentration
B. Reaction rate
C. Michaelis constant
D. Pressure

18. Lock and key hypothesis of enzyme action was given by __________

A. Koshland
B. Buchner
C. Kuhne
D. Fischer

19. Zymogen or proenzyme is a __________

A. Enzyme precursor
B. Modulator
C. Vitamin
D. Hormone

20. Which enzyme was first isolated and purified in the form of crystals?

A. Peptidase
B. Urease
C. Pepsin
D. Ribonuclease

21. Lyases are used for __________

A. Hydrolysis
B. Association of enzymes
C. Breaking of bonds in enzyme
D. Redox reactions

22. __________ are the enzymes which gives signals and are helpful in transportation.

A. Marker enzymes
B. Apoenzymes
C. Holoenzymes
D. Isoenzymes

23. The very first enzyme elevated in serum in myocardial infarction __________

A. SGOT
B. Alkaline phosphatase
C. Lactate dehydrogenase
D. Creatine phosphokinase

24. The enzyme streptokinase is used for __________

A. Blood clotting
B. Hepatitis
C. Skin allergy
D. Leukaemia

25. Coenzymes are __________

A. Organic part of apoenzyme
B. Inorganic part of factor
C. Organic part of factor
D. Inorganic part of apoenzyme

26. TPP is synthesized from __________

A. Oxidation
B. Thiamine
C. Translation
D. Deamination

27. Optimum pH value of pepsin is __________

A. 5
B. 1.5
C. 2
D. 3.5

28. __________ is a cleft or depression upon the enzyme molecule at which substrate molecule attaches to enzyme.

A. Activators
B. Active site
C. Inactive site
D. Inhibitors

29. The enzyme that digests fat is __________

A. Sucrase
B. Maltase
C. Lipase
D. Fructose

30. __________ are the enzymes which are present in its inactive forms.

A. Holoenzymes
B. Apoenzymes
C. Zymogens
D. Allosteric enzymes

31. In human body optimum temperature for enzymatic activities is __________

A. 30°C
B. 37°C
C. 24°C
D. 31°C

32. Inactive enzymes which are not bound to their cofactors are called __________

A. Holoenzymes
B. Enzyme inhibitors
C. Apoenzymes
D. Coenzymes

33. **The 'lock and key hypothesis' mechanism is related with ___________**
   A. For the formation of vacuole
   B. Explosives
   C. Digestion of fat in the body
   D. Enzyme specificity

34. **Non-protein component of enzymes are known as ___________**
   A. Coenzyme **B.** Cofactor
   C. Activator **D.** All of the above

35. **The coenzyme is ___________**
   A. Often a vitamin
   B. Often a metal
   C. Always a protein
   D. Always an inorganic compound

36. **Gamma-glutamyl transpeptidase activity in serum is elevated in ___________**
   A. Pancreatitis
   B. Alcoholism
   C. Muscular dystrophy
   D. Myocardial infarction

37. **Pepsin is an example for the class of enzymes, namely ___________**
   A. Ligases **B.** Oxidoreductases
   C. Transferases **D.** Hydrolases

38. **Enzymes are polymers of ___________**
   A. Amino acid **B.** Hexose sugar
   C. Inorganic phosphate **D.** Fatty acids

39. **An enzyme that joins the ends of two strands of nucleic acid is ___________**
   A. Helicase **B.** Polymerase
   C. Ligase **D.** Synthetase

40. **CPK means ___________**
   A. Creatinine pure kinase
   B. Creatinine phosphokinase
   C. Creatinine polymerase kinase
   D. Creatinine polymer kinase

Answer Key

1 C	2 D	3 A	4 C	5 B	6 B	7 C	8 B	9 C	10 D
11 C	12 C	13 B	14 D	15 B	16 A	17 C	18 D	19 A	20 B
21 C	22 A	23 D	24 A	25 D	26 B	27 B	28 B	29 C	30 C
31 B	32 C	33 D	34 D	35 A	36 B	37 D	38 A	39 C	40 B

CHAPTER 7

Vitamins

1. **Vitamins A, D, E, K are __________ vitamins.**
   A. Water soluble
   B. Fat soluble
   C. Both A and B
   D. None of the above

2. **__________ deficiency causes beriberi**
   A. Vitamin B_6 B. Vitamin B_1
   C. Vitamin B_2 D. Vitamin B_{12}

3. **Deficiency of vitamin A leads to __________**
   A. Dermatitis and pellagra
   B. Anaemia and polycythemia
   C. Night blindness and xerophthalmia
   D. None of the above

4. **__________ is a cobalt containing vitamin.**
   A. Vitamin A B. Vitamin E
   C. Vitamin B_1 D. Vitamin B_{12}

5. **Thiamine deficiency leads to __________**
   A. Scurvy B. Night blindness
   C. Beriberi D. Pellagra

6. **Pantothenic acid is important for __________**
   A. Gluconeogenesis
   B. Fatty acid synthesis
   C. Pyruvate carboxylase
   D. Glycolysis

7. **THF is a coenzyme of __________**
   A. Riboflavin B. Folic acid
   C. Ascorbic acid D. Niacin

8. **________ deficiency causes megaloblastic anaemia.**
   A. Cobalamin B. Folic acid
   C. Niacin D. Pyridoxine

9. **The vitamin that helps in blood clotting is __________**
   A. Vitamin A B. Vitamin K
   C. Vitamin C D. Vitamin D

10. **Vitamin A is the structural part of retinal pigment called __________**
    A. Calcitriol B. Rhodopsin
    C. Calciferol D. Tocoferol

11. **The deficiency of Niacin causes __________**
    A. Pernicious anaemia B. Scurvy
    C. Rickets D. Pellagra

12. **The following is a water-soluble vitamin __________**
    A. Vitamin B_2 B. Vitamin B_1
    C. Vitamin C D. All of the above

13. **__________ is a disorder caused due to deficiency of biotin.**
    A. Goitre B. Egg white injury
    C. Pellagra D. Night blindness

14. **Which of the following vitamins has a coenzyme function?**
    A. Vitamin B
    B. Vitamin A
    C. Vitamin C
    D. All of the above

15. **Vitamin B_2 is involved in the formation of coenzyme __________**
    A. NADP, FMN B. NAD, NADP
    C. FMN, FAD D. NAD, FAD

16. **________ is required in the synthesis of DNA and RNA.**
    A. Ascorbic acid B. Folic acid
    C. Thiamine D. Niacin

17. Fat-soluble vitamins are stored in ___________

A. Blood B. Liver
C. Skin D. Pancreas

18. Vitamin D is also called ___________

A. Retinol B. Calciferol
C. Thiamine D. Riboflavin

19. Liver damage is caused due to the overdose of _______

A. Vitamin B_3 B. Vitamin B_{12}
C. Vitamin B_6 D. Vitamin B_2

20. Beriberi is due to deficiency of ___________

A. Vitamin B_1 B. Vitamin D
C. Vitamin E D. Vitamin B_2

21. Which vitamin is required for RBC synthesis?

A. Vitamin B_{12}
B. Vitamin A
C. Vitamin B
D. Vitamin E

22. Folate deficiency causes ___________

A. Microcytic anaemia
B. Megaloblastic anaemia
C. Haemolytic anaemia
D. Iron deficiency anaemia

23. ___________ is also known as antihemorrhagic factor.

A. Vitamin C B. Vitamin A
C. Vitamin K D. Vitamin D

24. Which one of the following is a component of the coenzyme-A?

A. Pantothenic acid B. Retinol
C. Pyridoxine D. Retinoic acid

25. Which of the following vitamins serves as a hormone precursor?

A. Vitamin K B. Vitamin A
C. Vitamin C D. Vitamin D

26. What is the richest source of vitamin A?

A. Apple B. Orange
C. Carrot D. Spinach

27. Which vitamin is a major lipid-soluble antioxidant in cell membranes?

A. Vitamin E B. Vitamin A
C. Vitamin D D. Vitamin K

28. Which of the following water-soluble vitamin that can be stored in the liver for many years?

A. Vitamin B_6 B. Vitamin B_2
C. Vitamin B_1 D. Vitamin B_{12}

29. Vitamins are ___________

A. Proteins in nature
B. Accessory food factors
C. Generally synthesized in the body
D. Produced in endocrine glands

30. Which vitamin is essential for the health of brain?

A. Vitamin B_6 B. Vitamin B_9
C. Vitamin B_{12} D. All of the above

31. Which of the following is the richest source of vitamin C?

A. Dates
B. Citrus fruits and black currants
C. Eggs
D. Pulses

32. The tocopherols prevent the oxidation of ___________

A. Vitamin K B. Vitamin A
C. Vitamin D D. All of the above

33. The symptoms of scurvy is ___________

A. Dermatitis B. Loosening of teeth
C. Anorexia D. All of the above

34. Vitamin B_1 coenzyme (TPP) is involved in ___________

A. Hydroxylation
B. Transamination
C. Oxidative decarboxylation
D. Carboxylation

35. Kwashiorkor results from ___________

A. Protein and caloric deficiency in diet
B. Vitamin A deficiency
C. Vitamin D deficiency
D. Deficiency of minerals in diet

36. Rickets is caused due to the deficiency of ___________

A. Vitamin B_{12} B. Vitamin A
C. Vitamin C D. Vitamin D

37. Which among the following fatty acids is an essential fatty acid for man?

A. Linoleic acid B. Palmitic acid
C. Oleic acid D. None of the above

38. Vitamin K regulates the synthesis of blood clotting factors ___________

A. IX B. VII
C. X D. All of the above

39. The vitamin that increases the absorption of iron from the gut is ___________

A. Vitamin E B. Vitamin C
C. Vitamin K D. Vitamin D

40. Avidin is present in __________

A. Carrots
B. Cow's milk
C. Raw egg
D. Green leafy vegetables

41. Marasmus is due to malnutrition of __________

A. Proteins and minerals
B. Proteins
C. Proteins and calories
D. Proteins and vitamins

42. Energy value in kilocalorie per gram of fat in the body is __________

A. 9 B. 1
C. 4 D. 10

43. The functionally active form of vitamin D is _______

A. Cholecalciferol
B. Calcitriol
C. Ergocalciferol
D. Dehydrocholesterol

44. Which among the following is an essential amino acid for man?

A. Valine B. Alanine
C. Serine D. Glutamic acid

45. Under what condition basal metabolic rate goes up?

A. Hypothyroidism
B. Cold environment
C. Hot environment
D. Intake of base forming foods

46. Fibre in the diet is beneficial in __________

A. Colon cancer B. Hyperglycaemia
C. Hypercholesterolemia D. All of the above

47. Vitamin D is also called __________

A. Tocopherol B. Calciferol
C. Pantothenic acid D. Biotin

48. Which of the following is the most essential nutrient for a woman during her initial stages of pregnancy to prevent birth defects?

A. Vitamin E B. Thiamine
C. Folic acid D. Vitamin C

49. FAD and FMN are the coenzymes of __________

A. Riboflavin B. Niacin
C. Pantothenic acid D. Folic acid

50. Milk contains very poor amounts of __________

A. Riboflavin B. Calcium
C. Phosphate D. Iron

Answer Key

1 B	2 B	3 C	4 D	5 C	6 B	7 B	8 A	9 B	10 B
11 D	12 D	13 B	14 D	15 C	16 B	17 B	18 B	19 C	20 A
21 A	22 B	23 C	24 A	25 D	26 C	27 A	28 D	29 B	30 D
31 B	32 B	33 B	34 C	35 A	36 D	37 A	38 D	39 B	40 C
41 C	42 A	43 B	44 A	45 B	46 C	47 B	48 C	49 A	50 D

CHAPTER 8

Metabolism

1. ___________ is the degradative phase of metabolism which provides metabolic fuel and the building blocks for the cell.

   A. Anabolism B. Catabolism
   C. Transamination D. Ketosis

2. The process of conversion of glucose into glycogen in the liver is called ___________

   A. Glycogenolysis
   B. Glycogenesis
   C. Neo-glucogenesis
   D. Glycolysis

3. Total number of ATPs formed in Krebs cycle is ___________

   A. 10 B. 20
   C. 30 D. 40

4. ___________ is a peptide which plays an important role in glucose metabolism.

   A. Inulin B. Insulin
   C. Glucagaon D. pyruvate

5. Obesity increases the risk of ___________

   A. Cardiovascular disease
   B. Hypertension
   C. Diabetes mellitus
   D. All of the above

6. ___________ is the process of breakdown of glycogen into glucose in the liver.

   A. Glycogenolysis
   B. Glycogenesis
   C. Neo-glucogenesis
   D. Glycolysis

7. Restriction of salt intake is generally recommended in ___________

   A. Peptic ulcer B. Diabetes mellitus
   C. Hypertension D. Cirrhosis of liver

8. ETC stands for ___________

   A. Electron terminal chain
   B. Electron transport chain
   C. Electron triangular chain
   D. Electron triple chain

9. Normal specific gravity of urine is ___________

   A. 1.012–1.024
   B. 1.025–1.034
   C. 1.035–1.045
   D. 1.000–1.010

10. Heavy proteinuria occurs in ___________

    A. Nephrotic syndrome
    B. Acute glomerulonephritis
    C. Acute pyelonephritis
    D. Nephrosclerosis

11. The number of isomers of glucose is ___________

    A. 4 B. 16
    C. 8 D. 12

12. The pathway of breakdown of glucose into pyruvic acid is known as ___________

    A. Glycogenolysis
    B. Glycogenesis
    C. Glycolysis
    D. Neo-gluconeogenesis

13. Honey contains the hydrolytic product of ___________

    A. Starch B. Lactose
    C. Maltose D. Inulin

14. Cori cycle is designed for recycling of __________
A. Acetic acid
B. Lactic acid
C. Pyruvic acid
D. Malic acid

15. Insulin is secreted by __________
A. Pancreas
B. Liver
C. Kidney
D. Thyroid

16. Serum transaminases are significant markers for __________
A. Heart diseases
B. Liver diseases
C. Both A and B
D. None of the above

17. In glycolysis total __________ ATPs are synthesized.
A. 2
B. 3
C. 6
D. 8

18. The lipolysis is a __________
A. Formation of lipids
B. Breakdown of ketone bodies
C. Hydrolysis of triacylglycerol
D. Formation of ketone bodies

19. Which one of the following is a rate limiting enzyme of gluconeogenesis?
A. Pyruvate kinase
B. Hexokinase
C. Phosphofructokinase
D. Pyruvate carboxylase

20. TCA stands for __________
A. Tricarbolic acid
B. Tricarboxylic acid
C. Tetracarboxylic acid
D. Trans-carbonyl acid

21. An inborn error, maple syrup urine disease is due to deficiency of the enzyme __________
A. Adenosyl transferase
B. Alpha-keto acid decarboxylase
C. Isovaleryl-CoA-anhydrogenase
D. Phenylalanine hydroxylase

22. Gluconeogenesis occurs in __________ organ.
A. Fat
B. Kidney
C. Muscle
D. Liver

23. The end product of glycolysis under anaerobic condition is __________
A. Oxaloacetic acid
B. Lactic acid
C. Pyruvic acid
D. Acetoacetic acid

24. The cause of fatty liver includes __________
A. High fat intake
B. Alcoholism
C. Starvation
D. All of the above

25. Which of the following is tricarboxylic acid?
A. Citric acid
B. Acetic acid
C. Succinic acid
D. Pyruvic acid

26. How many ATPs are formed in case of palmitic acid by beta oxidation?
A. 147
B. 7
C. 129
D. 56

27. The process of formation of ketone bodies is known as __________
A. Ketolysis
B. Ketoacidosis
C. Ketogenesis
D. None of the above

28. In deamination, amino acid is converted to _______
A. Keto acid
B. Aldo acid
C. Hydrochloric acid
D. Citric acid

29. The process of transamination is catalysed by _______
A. Dehydrogenases
B. Transferases
C. Amino transferases
D. Hydrogenases

30. How many ATP molecules are generated during anaerobic glycolysis?
A. 8
B. 2
C. 10
D. 6

31. Which of the following are ketone bodies?
A. Acetone
B. Acetoacetate
C. Beta-hydroxy butyric acid
D. All of the above

32. Which of the following hormones is responsible for increasing gluconeogenesis in the liver during prolonged starvation?
A. Glucagon
B. TSH
C. Insulin
D. Thyroxine

33. Insulin is produced by __________ of the islets of Langerhans.
A. Gamma-cells
B. Beta-cells
C. Delta-cells
D. Alpha-cells

34. Glycolysis is also known as __________
A. HMP shunt
B. EMP pathway
C. Krebs cycle
D. ETC

35. Glycogen synthesis is increased by __________

A. Epinephrine B. Cortisone
C. Insulin D. GH

36. Enzymes concerned with the citric acid cycle are found in the __________

A. Mitochondria
B. Nucleus
C. Ribosomes
D. Non-particulate cytoplasm

37. Which of the following is a tricarboxylic acid?

A. Acetic acid B. Citric acid
C. Succinic acid D. Oxaloacetic acid

38. Serum cholesterol is decreased in __________

A. Thyrotoxicosis B. Myxoedema
C. Endemic goitre D. Cretinism

39. Which of the following is a ketone body?

A. Acetyl-CoA B. Carnitine
C. Acetoacetate D. Oxaloacetate

40. The first product of glycogenolysis is __________

A. Glucose-1-phosphate
B. Glucose-6-phosphate
C. Glucose-1,6-diphosphate
D. Fructose-1-phosphate

41. Fatty acid synthesis occurs in __________

A. Mitochondria
B. Endoplasmic reticulum
C. Cytosol
D. All of the above

42. In deamination the amino acid is converted to ________

A. Keto acid B. Aldol acid
C. Hydrochloric acid D. Citric acid

43. Specific gravity of urine is raised in all of the following *except* __________

A. Diabetes mellitus
B. Acute glomerulonephritis
C. Diabetes insipidus
D. Dehydration

44. The process of transamination is catalysed by _______

A. Dehydrogenases
B. Transferases
C. Amino transferases
D. Hydrogenases

45. __________ ATP consumed in glycolysis reaction.

A. 5 B. 2
C. 3 D. 4

46. Cause of hypercholesterolemia is __________

A. Stress B. Diabetes mellitus
C. Obesity D. All of the above

47. Total number of ATP formed in aerobic oxidation is __________

A. 20 B. 38
C. 40 D. 50

48. Symptoms of fatty liver is __________

A. Hypertension
B. Diabetes mellitus
C. Weakness
D. All of the above

49. __________ is a sequential removal of two carbon units as acetyl-CoA from carboxyl terminal of fatty acids by oxidation.

A. Beta-oxidation
B. Terminal oxidation
C. Peroxidation
D. Anerobic oxidation

50. Enzymes required for citric acid cycle are found in the __________

A. Cytoplasm B. Nucleus
C. Ribosomes D. Mitochondria

51. Consumption of iodised salt is recommended for the prevention of __________

A. Endemic goitre
B. Hypertension
C. Hyperthyroidism
D. None of the above

52. Hypercholesterolemia refers to a condition with high cholesterol with a serum cholesterol level of _______

A. >280 mg/dl B. >160 mg/dl
C. >200 mg/dl D. >240 mg/dl

53. Which of the following hormones is responsible for increasing gluconeogenesis in the liver during prolonged starvation?

A. Glucagon B. TSH
C. Insulin D. Thyroxine

54. Which of the following is non-essential amino acid?

A. Leucine B. Lysine
C. Serine D. Methionine

55. Electron transport system (ETS) is present in which of the following parts of mitochondria?

A. Stroma B. Inner membrane
C. Outer membrane D. Matrix

56. Fatty acid synthesis occurs in __________

A. Endoplasmic reticulum
B. Cytosol
C. Mitochondria
D. All of the above

57. The full form of NAD is __________

A. Nicotinamide adrenaline dinucleotide
B. Nucleotide adenine diamide
C. Nicotinamide adenine dinucleotide
D. None of the above

58. Urea cycle provides intermediate for which pathway?

A. Gluconeogenesis
B. Glycolysis
C. HMP-shunt
D. TCA cycle

59. Which of the following compounds are formed in urea cycle?

A. Fumarate
B. Arginosuccinate
C. Ornithine
D. All of the above

60. ETC is also known as __________

A. Beta-oxidation
B. Terminal oxidation
C. Peroxidation
D. Anerobic oxidation

Answer Key

1 B	2 B	3 C	4 B	5 D	6 À	7 C	8 B	9 A	10 C
11 B	12 C	13 D	14 B	15 A	16 B	17 D	18 C	19 C	20 B
21 B	22 D	23 B	24 D	25 A	26 C	27 C	28 A	29 C	30 B
31 D	32 A	33 B	34 B	35 C	36 A	37 B	38 A	39 C	40 A
41 C	42 A	43 B	44 C	45 B	46 D	47 B	48 A	49 A	50 D
51 A	52 D	53 A	54 C	55 B	56 B	57 C	58 D	59 D	60 B

CHAPTER 9

Minerals

1. **The minerals constituents about __________ of all inorganic material in the body.**
   A. 10% B. 40%
   C. 60% D. 80%

2. **Iodine is essential for the prevention of __________**
   A. Fever
   B. Goitre
   C. Weakness
   D. Diarrhoea

3. **__________ helps in the regulation of blood volume and blood pressure.**
   A. Phosphorous B. Iron
   C. Iodine D. Sodium

4. **Which of the following minerals controls growth and body weight?**
   A. Phosphorus B. Iodine
   C. Calcium D. All of the above

5. **____________ helps in the maintenance of osmotic pressure.**
   A. Iodine B. Iron
   C. Sodium D. Phosphorus

6. **Which one of the following is an example of macro minerals?**
   A. Sodium B. Chloride
   C. Calcium D. All of the above

7. **The deficiency of which mineral may result into impaired growth and development, skin lesions and loss of appetite?**
   A. Magnesium B. Zinc
   C. Cobalt D. Iron

8. **The mineral necessary for the clotting of blood is __________**
   A. Iron B. Calcium
   C. Cobalt D. Zinc

9. **__________ is condition in which the serum sodium level falls below the normal range.**
   A. Hypercalcemia
   B. Hypernatremia
   C. Hyponatremia
   D. Hyperkalaemia

10. **Which among the following is macro mineral?**
    A. Cobalt B. Calcium
    C. Copper D. Iodine

11. **Wilson's disease is due to abnormal metabolism of __________**
    A. Iodine B. Copper
    C. Calcium D. Iron

12. **A daily intake of selenium has been recommended for adults is __________**
    A. 50–210 mg B. 50–200 gm
    C. 50–200 mg D. 50–210 gm

13. **Polycythemia means __________**
    A. Decreased RBC in blood
    B. Decreased WBC in blood
    C. Increased WBC in blood
    D. Increased RBC in blood

14. **Which of the following minerals controls growth and body weight?**
    A. Phosphorous B. Iodine
    C. Calcium D. All of the above

15. Excessive intake of calcium in our diet results in __________

A. Gout B. Stroke
C. Diarrhoea D. Constipation

16. Calcium content in the body is about __________ body weight

A. 20 g/kg B. 25 g/kg
C. 22 g/kg D. 23 g/kg

17. What condition is caused by iodine deficiency during pregnancy and is characterized by stunted growth, deafness, and mental retardation?

A. Crohn's disease
B. Cretinism
C. Keshan disease
D. Multiple sclerosis

18. Which of the following are examples of macro minerals?

A. Sodium B. Calcium
C. Chloride D. All of the above

19. Which of the following vitamins is essential for the absorption of calcium from the intestinal tract?

A. Vit. C B. Vit. A
C. Vit. D D. Vit. E

20. Hyponatremia condition occurs due to __________

A. Increase in amount of sodium
B. Decrease in amount of sodium
C. Increase in amount of potassium
D. Decrease in amount of potassium

21. Chlorine maintains acid–base balance in association with __________

A. Zinc B. Sodium
C. Cobalt D. Iron

22. Calcium is excreted by ________

A. Kidney and pancreas
B. Kidney
C. Kidney and intestine
D. Kidney and liver

23. Daily requirement of potassium is about ________

A. 3.5 to 4.5 gm B. 1.5 to 4.5 gm
C. 2.5 to 4.5 gm D. 1.5 to 3.5 gm

24. Iron is a component of ________

A. Transaminase B. Transferase
C. Haemoglobin D. Ceruloplasmin

25. The daily requirement of iron for normal adult male is about ________

A. 5 mg B. 15 mg
C. 20 mg D. 8 mg

26. ________ is/ are essential trace elements.

A. Chromium B. Nickel
C. Vanadium D. All of the above

27. The total iron content of the human body is ______

A. 2–3 g B. 400–500 mg
C. 1–2 g D. 3–5 g

28. Iron is mainly absorbed from ________

A. Colon
B. Stomach and duodenum
C. Ileum
D. Caecum

29. Tetany can occur in ________

A. Alkalosis
B. Hypocalcaemia
C. Hypercalcaemia
D. Hypocalcaemia and alkalosis

30. The daily calcium requirement of an adult man is about __________

A. 800 mg B. 400 mg
C. 600 mg D. 1,000 mg

31. Iron is stored in the form of ________

A. Ferritin and transferrin
B. Ferritin and haemosiderin
C. Transferrin and haemosiderin
D. Haemoglobin and myoglobin

32. Iron is transported in blood in the form of ________

A. Transferrin
B. Ferritin
C. Haemoglobin
D. Haemosiderin

33. The normal serum level of phosphorus in human adult is ________

A. 5–7 mg B. 1–2 mg
C. 2–3 mg D. 3–4.5 mg

34. Hypocalcaemia affects ________

A. Cardiac muscles
B. Skeletal muscles
C. Smooth muscles
D. All of the above

35. Average concentration of chloride ions in cerebrospinal fluid per 100 ml is ________

A. 440 mg B. 365 mg
C. 40 mg D. 160 mg

36. Iron therapy is ineffective in which of the following conditions?

A. Chronic blood loss
B. Hypochromic anaemia of pregnancy
C. Inadequate Fe intake
D. Thalassemia minor

37. Zinc is a constituent of the enzyme ________

A. Succinate dehydrogenase
B. Carbonic anhydrase
C. Aldolase
D. Mitochondrial superoxide dismutase

38. ________ maintains water balance of the body.

A. TSH
B. ADH
C. ACTH
D. FSH

39. Which of the following are macro-minerals?

A. Sodium
B. Potassium
C. Calcium
D. All of the above

40. ________ is useful for synthesis of melanin.

A. Calcium
B. Chromium
C. Copper
D. Cobalt

Answer Key

1 D	2 B	3 D	4 B	5 C	6 D	7 B	8 B	9 C	10 B
11 B	12 C	13 D	14 B	15 B	16 C	17 B	18 D	19 C	20 B
21 B	22 C	23 B	24 C	25 D	26 D	27 A	28 B	29 D	30 A
31 B	32 A	33 D	34 D	35 A	36 B	37 C	38 B	39 D	40 C

CHAPTER

10

Water and Electrolytes

1. **Total body water is ________%.**
   A. 20 B. 60
   C. 80 D. None of the above

2. **The loss of water from the body is called ________**
   A. Semi-hydration
   B. Rehydration
   C. Dehydration
   D. None of the above

3. **Body water is regulated by the hormone ________**
   A. Epinephrine B. ADH
   C. ACTH D. FSH

4. **Principal electrolyte of intracellular cation fluid compartment ________**
   A. Sodium B. Calcium
   C. Potassium D. Magnesium

5. **The substances dissolved in water as ions with positive and negative charge are called ________**
   A. TBW
   B. Electrolytes
   C. Water
   D. None of the above

6. **________ being the only cation to exert significant osmotic pressure.**
   A. K B. Ca
   C. Na D. All of the above

7. **The extracellular fluid comprises ________**
   A. Interstitial fluid
   B. Tissue cells
   C. Plasma
   D. Plasma and interstitial fluid

8. **Water reabsorption is promoted by ________**
   A. Epinephrine
   B. ADH
   C. Prolactin
   D. Renin

9. **In healthy 70 kg adult male, the intracellular fluid volume is ________**
   A. 3.5 litres B. 42 litres
   C. 28 litres D. 14 litres

10. **The metabolism of sodium is regulated by the hormone ________**
    A. Somatostatin B. Insulin
    C. Aldosterone D. PTH

11. **The most predominant anion in the extracellular fluid is ________**
    A. Sodium
    B. Chloride
    C. Potassium
    D. Bicarbonate

12. **ORT (oral rehydration therapy) is commonly used to treat ________**
    A. Dehydration
    B. Cholera
    C. Diarrhoea
    D. All of the above

13. **The oral rehydration salt contains ________**
    A. Sodium chloride
    B. Anhydrous glucose
    C. Potassium chloride
    D. All of the above

14. _________ ml water is excreted through kidney.

A. 1200 ml B. 400 ml
C. 1500 ml D. 500 ml

15. Total body water accounts for __________ of body weight.

A. 71% B. 70%
C. 75% D. 60%

16. The oral rehydration fluid contains _________

A. Sodium B. Glucose
C. Both A and B D. Calcium

17. ORT stands for _________

A. Oral regular therapy
B. Oral rehydration therapy
C. Oral rebound therapy
D. Oral rinsing therapy

18. The daily requirement of magnesium in adults is about _________

A. 500 mg B. 300–400 mg
C. 100 mg D. 200–300 mg

19. Women have less fluids than men because they have more _________

A. Calcium B. Fat
C. Muscles D. Water

20. Sodium is the major cation in _________

A. ECF
B. Both ECF and ICF
C. Full body
D. ICF

21. ____________ ml of water is formed daily within the body itself by way of oxidation.

A. 300 B. 400
C. 500 D. 300–400

22. Fluid contained within a cell represents about two-thirds of all body fluids called _________

A. Oedema
B. Extracellular fluids
C. Intracellular fluids
D. Basophils

23. Abnormal accumulation of water in normally existing space in the body is called _________.

A. Water
B. TBW
C. Thrombocytes
D. Oedema

24. Compound sodium chloride injections IP is known as _________

A. Orange solution
B. Iodine solution
C. Ringer solution
D. Fehling's solution

25. _________ is a condition in which sodium (salt) levels become dangerously low.

A. Hyponatremia
B. Hypernatremia
C. Sickle cell anaemia
D. Diabetes insipidus

26. ICF constitutes about ___________ of the total body weight.

A. 25% B. 40%
C. 20% D. 10%

27. _________ is the sum of the water that is contained in arbitrary divisions of its distribution between the intracellular and extracellular compartments.

A. Total body water
B. Water
C. Electrolytes
D. None of the above

28. ___________ is a type of fluid replacement used as a treatment for dehydration.

A. Hypernatremia
B. Overhydration
C. ORT
D. Oedema

29. All the following are important electrolytes in the body *except* _________

A. Sodium ions
B. Potassium ions
C. Carbon ions
D. Chloride ions

30. Normal pH of venous blood and interstitial fluid is ___________.

A. 7.0 B. 7.35
C. 7.4 D. None of the above

31. The intracellular fluid compartment refers to all the water found in _________.

A. The bones of the body
B. All cells of the body
C. Areas outside the body cells
D. Areas within the gastrointestinal tract

32. **Approximately one-third of the body water exists in the _________.**
    A. Transcellular fluid compartment
    B. Kidneys and urinary bladder
    C. Blood
    D. Extracellular fluid compartment

33. **The interstitial fluid is generally poor while the plasma is generally rich in _________.**
    A. Protein
    B. Hydrogen ions
    C. Sodium and chloride ions
    D. Carbohydrates

34. **_________ results due to excess intake of water.**
    A. Dehydration
    B. Overhydration
    C. Oedema
    D. Electrolytes

35. **90% of the cations in the extracellular fluids consists of _________.**
    A. Bicarbonate ions
    B. Hydroxyl ions
    C. Calcium ions
    D. Sodium ions

36. **Electrolyte balance in the body usually refers to the balance of _________.**
    A. Acids B. Bases
    C. Salts D. Organic molecules

37. **The solute that contributes the most to the total serum osmolality is _________.**
    A. Urea B. Glucose
    C. Chloride D. Sodium

38. **The regulation of water balance is influenced by the hormones _________.**
    A. TSH and FSH
    B. ACTH and LDH
    C. ADH and aldosterone
    D. None of the above

39. **UNICEF means _________.**
    A. United Nations Inter-related Children's Fund
    B. United Nations International Children's Fund
    C. United Nations International Core Fund
    D. United Nations International Charity Fund

40. **The electrolytes are expressed as _________.**
    A. Milliequivalents B. Milligrams
    C. Micrograms D. Millilitres

Answer Key

1 B	2 C	3 B	4 C	5 B	6 C	7 D	8 B	9 C	10 C
11 B	12 D	13 D	14 C	15 B	16 C	17 B	18 D	19 B	20 A
21 D	22 C	23 D	24 C	25 A	26 B	27 A	28 C	29 C	30 B
31 B	32 D	33 A	34 B	35 D	36 C	37 D	38 C	39 B	40 A

CHAPTER 11

Introduction to Biotechnology

1. **The term biotechnology was coined in 1919 by _______ to describe a process for large scale production of pigs.**
   A. Francis Crick
   B. Karl Ereky
   C. Alexander Fleming
   D. James Watson

2. **OECD means _________**
   A. Organization for environmental corporation and development
   B. Organization for economic corporation and development
   C. Opportunity for economic corporation and development
   D. Organization for epidemic corporation and development

3. **Who gave the definition of biotechnology?**
   A. The European Federation of Biotechnology (EFB)
   B. National Center for Biotechnology Information (NCBI)
   C. National Institutes of Health (NIH)
   D. National Centre for Cell Science (NCCS)

4. **Application of biotechnology procedures in medical processes is classified as _________**
   A. Blue biotechnology
   B. White biotechnology
   C. Red biotechnology
   D. Green biotechnology

5. **_________ is a product of interaction between the biological science and technology.**
   A. Pharmacovigilance
   B. Phytochemistry
   C. Bio-taxonomy
   D. Biotechnology

6. **_________ is a product of biotechnology.**
   A. Vaccine
   B. Bacteria
   C. Skin
   D. Plants

7. **______________ is applied to agriculture and food production.**
   A. White biotechnology
   B. Red biotechnology
   C. Blue biotechnology
   D. Green biotechnology

8. **_________ is the technique of overcomes the limitation of traditional hybridization procedures.**
   A. Genetic engineering
   B. Immunology
   C. Cell biology
   D. Modern hybridization

9. **Field of biotechnology which is applied to industrial processes is known as ____________**
   A. Red biotechnology
   B. Blue biotechnology
   C. Green biotechnology
   D. White biotechnology

10. **Which of the following is an example of green biotechnology?**
    A. Industrial chemicals
    B. Industrial antibiotics
    C. BT corn and pesticides
    D. Industrial catalysts

11. **The science of use of living organisms to serve humans is _________**
    A. Service biology
    B. Biotechnology
    C. Social biology
    D. Human biology

12. Tissue culture is also known as ________

A. Soft biotechnology B. Hard biotechnology
C. Both of the above D. None of these

13. In ________ Alexander Fleming discovered the mold Penicillium.

A. 1929 B. 1930
C. 1931 D. 1928

14. Plant biotechnology is the combination of ________

A. Genetic engineering B. Plant tissue
C. Tissue culture D. Both A and B

15. ________ is the application of science and technology to living aquatic organisms for the production of knowledge, goods and services.

A. Blue biotechnology
B. White biotechnology
C. Red biotechnology
D. Green biotechnology

16. ________ is a technique in which fragments of plants are cultured and grown in a laboratory.

A. Cloning
B. Tissue culture
C. Genetic engineering
D. All of these

17. The process of using living organisms to develop products is known as ________

A. Bioengineering
B. Genome engineering
C. Medical engineering
D. Biotechnology

18. The golden rice variety is rich in ________

A. Vitamin D
B. Beta-carotene and ferritin
C. Vitamin C
D. Biotin

19. Which one of the following is a genetically modified crop?

A. Golden rice B. Bt-cotton
C. Bi-brinjal D. All of the above

20. Antibiotics is an example of ________

A. Green biotechnology
B. Red biotechnology
C. White biotechnology
D. Blue biotechnology

Answer Key

1 B	2 B	3 A	4 C	5 D	6 A	7 D	8 A	9 D	10 C
11 B	12 A	13 D	14 D	15 A	16 B	17 D	18 B	19 D	20 B

CHAPTER 12

Organ Function Tests

1. **The kidney function test measures ________________ function.**
   A. Sodium and calcium
   B. Extracellular and intracellular fluids
   C. Glomerular and tubular
   D. NaCl and KCl

2. **__________ is intravenously administered to measure glomerular filtration rate.**
   A. Insulin B. Inulin
   C. Mannitol D. Urea

3. **Modified Gmelin's test is used for detection of_______.**
   A. Bile pigments
   B. Ketone bodies
   C. Sugars
   D. Pus

4. **__________ test is used to assess liver function.**
   A. Bilirubin
   B. ALT
   C. AST
   D. All of the above

5. **Protein responsible for muscle contraction and relaxation are __________.**
   A. Elastin
   B. Myosin
   C. Actin
   D. Both A and B

6. **ALT is also known as __________.**
   A. Aspartate aminotransferase
   B. Alanine aminotransferase
   C. Amino leucine transferase
   D. None of the above

7. **GFR means __________.**
   A. Glomerular fastest rate
   B. Glomerular filtration rate
   C. Glomerulus forward rate
   D. Glomerular further rate

8. **Total serum T3 and T4 can be determined by _______.**
   A. Chemiluminescence method
   B. Immunoassay (RIA or ELISA)
   C. Both A and B
   D. None of the above

9. **TBG is __________.**
   A. Thyroid stimulating hormone
   B. Thyroid binding globulin
   C. Thyroid releasing hormone
   D. None of the above

10. **In which condition there is yellow coloration of the eye and some parts of the skin?**
    A. Cirrhosis
    B. Anaemia
    C. Jaundice
    D. Uraemia

11. **In an adult GFR is about __________.**
    A. 30 ml/min B. 200 ml/min
    C. 120 ml/min D. 50 ml/min

12. **The lipoprotein particles that have the highest percentage concentration of cholesterol is __________.**
    A. HDL
    B. Chylomicron
    C. VLDL
    D. LDL

13. Presence of sugar in urine indicates __________.

A. Proteinuria **B.** Kidney stone
C. Diabetes **D.** Hepatitis

14. Most useful test to assess renal function is __________.

A. Glomerular filtration rate
B. Clearance test
C. Both A and B
D. None of the above

15. Which of the following test is used to measure glomerular filtration rate?

A. Urine acidification test
B. Clearance test
C. Urine concentration test
D. Urine dilution test

16. The highest elevation with AST is seen in viral _______.

A. Meningitis **B.** Influenza
C. Hepatitis **D.** Pneumonia

17. ____________ is an enzyme found in your bones, bile ducts and liver.

A. Alkaline phosphatase (ALP)
B. Alanine transaminase (ALT)
C. Aspartate aminotransferase (AST)
D. Albumenise

18. Creatinine is most commonly measured in laboratories calorimetrically by ____________.

A. Oswald method
B. Jaffe's method
C. Kinetic method
D. None of the above

19. Parameters used in diagnosis of liver cell damage are __________.

A. ALP **B.** AST
C. ALT **D.** All of the above

20. Impaired liver function is diagnosed by __________.

A. Bilirubin
B. Serum protein
C. Both A and B
D. None of these

21. Normal range of urea in serum or plasma is mg/dl.

A. 5 to 15 **B.** 15 to 45
C. 20 to 30 **D.** None of the above

22. LDL means __________.

A. High cholesterol
B. Good cholesterol
C. Bad cholesterol
D. None of the above

23. ____________ rate can be used to measure glomerular filtration rate.

A. Clearance
B. ALT
C. Creatinine clearance
D. AST

24. Diseases associated with abnormal metabolism of lipids are

A. Fatty liver
B. Obesity
C. Diabetes mellitus
D. All of the above

25. Normal range of urea in serum or plasma is _________ mg/dl.

A. 5–15 **B.** 15 to 45
C. 30–20 **D.** None of the above

26. The lipid test is known as __________.

A. Coronary risk panel
B. Cholesterol test
C. ALP test
D. Both A and B

27. Aspartate transaminase is an enzyme present in ______.

A. Spleen **B.** Bile duct
C. Liver **D.** Pancreatic duct

28. Renin is an enzyme used for __________.

A. Decrease urine production
B. Controlling BP
C. Increase urine production
D. None of the above

29. __________ is also named a bad cholesterol.

A. TC **B.** LDL
C. HDL **D.** None of the above

30. Red brown colour of urine is due to presence of _____.

A. Haemoglobin
B. RBC
C. Myoglobin
D. All of the above

31. Alkaline phosphatase is found in __________.

A. Liver **B.** Spleen
C. Lungs **D.** Heart

32. Normal range of total bilirubin is __________.

A. 2.0–10.0
B. 0.2–1.0
C. 1–1.3
D. None of the above

33. Which test is used to detect lipid dysfunction?

A. Alkaline phosphatase
B. Urine glucose
C. Total cholesterol
D. SGOT

34. Which colour of urine indicates rise in bilirubin level?

A. Yellow **B.** Pink
C. Orange **D.** Red

35. The pH of normal random sample of urine is _______.

A. 1–2.2 **B.** 3.5–4
C. 5–6 **D.** 4.5–8.0

36. Protein present in the urine indicates __________ disease.

A. Heart
B. Liver
C. Kidney
D. All of the above

37. Normal range of HDL in men should be __________.

A. 15–25 mg/dl **B.** 35–65 mg/dl
C. 25–35 mg/dl **D.** 65–85 mg/dl

38. The rise in the level of __________ indicates biliary tree due to cholestasis.

A. Urea
B. Cholesterol
C. Alkaline phosphatase
D. Creatinine

39. Ketone bodies is composed of __________.

A. Beta-hydroxybutyric acid
B. Acetone
C. Acetoacetic acid
D. All of the above

40. __________ is the type of cholesterol that is known as 'good cholesterol'.

A. HDL **B.** LDL
C. VLDL **D.** Triglyceride

Answer Key

1 C	2 B	3 A	4 D	5 D	6 B	7 B	8 C	9 B	10 C
11 C	12 D	13 C	14 C	15 B	16 C	17 A	18 B	19 D	20 C
21 B	22 C	23 C	24 D	25 B	26 D	27 A	28 B	29 B	30 D
31 A	32 B	33 C	34 B	35 D	36 C	37 B	38 C	39 D	40 A

CHAPTER 13

Pathology of Blood and Urine

1. **The scientific study of disease which deals with causes, effects, mechanism, and nature of the disease is called __________.**
   A. Physiology
   B. Pathology
   C. Biology
   D. Biochemistry

2. **The study of blood and its disease is known as ______.**
   A. Parasitology
   B. Haematology
   C. Zoology
   D. None of the above

3. **The average life span of platelets is __________.**
   A. 1 to 2 days
   B. 5 to 10 days
   C. 20 to 40 days
   D. 40 to 60 days

4. **Lymphocytes are the types of __________.**
   A. Platelets
   B. RBC
   C. WBC
   D. All of the above

5. **__________ is a hereditary disease also known as bleeding disease.**
   A. Haematuria
   B. Haemoglobinuria
   C. Haemophilia
   D. Haemolysis

6. **The size of lymphocytes ranges from __________ micrometre in diameter.**
   A. 7–8
   B. 7–20
   C. 5–10
   D. 0–5

7. **Platelets are also called __________.**
   A. Erythrocytes
   B. Basophils
   C. Lymphocytes
   D. Thrombocytes

8. **__________ is a disease caused by the decrease in the normal platelet count.**
   A. Leukaemia
   B. Leucopenia
   C. Purpura
   D. Anaemia

9. **High level of bilirubin in the urine indicates ______.**
   A. Cancer
   B. Jaundice
   C. Diabetes
   D. Hypertension

10. **The increased amount of uric acid in the urine indicates __________.**
    A. Diabetes
    B. Gout
    C. Inflammation
    D. Liver disorder

11. **Haematuria indicates the presence of __________ in the blood.**
    A. Blood
    B. Bile
    C. Bilirubin
    D. All of the above

12. **Pyuria refers to presence of __________ in urine**
    A. Bile
    B. Pus
    C. Blood
    D. Cancerous cell

13. **The Glycosuria is seen in __________.**
    A. Diabetes insipidus
    B. Diabetes mellitus
    C. Hepatitis
    D. Both A and C

14. The lifespan of a red blood cell is around __________.

A. 100 days **B.** 130 days
C. 120 days **D.** 140 days

15. __________ can identify viruses and microorganisms from the antigens.

A. Monocytes **B.** T-cells
C. B-cells **D.** Matter platelets

16. Benzidine test is used for detection of __________.

A. Ketone bodies in urine
B. Protein in urine
C. Blood in urine
D. Glucose in urine

17. Decrease in numbers of platelets below the normal range and is observed in __________.

A. Dengue
B. Aplastic anaemia
C. Megaloblastic anaemia
D. All of the above

18. Abnormal constituent present in urine is __________.

A. Ketone bodies **B.** Urea
C. Uric acid **D.** Creatinine

19. Destruction of red bone marrow results in a condition called __________.

A. Megaloblastic anaemia **B.** Aplastic anaemia
C. Haemolytic anaemia **D.** All of the above

20. Rothera's test is used for the detection of __________ in the urine.

A. Lipids **B.** Ketones
C. Proteins **D.** Sugar

21. Leucocytosis is increase in number of __________.

A. WBCs **B.** RBCs
C. Platelets **D.** None of these

22. The name of the iron-containing protein that gives red blood vessels their colour is

A. Myoglobin **B.** Hemocyanin
C. Haemoglobin **D.** Pyrite

23. Red cell count is carried out by __________.

A. Electrogram **B.** Haemocytometer
C. Haemoglobinometer **D.** Sphygmomanometer

24. An increased white blood cell count is indicative of which disease?

A. Melanoma **B.** Haemophilia
C. Anaemia **D.** Leukaemia

25. The blood cells that secrete antibodies are __________

A. Neutrophils
B. Eosinophils
C. Lymphocytes
D. Monocytes

26. Absence of ______________ clotting factor leads to haemophilia.

A. Factor X **B.** Factor VII
C. Factor IX **D.** Factor VIII

27. Orange colour of urine indicates __________.

A. Brain infections
B. Liver disease
C. Kidney diseases
D. None of the above

28. Destruction of red bone marrow results in a condition called __________.

A. Haemolytic anaemia
B. Megaloblastic anaemia
C. Aplastic anaemia
D. All of the above

29. __________ means decrease in number of erythrocytes.

A. Anaemia **B.** Leukaemia
C. Anuria **D.** Leucopenia

30. Leukopenia is __________ in white blood cell count.

A. Elevated **B.** Decrease
C. Increase **D.** All of the above

31. The normal volume of urine is ________ ml/24 hours.

A. 5000–6000 **B.** 600–2500
C. 1200–2400 **D.** None of the above

32. Normally odour of urine is __________.

A. Characteristic
B. Slightly "nutty"
C. Aromatic
D. Both A and B

33. Urine glucose is detected by __________.

A. The copper sulphate method
B. Dipstick
C. Both A and B
D. None of these

34. Rothera's test is for the detection of ____________ in the urine.

A. Sugar **B.** Ketones
C. Proteins **D.** None of the above

35. The disorder of platelets results into _________.

A. Thalassemia
B. Thrombocytopenia
C. Leukocytes
D. Leukopenia

36. The disorder of red blood cells results into ________.

A. Aplastic anaemia
B. Thalassemia
C. Sickle cell anaemia
D. All of the above

37. The most important organic substances in urine is __________.

A. Creatinine
B. Calcium
C. Iron
D. All of the above

38. ____________ is used for the detection of albumin and globulin in urine.

A. Fouchet's test
B. Heat coagulation test
C. Benzidine test
D. Hay's test

39. The following are an abnormal constituents of urine *except* __________.

A. Bile
B. Ammonia
C. Pus
D. Ketone bodies

40. Hay's test performs for the detection of __________.

A. Albumin **B.** Bile salt
C. Glucose **D.** Fructose

Answer Key

1 B	2 B	3 B	4 C	5 C	6 B	7 D	8 C	9 B	10 B
11 A	12 B	13 B	14 C	15 B	16 C	17 D	18 A	19 A	20 B
21 A	22 C	23 B	24 D	25 C	26 D	27 B	28 C	29 A	30 B
31 B	32 B	33 C	34 B	35 B	36 D	37 A	38 B	39 B	40 B

Section IX

Pharmacotherapeutics

1. Introduction to Pharmacotherapeutics
2. Cardiovascular System
3. Respiratory System
4. Endocrine System
5. Central Nervous System
6. Gastrointestinal Disorders
7. Haematological Disorders
8. Infectious Diseases
9. Musculoskeletal Disorders
10. Dermatology
11. Psychiatric Disorders
12. Ophthalmology
13. Anti-microbial Resistance
14. Women's Health

Syllabus (As Per ER 2020) Pharmacotherapeutics

Chapter	Topics
1	**Pharmacotherapeutics:** Introduction, scope, and objectives. Rational use of Medicines, Evidence Based Medicine, Essential Medicines List, Standard Treatment Guidelines (STGs)
2	Definition, etiopathogenesis, clinical manifestations, non-pharmacological and pharmacological management of the diseases associated with: **(a) Cardiovascular System** ■ Hypertension ■ Hyperlipidaemia ■ Angina and Myocardial infarction ■ Congestive Heart Failure **(b) Respiratory System** ■ Asthma ■ COPD **(c) Endocrine System** ■ Diabetes ■ Thyroid disorders—Hypo and Hyperthyroidism **(d) Central Nervous System** ■ Epilepsy ■ Alzheimer's disease ■ Migraine ■ Parkinson's disease ■ Stroke **(e) Gastrointestinal Disorders** ■ Gastro-oesophageal reflux disease ■ Peptic ulcer disease ■ Alcoholic liver disease ■ Inflammatory Bowel Diseases (Crohn's Disease and Ulcerative Colitis) **(f) Haematological Disorders** ■ Iron deficiency anaemia ■ Megaloblastic anaemia **(g) Infectious Diseases** ■ Tuberculosis ■ Urinary tract infections ■ Gonorrhoea and syphilis ■ HIV and opportunistic infections ■ Pneumonia ■ Hepatitis ■ Malaria ■ Viral Infections (SARS, CoV2) **(h) Musculoskeletal Disorders** ■ Rheumatoid arthritis ■ Osteoarthritis **(i) Dermatology** ■ Psoriasis ■ Scabies ■ Eczema **(j) Psychiatric Disorders** ■ Depression ■ Anxiety ■ Psychosis **(k) Ophthalmology** ■ Conjunctivitis (bacterial and viral) ■ Glaucoma **(l) Anti-microbial Resistance** **(m) Women's Health** ■ Polycystic Ovary Syndrome ■ Dysmenorrhea ■ Premenstrual Syndrome

CHAPTER 1

Introduction to Pharmacotherapeutics

1. The study of quality use of ________________ imparts knowledge and skills necessary for contribution quality use of medicines.

A. Pharmaceutics
B. Pharmacotherapeutics
C. Pharmacokinetics
D. Pharmacovigilance

2. The objective of study of pharmacotherapeutics is ______

A. To ensure patient compliance
B. To avoid medical errors
C. To maximize the effect
D. All of the above

3. Pharmacotherapeutics is the study of __________

A. Effect of drugs
B. Therapeutic uses
C. Both A and B
D. None of the above

4. Which of the following medicines satisfy the priority healthcare needs of the population?

A. Non-essential medicines
B. Essential medicines
C. Unethical medicines
D. Toxic medicines

5. EBM stands for __________

A. Economic based medicines
B. Evidence based medicines
C. Everyone based medicines
D. Eternal based medicines

6. The following is a feature of standard treatment guideline (STG) manual __________

A. Simplicity **B.** Credibility
C. User friendly **D.** All of the above

7. _______________ become the first country to prepare Essential Medicine List (EML).

A. Ethiopia **B.** Tanzania
C. Malaysia **D.** Uganda

8. The WHO model list of Essential Medicines is updated every __________ years.

A. 03 **B.** 04
C. 02 **D.** 05

9. Pharmacotherapy is therapy using __________

A. Radiation therapy
B. Pharmaceutical drugs
C. Surgical therapy
D. All of the above

10. __________ are the experts responsible for application of good pharmacotherapeutics practices.

A. Nurses
B. Physicians
C. Pharmacists
D. None of the above

11. EML stands for __________

A. Economic Medicine List
B. Essential Medicine List
C. Earliest Medicine List
D. Easy Medicine List

12. Which of the following is a reason for irrational use of medicines?

A. Demand from the patient
B. Role models of seniors
C. Self medication
D. All of the above

13. The prescriber should have the following aim?
- **A.** Minimize the effectiveness
- **B.** Minimize the risk
- **C.** Maximize the cost
- **D.** All of the above

14. __________ revises and publishes NLEM in India.
- **A.** IJPER
- **B.** JJPER
- **C.** ICMR
- **D.** IDMA

15. Impact of irrational drug usage __________
- **A.** Drug resistance
- **B.** Morbidity and mortality
- **C.** ADRs
- **D.** All of the above

16. NLEM stands for __________
- **A.** Natural List of Essential Medicines
- **B.** National List of Essential Medicines
- **C.** Nominal List of Essential Medicines
- **D.** Numerical List of Essential Medicines

17. The first NLEM of India was released in the year _____
- **A.** 1986 **B.** 1996
- **C.** 2006 **D.** 2016

18. Selection criterion for essential drug list __________
- **A.** Drug safety
- **B.** Disease prevalence
- **C.** Cost effectiveness
- **D.** All of the above

19. Which of the following is not a qualitative research methodology?
- **A.** Grounded theory
- **B.** Ethnography
- **C.** Randomized control trial
- **D.** Phenomenology

20. Standard Treatment Guidelines are also termed ______
- **A.** Clinical protocol
- **B.** Clinical guidelines
- **C.** Both A and B
- **D.** None of the above

21. STGs stand for __________
- **A.** State Treatment Guidelines
- **B.** Standard Treatment Guidelines
- **C.** Single Treatment Guidelines
- **D.** Some Treatment Guidelines

22. Which of the following is an irrational use of medicines?
- **A.** Incorrect dosing
- **B.** Polypharmacy
- **C.** Unnecessary combination
- **D.** All of the above

23. The study of therapeutic uses and effects of drugs is __________
- **A.** Pharmacodynamics
- **B.** Pharmacology
- **C.** Pharmacotherapeutics
- **D.** Pharmacokinetics

24. NGOs stand for __________
- **A.** Non-governmental Organizations
- **B.** Near-governmental organizations
- **C.** Nine-governmental Organizations
- **D.** Non-governor Organizations

25. The use of at least five drugs daily by an individual is __________
- **A.** Pharmacy
- **B.** Polypharmacy
- **C.** Monopharmacy
- **D.** Monotherapy

26. Which of the following patient related factors leading to irrational drug usage?
- **A.** Inability to communicate problem
- **B.** Drug misinformation
- **C.** Misleading belief
- **D.** All of the above

27. ICMR stands for __________
- **A.** Indian Council of Medical Research
- **B.** Indian Corporation of Medical Research
- **C.** Indian Cadet of Medical Research
- **D.** Indian Component of Medical Research

28. The aim of ______________ is to generate data for optimum use of drugs and the practice 'evidence-based medicine'.
- **A.** Pharmacogenomics
- **B.** Pharmacotherapeutics
- **C.** Clinical pharmacology
- **D.** Pharmacovigilance

29. Find out the incorrect statement: Essential medicines list is prepared by considering __________
- **A.** Safety of medicines
- **B.** Disease prevalence
- **C.** Efficacy of medicines
- **D.** Manufacturer of medicines

30. **The updated WHO List of Essential Medicines and List of Essential Medicines for Children are published every __________**
    A. Five years B. One year
    C. Two years D. Three years

31. **Barrier to adherence is __________**
    A. Ran out of pills B. Slept in
    C. Away from home D. All of the above

32. **Which of the following does not affect CNS?**
    A. Anti-anxiety B. Anti-Parkinson drug
    C. Antianginal drugs D. Hypnotic drugs

33. **Drawbacks of irrational drug prescribing are _______**
    A. Prolong hospitalization
    B. Delay in cure
    C. More side effects
    D. All of the above

34. **The aim of _______ is to generate data for optimum use of drugs and the practice of evidences-based medicines.**
    A. Toxicology
    B. Clinical pharmacology
    C. Socioeconomics
    D. Clinical biology

35. **How many features are keys to the success of an STG?**
    A. 7 B. 4
    C. 5 D. 6

36. **The STGS are published as ________ pocket manuals, which makes them convenient to carry and use.**
    A. Small, endurable B. Small, durable
    C. Large, durable D. Large, endurable

37. **Who should present the new guidelines at a public forum?**
    A. Leading clinicians
    B. The Minister of Health
    C. The leaders of professional bodies
    D. All of the above

38. **Rational use of medicines includes __________**
    A. Right medicine B. Right dose
    C. Right indication D. All of the above

39. **__________ is use of medicine in treatment of disease, conditions and symptoms.**
    A. Pharmacokinetics
    B. Pharmacodynamics
    C. Pharmacotherapeutics
    D. None of the above

40. **Which of the following is not the key feature of standard treatment guidelines?**
    A. Medicine supply based on standards
    B. Complexity
    C. User friendly
    D. None of the above

Answer Key

1 B	2 D	3 C	4 B	5 B	6 D	7 B	8 C	9 D	10 C
11 B	12 D	13 B	14 C	15 D	16 B	17 B	18 D	19 D	20 C
21 B	22 D	23 C	24 A	25 B	26 D	27 A	28 C	29 D	30 C
31 D	32 C	33 D	34 B	35 A	36 B	37 D	38 D	39 C	40 B

CHAPTER 2

Cardiovascular System

Hypertension, Angina and Myocardial Infarction Hyperlipidemia, Congestive Heart Failure

1. The most common cause of heart failure is _________

A. Aortic stenosis
B. Ischemic heart failure
C. Hypertension
D. Sarcoidosis

2. Angina pectoris means __________

A. Pain below the abdomen
B. Low blood pressure
C. Chest pain caused by coronary heart disease
D. None of the above

3. __________ is commonly called silent killer.

A. Hypoglycemia **B.** Hypertension
C. Hyponatremia **D.** Hypotension

4. Which is the first line lipid lowering drug from the following?

A. Niacin **B.** Ezetimibe
C. Inclisiran **D.** Atorvastatin

5. The total cholesterol of higher than 240 mg/dl is _____

A. Normal **B.** Abnormal
C. Moderate **D.** None of the above

6. The following is not a type of heart failure?

A. Congestive heart failure
B. Right-sided heart failure
C. Myocardial heart failure
D. Left-sided heart failure

7. Which of the following may cause heart failure?

A. Untreated hypertension
B. Myocardial infarction
C. Both A and B
D. None of the above

8. The blood clot that lodges the cerebral artery cause __________

A. Depression **B.** Stroke
C. Insomnia **D.** Anxiety

9. The angina which is usually provoked by physical exertion or emotional stress is

A. Prinzmetal angina
B. Stable angina
C. Unstable angina
D. Vasospastic angina

10. ______ measure of myocardial oxygen consumption.

A. Heart rate
B. Blood pressure
C. Angina index
D. Body mass index

11. Angina index can be calculated as

A. Angina index = pulse rate × diastolic BP
B. Angina index = heart rate × systolic BP
C. Angina index = heart rate × diastolic BP
D. Angina index = pulse rate × systolic BP

12. Which type of angina attacks are unpredictable and almost always occur at rest or during sleep?

A. Stable angina
B. Prinzmetal angina
C. Classical angina
D. Cardiac syndrome

13. The normal range of blood pressure is __________

A. 90/100 mmHg
B. 70/110 mmHg
C. 150/90 mm/Hg
D. 120/80 mmHg

14. Crescendo angina is __________

A. Classical angina
B. Cardiac syndrome
C. Unstable angina
D. Stable angina

15. The blood pressure is measured by an instrument known as __________

A. Glucometer
B. Spirometer
C. Peak flow meter
D. Sphygmomanometer

16. Full form of NSTEMI is __________

A. Native-ST-Section Elevation Myocardial Infarction
B. Native-ST-Segment Elevation Myocardial Infarction
C. Non-ST-Segment Elevation Myocardial Infarction
D. Null-ST-Segment Elevation Myocardial Infarction

17. CCF means __________

A. Congestive column failure
B. Congestive heart failure
C. Congestive cardiac failure
D. Congestive critical failure

18. Which one of the following is non-pharmacological management of angina?

A. Smoking cessation
B. Avoid alcohol consumption
C. Weight loss
D. All of the above

19. The condition in which there is an inadequate supply of oxygen to a portion of the myocardium is known as __________

A. Toxemia B. Anaemia
C. Ischemia D. Septicemia

20. Which is the most common type of angina?

A. Microvascular angina
B. Stable angina
C. Unstable angina
D. Coital angina

21. Hypertension is systolic blood pressure greater than __________ and/or diastolic blood pressure greater than __________

A. 130 mmHg: 90 mmHg
B. 120 mmHg: 80 mmHg
C. 140 mmHg; 90 mmHg
D. 140 mmHg: 80 mmHg

22. What are the two categories of angina?

A. Arterial and venous
B. Stable and unstable
C. Chronic and acute
D. Severe and mild

23. Hyperlipidaemia is a condition of having serum concentrations of total cholesterol __________

A. >200 kg/dl B. <200 mg/dl
C. >200 mg/dl D. >200 mg/ml

24. Which is the common sign and symptom of heart failure?

A. Fatigue
B. Swelling
C. Shortness of breath or trouble breathing
D. All of the above

25. Angina pectoris is a major symptom of __________

A. Low blood pressure
B. Myocardial infarction
C. Cyanosis
D. High blood pressure

26. Which of the following medications is not used to treat angina?

A. Anti-anxiety drugs
B. Beta blockers
C. Nitro-glycerine
D. Calcium channel blockers

27. Which of the following is not a cause of angina?

A. Atheroma
B. Plaque disruption–thrombus
C. Severe anaemia
D. Oversensitivity to vasoconstrictors

28. The myocardial infarction is also known as _______

A. Hypertension
B. Diabetes
C. Heart attack
D. Endocarditis

29. Which of the following is the most common symptom of myocardial infarction?

A. Dyspnea B. Edema
C. Chest pain D. Palpitations

30. What is not a primary cause of congestive heart failure?

A. Coronary artery disease
B. Poliomyelitis
C. Cardiomyopathy
D. High blood pressure

31. Which of the following is an example of ACE inhibitor?

A. Losartan B. Amlodipine
C. Thiazide D. Captopril

32. Which of these can cause angina?

A. Old age B. Tobacco
C. Stress D. All of the above

33. ________________ is not used in CHF.

A. Calcium channel blocker
B. Selective beta-blocker
C. Non-selective beta-blocker
D. Mixed blocker

34. Which one of this drug is not prescribed routinely for the treatment of congestive heart failure (CHF)?

A. Digitalis B. Diuretics
C. ACE inhibitors D. Benzodiazepine

35. Angina where there is no coronary artery blockage is __________.

A. Unstable angina B. Classical angina
C. Stable angina D. Microvascular angina

36. Which of the following is an agonist in hypertension?

A. Nifedipine B. Clonidine
C. Ivabradine D. Ticlopidine

37. Identify the drug which is not a thiazide diuretic.

A. Hydrochlorothiazide
B. Torsemide
C. Metolazone
D. Indapamide

38. The heart attack occurs when there is blood clotting in __________

A. Renal arteries B. Coronary arteries
C. Mesenteric arteries D. Hepatic arteries

39. ______________ is an example of non-selective alpha-blocker.

A. Clonidine B. Pheniramine
C. Phentolamine D. Prazosin

40. Inotropic effect is seen with __________.

A. Amlodipine B. Digoxin
C. Minoxidil D. Propranolol

Answer Key

1 C	2 C	3 B	4 D	5 B	6 C	7 C	8 B	9 B	10 C
11 B	12 B	13 D	14 C	15 D	16 C	17 C	18 D	19 C	20 B
21 C	22 B	23 C	24 D	25 B	26 A	27 C	28 C	29 C	30 D
31 D	32 D	33 A	34 D	35 D	36 B	37 B	38 B	39 C	40 B

CHAPTER 3

Respiratory System
Asthma, COPD

1. Asthma is caused due to the inflammation of ________
- A. Lungs
- B. Bronchi and bronchioles
- C. Pharynx
- D. Larynx

2. The following drug can cause drug-induced asthma?
- A. Kanamycin
- B. Aspirin
- C. Streptomycin
- D. Erythromycin

3. COPD stands for __________
- A. Chronic occlusion pulmonary disease
- B. Chronic obstructive pulmonary disease
- C. Chronic obsessive pulmonary disease
- D. Chronic open pulmonary disease

4. The phenomenon in which alveolar walls are vanished due to damage and sac space increase with decrease in surface area is called __________
- A. Chronic bronchitis
- B. Asthma
- C. Emphysema
- D. Status asthmaticus

5. The antibiotics help in COPD __________
- A. Making mast cell release
- B. By preventing infection
- C. As bronchodilator
- D. By improving inflammation

6. Swelling and itching of the bronchi is a symptom of __________
- A. Bronchioles
- B. Bronchitis
- C. Bronchoconstriction
- D. Bronchodilatation

7. Most patients with COPD have a history of_________
- A. Sugar intake
- B. Cigarette smoking
- C. Vitamin intake
- D. Mineral intake

8. Which of the following is used as inhaled corticosteroid?
- A. Budesonide
- B. Prednisone
- C. Fluticasone
- D. Prednisolone

9. An asthma __________ occurs when asthma symptoms become worse than usual.
- A. Event
- B. Crisis
- C. Attack
- D. All of the above

10. Which of the following symptoms do COPD sufferers often experience?
- A. Lack of energy
- B. Shortness of breath
- C. A chronic cough that produces phlegm
- D. All of the above

11. Medically speaking, breathlessness or being short of breath is called __________
- A. Bronchitis
- B. Dyspnoea
- C. Asthma
- D. Winded

12. Which of the following is not used in COPD?

A. Corticosteroids
B. Methylxanthines
C. LAMA
D. Mast cell stabilizers

13. Identify the chronic inflammatory disease among the following:

A. Cancer
B. Diabetes mellitus
C. Asthma
D. Myasthenia gravis

14. Bullectomy in COPD is carried out to __________

A. Replace bronchi
B. Remove non-functional alveoli
C. Create positive pressure
D. Increase lung volume

15. The asthma in which symptoms occur daily and at least one night every week is __________

A. Severe persistent asthma
B. Mild intermittent asthma
C. Mild persistent asthma
D. Moderate persistent asthma

16. Which one of the following drug is trigger factor for asthma?

A. Vitamin K
B. Insulin select the short-acting β_2 agonist
C. Aspirin
D. Salbutamol

17. What is a common symptom of asthma?

A. Snoring
B. Wheezing
C. Whistling
D. Full breaths

18. Select the short-acting β_2 agonist among the following drugs:

A. Terbutaline
B. Atropine
C. Tiotropium
D. Prednisone

19. Which medication helps relieve airway inflammation caused by severe asthma?

A. Methylprednisolone
B. Prednisone
C. Both A and B
D. None of the above

20. Which of the following is not used as immunosuppressant in asthma?

A. Ipratropium B. Omalizumab
C. Cromolyn D. Monteleukast

21. Signs and symptoms that interfere with asthma are __________.

A. Exercise
B. Sleep
C. Work
D. All of the above

22. The air passages in the lungs become narrow due to __________ of the muscles around the small airways.

A. Loosening and tightening
B. Inflammation and tightening
C. Inflammation and swelling
D. Inflammation and loosening

23. In what age group is the asthma incidence rate the highest?

A. Children
B. Adult
C. Elderly
D. All of the above

24. Which of the antiasthmatic drugs act as bronchodilators?

A. Theophylline
B. Salbutamol
C. Ipratropium
D. All of the above

25. __________ affects the air sacs in the lungs, as well as the walls between them. They become damaged and are less elastic.

A. Chronic bronchitis
B. Emphysema
C. Both A and B
D. Asthma

26. __________ is a PDE-4 inhibitor.

A. Ipratropium bromide
B. Theophylline
C. Roflumilast
D. None of the above

27. The COPD is treated by __________

A. Supplemental oxygen
B. Bronchodilators
C. Inhaled corticosteroids
D. All of the above

28. Late-phase asthmatic response results in __________

A. Hyper responsiveness of bronchial smooth muscles
B. Epithelial damage
C. Airway edema
D. All of the above

29. The asthma which is diagnosed for the first time in adult years is __________

A. Non-allergic asthma
B. Late-onset asthma
C. Allergic asthma
D. Asthma with fixed airflow limitation

30. The cause of an asthma attack is __________

A. Irritants
B. Allergens
C. Smoke
D. All of the above

Answer Key

1 B	2 B	3 B	4 C	5 B	6 B	7 B	8 C	9 C	10 D
11 B	12 D	13 C	14 B	15 D	16 C	17 B	18 A	19 C	20 A
21 D	22 B	23 B	24 D	25 B	26 C	27 D	28 A	29 B	30 D

CHAPTER 4

Endocrine System

Diabetes, Thyroid Disorders: Hypo and Hyperthyroidism

1. **Diabetes disease is known as __________**
   - A. Graves disease
   - B. Hensen's disease
   - C. Madhumeha
   - D. Madhu leha

2. **The hormone that is secreted by the alpha cells of the pancreas that raises blood glucose when levels are low is __________**
   - A. Epinephrine
   - B. Glucagon
   - C. Insulin
   - D. Cortisol

3. **The duration of rapid acting insulin is _______ hours.**
   - A. 1 to 2
   - B. 2 to 3
   - C. 3 to 4
   - D. 6 to 8

4. **What are the symptoms of too much release of T3 and T4 hormones?**
   - A. Hair loss
   - B. Anxiety
   - C. Nervousness
   - D. All of the above

5. **Insulin _____________ the amount of sugar in blood stream.**
   - A. Lowers
   - B. Raises
   - C. Does not changes
   - D. Elevates

6. **Deficiency of iodine produce __________**
   - A. Gangrene
   - B. Goitre
   - C. Gout
   - D. Gingivitis

7. **__________ promote the release of insulin from Beta-cells of Islets of Langerhans.**
   - A. Biguanides
   - B. Sulfonyl ureas
   - C. Nonsulfonylurea
   - D. Alpha-glucosidase inhibitors

8. **Oral hypoglycaemic agents are never indicated for __________**
   - A. Type II diabetes mellitus
   - B. Type I diabetes mellitus
   - C. Both A and C
   - D. All of the above

9. **Which of the following is not a common physical sign of hypothyroidism?**
   - A. Jaundice
   - B. Ascites
   - C. Bradycardia
   - D. Slowed speech and movements

10. **__________ mainly controls and regulates the thyroid activity.**
    - A. Pituitary gland
    - B. Parathyroid gland
    - C. Adrenal gland
    - D. Pineal gland

11. **The main hormone secreted by the thyroid gland______**
    - A. T3
    - B. T4
    - C. Both A and B
    - D. TSH

12. **Medications for hypothyroidism include treatment that:**
    - A. Replaces surfactant
    - B. Replaces insulin
    - C. Replaces ADH
    - D. Replaces TH

13. **Which of the following is a clinical manifestation of diabetes mellitus?**
    - A. Polyuria
    - B. Hyperglycemia
    - C. Polyphagia
    - D. All of the above

14. **Which drug may have comparatively high risk to cause hypothyroidism?**
A. Digoxin B. Amiodarone
C. Verapamil D. Spironolactone

15. **Thiazolidinediones are also known as __________**
A. Acarbose B. Glipizide
C. Glyburide D. Glitazones

16. **Rapid heart rate, weight loss, heat sensitivity are most likely the symptoms of**
A. Hyperthyroidism B. Thyroid cancer
C. Hypothyroidism D. All of the above

17. **Which adrenergic blockers are used to manage hyperthyroidism?**
A. Carvedilol and Bisoprolol
B. Bisoprolol and Atenolol
C. Propranolol and Nadolol
D. Atenolol and Carvedilol

18. **The sign of hyperthyroidism is __________**
A. Tachycardia B. Weight loss
C. Tremor D. All of the above

19. **Identify type of diabetes which is commonly associated with overweight and obesity.**
A. Monogenic diabetes mellitus
B. Type 1 diabetes mellitus
C. Type 2 diabetes mellitus
D. Gestational diabetes mellitus

20. **Diagnostic parameter for diabetes is fasting plasma glucose level __________ mg/dl.**
A. >126 B. >200
C. <100 D. >100

21. **First choice pharmacotherapy for type 2 diabetes mellitus is __________**
A. Sitagliptin B. Metformin
C. Glipizide D. Acarbose

22. **Insulin aspart is an example of __________**
A. Ultra long-acting insulin
B. Rapid-acting insulin
C. Short-acting insulin
D. Intermediate-acting insulin

23. **Hashimoto's thyroiditis causes __________**
A. Diabetes mellitus B. Hyperglycaemia
C. Hypothyroidism D. Thyrotoxicosis

24. **Hyperthyroidism is caused by __________**
A. Thyroid hypoplasia B. Graves' disease
C. Hashimoto's thyroiditis D. Iodine deficiency

25. **Which of the following is a chronic complication of diabetes mellitus?**
A. Hypoglycaemia
B. Diabetic ketoacidosis
C. Nephritis
D. Retinopathy

26. **Myxoedema is a condition associated with __________**
A. Hypertension B. Hypothyroidism
C. Hyperthyroidism D. CHF

27. **Diagnostic parameter for prediabetes is Oral Glucose Tolerance Test (OGTT) __________ mg/dl**
A. 250–300 B. 100–125
C. 140–199 D. 200–250

28. **Too much release of thyroid hormone in the body causes __________**
A. Goitre B. Hypothyroidism
C. Hyperthyroidism D. None of the above

29. **The four small glands present in the thyroid gland are known as __________**
A. Adrenal glands
B. Pineal glands
C. Parathyroid glands
D. Endocrine and exocrine glands

30. **T_4 and T_3 are the hormones secreted by __________**
A. Parathyroid glands B. Adrenal glands
C. Thyroid glands D. Testes

Answer Key

1 C	2 B	3 C	4 D	5 A	6 B	7 B	8 B	9 B	10 A
11 C	12 D	13 D	14 B	15 D	16 A	17 C	18 D	19 C	20 A
21 B	22 B	23 C	24 B	25 D	26 B	27 C	28 C	29 C	30 C

CHAPTER 5

Central Nervous System
Epilepsy, Parkinson's Disease, Alzheimer's Disease, Stroke, Migraine

1. Migraine is ________ disorder.

A. A vascular
B. A neurovascular
C. A neuronal
D. A pulmonary

2. The first phase of migraine might last a few hours or even days. This phase is known as __________

A. Pre-aura
B. Prodrome
C. Aura
D. Pre-headache

3. What causes Parkinson's disease?

A. Depression
B. A severe blood infection
C. Loss of the brain chemical dopamine
D. Stroke

4. Alzheimer disease is the most common form of which of these?

A. Fatigue
B. Malnutrition
C. Dementia
D. Psychosis

5. Which is an ergot alkaloid, given in IV form for management of migraine headache?

A. Estradiol
B. Ergotamine
C. Carbidopa
D. Dihydroergotamine

6. Which is the most important differential diagnosis of 'first seizure'?

A. Syncope
B. Migraine without aura
C. Abdominal migraine
D. Migraine with aura

7. The classic features of Parkinson's disease are _____

A. Rigidity
B. Akinesia
C. Tremor at rest
D. All of the above

8. Which of the following neurotransmitters is low in Parkinson's disease?

A. Dopamine
B. Serotonin
C. Noradrenaline
D. All of the above

9. What is often the first symptom of Parkinson disease?

A. Turning of the head
B. Headache
C. Nausea
D. Shaking of a hand or foot

10. How is Parkinson disease diagnosed?

A. With an X-ray
B. With a blood test
C. With a neurological exam
D. All of the above

11. How is Parkinson disease treated?

A. Surgery
B. Medicine
C. Radiation
D. Both A and B

12. Which central neurotransmitters are affected by Alzheimer's disease?

A. Glutamate
B. Acetylcholine
C. Norepinephrine
D. All of the above

13. **Degeneration of dopaminergic neurones causes __________**
    A. Stroke
    B. Myasthenia gravis
    C. Parkinson's disease
    D. Migraine

14. **Which of the following is not an anti-epileptic drug?**
    A. Clonazepam B. Levothyroxine
    C. Clobazam D. Diazepam

15. **What are the stages of migraine?**
    A. Attack B. Prodrome
    C. Aura D. All of the above

16. **Which is not a symptom of Parkinson's disease?**
    A. Vision loss
    B. Tremor
    C. Writing changes
    D. Speech changes

17. **Another name of stroke is __________**
    A. Heart attack B. Brain attack
    C. Viral attack D. Bacterial attack

18. **Parkinson is induced by all drugs *except* __________**
    A. Amantadine
    B. Reserpine
    C. Metaclopramide
    D. Chlorpromazine

19. **As per AHA/ ASA guidelines, alteplase should be started within _________ hours of onset of ischemic stroke.**
    A. 4 B. 5
    C. 3 D. 6

20. **What is the most common type of seizure?**
    A. The simple seizure
    B. The grand mal seizure
    C. The absence seizure
    D. The complex seizure

21. **Which of the following is a trigger factor for migraine?**
    A. Physical triggers
    B. Emotional triggers
    C. Environmental triggers
    D. All of the above

22. **First symptoms of Parkinson's disease is __________**
    A. Postural instability
    B. Tremors
    C. Rigidity
    D. Bradykinesia

23. **Signs of Alzheimer disease include which of these symptoms?**
    A. Restlessness
    B. Loss of memory
    C. Increase in irritability
    D. All of the above

24. **Tonic-clonic seizure is also known as __________**
    A. Focal seizures
    B. Grand mal epilepsy
    C. Petit-mal epilepsy
    D. Absence seizures

25. **A sudden, brief, repetitive contraction of muscles of a limb or the whole body may be __________**
    A. Absence seizures
    B. Atonic seizures
    C. Myoclonic seizures
    D. Tonic seizures

26. **Valproate acts by __________**
    A. Inhibiting Na^+ channels
    B. Increasing GABA
    C. Decreasing GABA
    D. Blocking Ca^{++} channel

27. **The term migraine is originated from Greek word __________**
    A. Cranium B. Cranicoid
    C. Hermacoid D. Hermicrania

28. **Alzheimer disease appears before age.**
    A. 30 B. 40
    C. 50 D. 60

29. **Select the antiepileptic drug which acts by inactivating Na^+ channel.**
    A. Ethosuximide B. Valproate
    C. Phenytoin D. Levetiracetam

30. **The most serious side effect reported with valproic acid is __________**
    A. Pulmonary fibrosis
    B. Nephrotoxicity
    C. Hepatotoxicity
    D. Cardiac failure

31. **In Parkinson's disease, there is a predominant loss of dopaminergic neurons primarily in __________**
    A. Locus ceruleus
    B. Substantia nigra
    C. Cerebellar cortex
    D. Cerebral cortex

32. Parkinson's disease is caused by loss or degeneration of _________ neurons in the substantia nigra of the midbrain.

A. Dopaminergic
B. Adrenergic
C. Cholinergic
D. Histaminergic

33. The cardinal feature of Parkinson's disease among the following is _________

A. Sexual dysfunction
B. Rapid eye movement
C. Bradykinesia
D. Hyposmia

34. How is Alzheimer disease diagnosed?

A. Neurological tests
B. Mental-status tests
C. Blood tests
D. All of the above

35. Improvement of memory in Alzheimer's disease is brought about by drugs which increase transmission in _________

A. Cholinergic receptors
B. GABAergic receptors
C. Dopaminergic receptors
D. Adrenergic receptors

36. Onset of Parkinson's disease is usually between _________

A. 70 and 85 years of age
B. 20 and 30 years of age
C. 40 and 70 years of age
D. 30 and 40 years of age

37. Stroke characterized by the sudden obstruction of a blood vessel that supplies blood to an area of the brain is _________

A. Intracerebral haemorrhage stroke
B. Ischemic stroke
C. Haemorrhagic stroke
D. Subarachnoid haemorrhage stroke

38. Which one of the following is a thrombolytic drug?

A. Aspirin
B. Alteplase
C. Warfarin
D. Heparin

39. Ethosuximide is indicated for treatment of _________

A. Unclassified epilepsy
B. Focal epilepsy
C. Generalized tonic-clonic seizures
D. Generalized non-motor (absence) seizures

40. It is suggested that _________ is a key mediator in the pathogenesis of migraine.

A. Histamine
B. Acetylcholine
C. Serotonin
D. Adrenaline

Answer Key

1 B	2 B	3 C	4 C	5 D	6 A	7 D	8 A	9 D	10 C
11 D	12 B	13 C	14 B	15 D	16 A	17 B	18 A	19 C	20 B
21 D	22 B	23 D	24 B	25 C	26 B	27 D	28 D	29 C	30 C
31 B	32 A	33 C	34 D	35 B	36 C	37 B	38 B	39 D	40 C

CHAPTER 6

Gastrointestinal Disorders

Gastroesophageal Reflux Disease (GERD), Peptic Ulcer Disease, Alcoholic Liver Disease, Inflammatory Bowel Disease (IBD): Ulcerative Colitis and Crohn's Disease

1. People with GERD should avoid foods and beverages such as __________

A. Mint, tomato, mustard
B. Caffeine, alcoholic drinks, pepper
C. Orange, grapefruit, vinegar
D. All of the above

2. Which of the following is not a causative agent for a peptic ulcer?

A. *Helicobacter pylori*
B. NSAIDs
C. Augmentin
D. Physiological stress

3. __________ is associated with overproduction of stomach acid.

A. Crohn's disease B. Zollinger's disease
C. Graves disease D. Gastritis

4. Both gastric ulcers and *H. pylori* infection are highly associated with __________

A. Bloating
B. Gastric malignancy
C. Uveitis
D. Oesophageal neoplasms

5. IBD stands for __________

A. Intestine bowel disease
B. Induced bowel disease
C. Inflammatory bowel disease
D. Inflammatory Bowman's disease

6. Which of the following is the mainstay of treatment for alcohol-related liver disease?

A. A Disulfiram B. Abstinence
C. Naltrexone D. Baclofen

7. The adult dose of omeprazole in *H. pylori* eradication therapy is __________

A. 5 mg daily B. 10 mg daily
C. 20 mg twice daily D. 50 mg twice daily

8. Crohn's disease __________

A. Always affects the colon
B. May lead to intestinal obstruction
C. Is best treated surgically
D. Requires a gluten-free diet

9. A person who suffers from ulcerative colitis for a long period of time is at risk for __________

A. Haemorrhoids B. Colon cancer
C. Faecal incontinence D. Parkinson's disease

10. The condition in which gastric contents flow back into the oesophagus is __________

A. Asthma B. GERD
C. Peptic ulcer D. Appendicitis

11. PPIs stand for __________

A. Protein pump inhibitors
B. Proton pump inhibitors
C. Proteose pump inhibitors
D. Proguanil pump inhibitors

12. Hiatal hernia is a risk factor associated with ________

A. Peptic ulcer B. GERD
C. Asthma D. Angina pectoris

13. The long form ELISA is __________

A. Eco linked immunosorbent assay
B. Enzyme linked immunosorbent assay
C. Endo linked immunosorbent assay
D. Exeo linked immunosorbent assay

14. **Retrosternal pain is a symptom of ________.**
A. Epilepsy
B. GERD
C. Anaemia
D. Tuberculosis

15. **Which one of the following is extraoesophageal manifestation of GERD?**
A. Epigastric pain
B. Regurgitation
C. Heart burn
D. Otitis media

16. **Symptoms of ulcerative colitis can include ________**
A. Rectal bleeding
B. Abdominal pain
C. Diarrhoea
D. All of the above

17. **GERD is closely linked to ________**
A. Stomach cancer
B. Oesophageal cancer
C. Intestinal cancer
D. Anal cancer

18. **Select PPI drug among the following.**
A. Rabeprazole
B. Domperidone
C. Ranitidine
D. Metoclopramide

19. **Which one of the following drugs is contraindicated in peptic ulcer?**
A. Morphine
B. Ranitidine
C. Aspirin
D. Omeprazole

20. **Select the drug which is an irreversible inhibitor of H^+/K^+-ATPase pump ________**
A. Neostigmine
B. Captopril
C. Omeprazole
D. Sulphonamides

21. **Which of the following is a non-pharmacological management of peptic ulcer?**
A. Avoid alcohol
B. Avoid smoking
C. Avoid stress
D. All of the above

22. **Proton pump inhibitors are most effective when they are given ________**
A. After meals
B. Shortly before meals
C. Along with H blockers
D. During prolonged fasting periods

23. **Drug of choice for the treatment of peptic ulcer caused due to chronic use of NSAIDs is ________**
A. Pirenzepine
B. Loxatidine
C. Misoprostol
D. Esomeprazole

24. **Reflux is an alternative term for ________**
A. Vomiting
B. Acid erosion
C. Regurgitation
D. Salivating

25. **NSAID induced ulcers are treated by ________**
A. Antacids
B. H2 blockers
C. Misoprostol
D. PPI (proton pump inhibitors)

26. **Esomeprazole acts by inhibiting**
A. H^+/K^+-ATPase pump
B. H^+/Na^+-ATPase pump
C. H^+ pump
D. Any of the above

27. **All are H2 blockers *except* ________**
A. Omeprazole
B. Cimetidine
C. Famatodine
D. Ranitidine

28. **Which of the following is the drug of choice for treatment of peptic ulcer disease?**
A. Omeprazole
B. Pirenzepine
C. Ranitidine
D. Sucralfate

29. **Fundoplication is a surgical treatment for ________**
A. Asthma
B. GERD
C. Peptic ulcer
D. Appendicitis

30. **Urea breath test is used to confirm presence of ________**
A. *E. coli*
B. *S. typhi*
C. *H. pylori*
D. *Vibrio cholerae*

31. **________ is characterized by the deposition of fat in hepatocytes.**
A. Steatosis
B. Steatohepatitis
C. Cirrhosis
D. Hepatocellular carcinoma

32. **________ is the final stage of alcoholic liver disease.**
A. Alcoholic fatty liver
B. Alcoholic hepatitis
C. Alcohol-related cirrhosis
D. Hepatocellular carcinoma

33. **The cluster of swollen veins in abdomen is known as ____**
A. Jaundice
B. Ascites
C. Telangiectasia
D. Caput medusa

34. **Elevated __________ and __________ levels indicate recent excessive alcohol use.**
A. AST and GGT B. ALT and AST
C. ALT and GGT D. AST and GLDH

35. **A diffuse mucosal inflammation in GI tract which is limited to the rectum and colon is __________**
A. Ulcerative colitis B. Peptic ulcer
C. Crohn's disease D. GERD

36. **Ulcerative colitis that affects the entire colon is _______**
A. Ulcerative proctitis B. Distal colitis
C. Left-sided colitis D. Extensive colitis

37. **The adult oral dose of Omeprazole in *H. pylori* eradication therapy is __________**
A. 40 mg once daily B. 20 mg twice daily
C. 100 mg twice daily D. 100 mg once daily

38. **Drug not used in *H. pylori* is __________**
A. Metronidazole B. Omeprazole
C. Mosapride D. Amoxicillin

39. **A patchy, transmural inflammation of the gastro-intestinal tract that can affect any part, from the mouth to the anus is __________**
A. Ulcerative colitis B. Peptic ulcer
C. Crohn's disease D. GERD

40. **An indicative sign of liver disease is __________**
A. Hair loss B. Increased urination
C. Insomnia D. Jaundice

41. **Crohn's colitis is __________**
A. Inflammation of both the ileum and the large intestine (colon)
B. Inflammation and irritation of the ileum only
C. Inflammation of the colon only
D. Inflammation in the top half of the jejunum

42. **All of the following are signs and symptoms of Crohn's disease, *except* __________**
A. Fistulas B. Fever
C. Haematochezia D. Severe vomiting

43. **Chronic diarrhoea or constipation, bloody stool and iritis are some of the symptoms of __________**
A. GERD
B. Peptic ulcer
C. Alcoholic liver disease
D. Inflammatory bowel disease

44. **The feeling to pass stools is __________**
A. Nocebo B. Anorexia
C. Tenesmus D. Nausea

45. **Which of the following is a complication of peptic ulcer?**
A. Barrett's B. GI bleeding
C. Perforation D. Both B and C

46. **The first line of treatment for mild to moderate ulcerative colitis is __________**
A. Corticosteroids B. Amino salicylates
C. TNF-α inhibitors D. Thiopurines

47. **Sulpha drug used in inflammatory bowel disease includes __________**
A. Sulfasalazine B. Sulfamethoxazole
C. Sulfinpyrazone D. Solpadine

48. **Sulfasalazine is used in __________**
A. Ulcerative colitis
B. Osteoarthritis
C. Gouty arthritis
D. Irritable bowel syndrome

49. **Ulcerative colitis and Crohn's disease are types of ______**
A. Gastroesophageal reflux disease (GERD) intolerance
B. Peptic ulcer disease
C. Alcoholic liver disease
D. Inflammatory bowel disease

50. **Which amongst the following is a treatment of peptic ulcer disease?**
A. Proton pump inhibitors
B. Prostaglandin analogues
C. Anticholinergics
D. All of the above

51. ***Helicobacter pylori* (*H. pylori*) is a causative agent of which disease?**
A. Inflammatory bowel disease
B. Alcoholic liver disease
C. Peptic ulcer disease
D. GERD

52. **What are the risk factors of GERD?**
A. Smoking B. Eating large meals
C. Eating fried food D. All of the above

53. **GERD is a ____________ disorder that affect the ring of muscles.**
A. Respiratory B. Reproductive
C. Skeletal D. Digestive

54. **____________ is associated with overproduction of stomach acid.**
A. Crohn's syndrome
B. Graves disease
C. Polycystic ovary syndrome
D. Zollinger-Ellison syndrome

55. **The adult dose of omeprazole in *H. pylori* eradication therapy is ________**

A. 5 mg twice daily
B. 4 mg twice daily
C. 2 mg twice daily
D. 20 mg twice daily

56. **Continued consumption of a diet, rich in butter, red meat and eggs for longer period may cause ________**

A. Goitre
B. Hypocholesterolemia
C. Hypercholesterolemia
D. Hypoglycemia

57. **__________ is a digestive disorder that affects the ring of muscle, i.e. lower oesophageal sphincter between the oesophagus and your stomach.**

A. Inflammatory bowel disease
B. Alcoholic liver disease
C. Peptic ulcer disease
D. GERD

58. **What is the most common cause of chronic liver disease in the US?**

A. Genetics
B. Alcohol abuse
C. Bacteria
D. Viruses

59. ***Helicobacter pylori* can live in the stomach's acidic conditions because it secretes ______________ which neutralizes the acid.**

A. Ammonia
B. Urease
C. Carbon dioxide
D. Bicarbonate

60. **Which is a potential infectious agent responsible for occurrence of IBD?**

A. Protozoans
B. Mycobacteria
C. *Escherichia coli*
D. All of the above

Answer Key

1 D	2 C	3 B	4 B	5 C	6 B	7 C	8 B	9 B	10 B
11 B	12 A	13 B	14 B	15 D	16 D	17 B	18 A	19 C	20 C
21 D	22 B	23 D	24 C	25 D	26 B	27 A	28 A	29 B	30 C
31 A	32 C	33 D	34 A	35 A	36 D	37 B	38 C	39 C	40 D
41 C	42 D	43 D	44 C	45 D	46 B	47 A	48 D	49 D	50 D
51 C	52 D	53 D	54 D	55 D	56 C	57 D	58 B	59 A	60 D

CHAPTER 7

Haematological Disorders

Iron Deficiency Anaemia, Megaloblastic Anaemia

1. **The low haemoglobin signifies __________**
   A. Polycythemia B. Anaemia
   C. Leukaemia D. Leukopenia

2. **The substance in the diet which favours iron absorption is __________**
   A. Tannate B. Oxalate
   C. Ascorbic acid D. Phenate

3. **Which of the following is a symptom of megaloblastic anaemia?**
   A. Tonsillitis B. Glossitis
   C. Rhinitis D. Otitis

4. **Vitamin B_{12} deficiency results in __________**
   A. Microcytic red blood cell
   B. Large red blood cells
   C. Small and pale red blood cells
   D. Normal-sized red blood cells

5. **Identify the pathological condition associated with macrocytic anaemia __________**
   A. Myelofibrosis
   B. Sideroblastic anaemia
   C. Folic acid deficiency
   D. Autoimmune haemolytic anaemia

6. **Cobalt containing vitamin is __________**
   A. Vitamin C B. Vitamin K
   C. Vitamin A D. Vitamin B_{12}

7. **Iron deficiency anaemia is __________**
   A. Macrocytic, hypochromic
   B. Microcytic, hypochromic
   C. Microcytic, normochromic
   D. Macrocytic, normochromic

8. **Which of the following is a cause of anaemia?**
   A. Excessive blood loss
   B. Destruction of RBCs
   C. Failure of function of bone marrow
   D. All of the above

9. **The human body stores iron as __________ and hemosiderin in liver**
   A. Transferrin B. Haemoglobin
   C. Ferritin D. Erythropoietin

10. **Haemoglobin level (g/dl) that indicates severe anaemia in children of 12–14 years old is __________**
    A. >12 B. <8
    C. <9 D. <9.5

11. **Megaloblastic anaemia is a type of ________ anaemia.**
    A. Normochromic B. Microcytic
    C. Macrocytic D. Normocytic

12. **The life span of RBCs is __________ days.**
    A. 50 B. 60
    C. 100 D. 120

13. **The condition associated with increased demand of vitamin B_{12} is __________**
    A. Pregnancy
    B. Hypothyroidism
    C. Splenectomy
    D. Aplastic anaemia

14. **__________ is a most common symptom of megaloblastic anaemia.**
    A. Hypertension
    B. Sweating
    C. Fatigue
    D. Conjunctivitis

15. Consequence of vitamin B_{12} deficiency is impaired ________

A. Folic acid synthesjs
B. DNA synthesis
C. Production of intrinsic factor
D. Absorption of iron

16. Vitamin B_{12}-IF complex is absorbed in ________

A. Jejunum
B. First part of duodenum
C. Ileum
D. Second part of duodenum

17. The intrinsic factor is required for the absorption of ________

A. Magnesium **B.** Vitamin B_{12}
C. Zinc **D.** Iron

18. Di Guglielmo's syndrome is a cause of ________

A. Hypoplastic anaemia
B. Sickle cell anaemia
C. Megaloblastic anaemia
D. Haemolytic anaemia

19. Deficiency of intrinsic factor may be caused by ______

A. Gastrectomy
B. Crohn disease
C. Large bowel resection
D. Malabsorption syndrome

20. RBCs are produced in the red bone marrow by the process of ________

A. Fibrinolysis
B. Erythropoiesis
C. Haemolysis
D. Thrombosis

Answer Key

1 B	2 C	3 B	4 B	5 C	6 D	7 B	8 D	9 C	10 B
11 C	12 D	13 A	14 C	15 B	16 C	17 B	18 C	19 A	20 B

CHAPTER 8

Infectious Diseases

Tuberculosis, Pneumonia, Urinary Tract Infections, Hepatitis, Gonorrhoea and Syphilis, Malaria, HIV and Opportunistic Infections, Viral Infections—SARS-CoV-2

1. **Tuberculosis is also known as ___________**
   A. Graves disease
   B. Addison's disease
   C. Hansen's disease
   D. Koch's disease

2. **Pulmonary tuberculosis mainly affects ___________**
   A. Lungs B. Kidney
   C. Liver D. Pancreas

3. **Tuberculosis is the infectious _____________ born disease.**
   A. Food B. Water
   C. Air D. Insect bite

4. **First line drug used for TB treatment is ___________**
   A. Ethionamide
   B. Streptomycin
   C. Kanamycin
   D. Amikacin

5. **HIV stands for ___________**
   A. Human immunomodulatory virus
   B. Human integratory virus
   C. Human immunodeficiency virus
   D. Human immune enhancer virus

6. **___________ is the organ mainly affected by hepatitis.**
   A. Stomach B. Lungs
   C. Liver D. Oesophagus

7. **AIDS stands for ___________**
   A. Acquired Immunodeficiency syndrome
   B. Abnormal immunodeficiency virus
   C. Additional immunodeficiency virus
   D. Ancient immunodeficiency virus

8. **The major complications of falciparum malaria infection include ___________**
   A. Hypoglycaemia B. Seizures and coma
   C. Chronic renal failure D. Both A and B

9. **Urinary tract infection may also result due to the infection in the kidneys, the infection is also called ___________**
   A. Cystitis B. Urethritis
   C. Acute pyelonephritis D. Sinusitis

10. **The first person who discovered *Mycobacterium tuberculosis* was ___________**
    A. Louis Pasteur B. Robert Koch
    C. Edward Jenner D. None of the above

11. **MERS stands for ___________**
    A. Middle East Respiratory Syndrome
    B. More East Respiratory Syndrome
    C. Medium East Respiratory Syndrome
    D. Median East Respiratory Syndrome

12. **The chronic inflammation of the lining (synovial tissue) of joint capsule results in the proliferation of the tissue in ___________**
    A. Rheumatoid arthritis
    B. Osteoarthritis
    C. Both A and B
    D. None of the above

13. **___________ is an example of disease modifying anti-rheumatic drug (DMARD).**
    A. Prostaglandin
    B. Methotrexate
    C. Hyaluronic acid
    D. None of the above

14. ________ is a drug of treatment for both rheumatoid arthritis and osteoarthritis?
A. NASAIDs
B. DMARDs
C. Glucosamine and chondroitin
D. COX2

15. Intake of antacids should be restricted with drug______
A. Cyclomerize
B. Fluroquinolones
C. Bed aquiline
D. Ethionamide

16. Tuberculosis is treated with __________
A. Surgery
B. Antiviral medicines
C. Antibiotics
D. Monoclonal antibodies

17. The long form of RNTCP is __________
A. Rural National Tuberculosis Control Programme
B. Revised National Tuberculosis Control Programme
C. Research National Tuberculosis Cases Planning
D. Revised National Tuberculosis Cases Planning

18. NTEP stands for __________
A. National Tuberculosis Eradication Program
B. Novel Tuberculosis Eradication Program
C. National Tuberculosis Elimination Program
D. Non-Tuberculosis Existence Program

19. Recently, WHO recommended the ___________ for diagnosing TB.
A. Mantoux test
B. AFB test
C. ELISA
D. GeneXpert MTB/RIF assay

20. Which of the following bacterial pneumonia has the highest mortality rate?
A. *E. coli*
B. *P. aeruginosa*
C. Klebsiella spp.
D. *S. aureus*

21. Infection and inflammation of the urinary bladder is __________
A. Pyelonephritis
B. Urethritis
C. Cystitis
D. Prostatitis

22. Pyelonephritis is the inflammation of the__________
A. Prostate gland
B. Urethra
C. Bladder
D. Kidney

23. The bacteria responsible for more than 85% uncomplicated UTI is __________
A. *Klebsiella pneumoniae*
B. *Serratia marcescens*
C. *Escherichia coli*
D. *Staphylococcus saprophyticus*

24. ART stands for __________
A. Anti-rheumatic therapy
B. Anti-retroviral therapy
C. Anti-rhinitis therapy
D. Anti-rigorous therapy

25. The bacteria mainly responsible for nosocomial UTI is __________
A. *Klebsiella pneumonia*
B. *Serratia marcescens*
C. *Pseudomonas aeruginosa*
D. *Staphylococcus saprophyticus*

26. RT-PCR test is used for screening of __________
A. Malaria
B. Syphilis
C. Rabies
D. Covid-19

27. Bacteria mostly involved in complicated UTI is______
A. *Klebsiella pneumoniae*
B. *Enterococcus faecalis*
C. *Escherichia coli*
D. *Staphylococcus saprophyticus*

28. The assay uses quantitative real-time polymerase chain reaction (qRT-PCR) to detect both *M. tuberculosis* and rifampicin resistance within 2 hours is __________
A. RASQ
B. ELISA
C. GeneXpert MTB/RIF
D. GeneSupport

29. Serological detection of ___________ confirms the diagnosis of hepatitis A.
A. HBsAg
B. Anti-HCV antibodies
C. HBAg
D. Anti-HAV IgM antibodies

30. Which one of the following is DNA virus?
A. HCV
B. HAV
C. HBV
D. HDV

31. The route of transmission of hepatitis B virus is _____
A. Skin contact
B. Oral-faecal
C. HBV contaminated body fluids
D. Aerosol droplets

32. The incubation period for HCV is ___________

A. 15–60 days
B. 15–50 days
C. 30–180 days
D. 14–180 days

33. Which one of the following viruses is found only in patients with hepatitis B?

A. HAV
B. HCV
C. HBV
D. HEV

34. Remedesivir and Favipiravir are useful for the treatment of ___________

A. Gonorrhoea
B. Typhoid
C. Amoebiasis
D. Covid-19

35. The pregnant women are more prone to acute liver failure with ___________

A. Hepatitis B
B. Hepatitis E
C. Hepatitis C
D. Hepatitis D

36. The main causative agent of hepatitis is ___________

A. Viruses
B. Bacteria
C. Fungi
D. Autoimmune disorders

37. HIV is a ___________

A. Water borne virus
B. Blood borne virus
C. Air borne virus
D. Fomite borne virus

38. From the sample of blood ___________ elevated levels to confirm the hepatitis.

A. White blood cells
B. Interferon's
C. Calcium
D. Liver enzymes

39. Hepatitis C virus is ___________

A. Single-stranded RNA virus
B. Double-stranded RNA virus
C. Double-stranded DNA virus
D. Single-stranded DNA virus

40. Gonorrhoea is a ___________ disease.

A. Protozoal
B. Fungal
C. Viral
D. Bacterial

41. Diagnostic test for gonorrhoea is ___________

A. Liver function tests
B. Nucleic acid amplification testing
C. Venereal disease research laboratory (VDRL) slide test
D. GeneXpert MTB/RIF assay

42. Which of the following is STD disease?

A. Plague
B. Syphilis
C. Hepatitis A
D. Leprosy

43. Syphilis is complicated and organized sexually transmitted diseases where the causative agent is ________

A. A protozoan
B. A fungus
C. A virus
D. A bacterium

44. Drug of choice for syphilis in a pregnant lady is ______

A. Ceftriaxone
B. Penicillin
C. Azithromycin
D. Tetracycline

45. RT-PCR stands for ___________

A. Reverse transcription – polymerised chain reaction
B. Reverse transport – polymerised chain reaction
C. Reverse transit – polymerised chain reaction
D. Reverse tension polymerised chain reaction

46. Drug of choice for primary syphilis is ___________

A. Tetracycline
B. Ampicillin
C. Benzathine penicillin
D. Erythromycin

47. First line drug for falciparum malaria in pregnancy is ___________

A. Tetracycline
B. Chloroquine
C. Quinine
D. Primaquine

48. Dosage of benzyl penicillin in treatment of primary syphilis is ___________

A. 4.8 MU single IM
B. 1.2 MU single IM
C. 1.2 MU single IV
D. 2.4 MU single IM

49. Bite of mosquito causes malaria is ___________

A. Female *Aedes aegypti*
B. Female anopheles
C. Male anopheles
D. Male *Aedes aegypti*

50. Incubation period for falciparum malaria is _______

A. 10–30 days
B. 9–14 days
C. 8–17 days
D. 30–180 days

51. The sexual stage of malarial parasites occurs in ______

A. Human liver
B. Erythrocytes
C. Mosquito
D. All of the above

52. NVBDCP stands for ___________

A. National Vector Borne Drug Control Programme
B. National Vector Borne Disease Control Programme
C. National Viral Borne Disease Control Programme
D. National Vehicle Borne Disease Control Programme

53. Which of the following can cause hypoglycaemia in a patient of severe cerebral malaria on treatment?

A. Mefloquine
B. Quinine
C. Chloroquine
D. Halofantrine

54. Drug of choice for the treatment of a pregnant woman with *P. vivax* malaria is __________

A. Paracetamol B. Quinine
C. Chloroquine D. Artemether

55. Syphilis is a STD infection caused by __________

A. Spirochete
B. Fungi
C. Bacteria
D. Arthropod

56. Tuberculosis and *Candida albicans* infection generally develops at CD4 counts of __________

A. 2000–5000 cells/mm^3
B. Below 100 cells/mm^3
C. Below 200 cells/mm^3
D. 200–500 cells/mm^3

57. Aspergillosis is an opportunistic infection of ______

A. CNS
B. Respiratory system
C. Gastrointestinal system
D. Skin and mucous membranes

58. Opportunistic infections and cancers start to appear in __________ stage of HIV disease.

A. AIDS B. Primary
C. Asymptomatic D. Symptomatic

59. NACO stands for __________

A. National AIDS Core Organisation
B. National AIDS Co-ordination Organisation
C. National AIDS Control Organisation
D. National AIDS Caring Organisation

60. Which one of the following anti-malarial drugs is safe for use in pregnancy?

A. Quinine
B. Primaquine
C. Atovaquone
D. Tetracycline

61. NACP stands for __________

A. National AIDS Caring Programme
B. National AIDS Control Programme
C. National AIDS Co-ordination Programme
D. National AIDS Core Programme

62. SARS stands for __________

A. Serious Acute Respiratory Syndrome
B. Severe Acute Rotavirus Syndrome
C. Severe Acute Respiratory Syndrome
D. Serious Acute Rotavirus Syndrome

63. The causative agent of SARS is __________

A. Cytomegalovirus
B. SARS-CoV
C. SARS-COV-2
D. H1N1 influenza virus

64. What are the main causes of megaloblastic anaemia?

A. Cobalamin deficiency
B. Folate deficiency
C. None of the above
D. Both A and B

65. What is the main clinical feature of folate deficiency megaloblastic anaemia?

A. Anaemic symptoms, pallor
B. Muscle weakness
C. Spasticity
D. Optic neuropathy

66. Megaloblastic anaemia is a general term used to describe a group of anaemias caused by impaired __________ synthesis.

A. Ribosome
B. DNA
C. RNA
D. None of the above

67. The causative agent of COVID-19 is __________

A. SARS-CoV
B. SARS-CoV-2
C. H1N1 influenza virus
D. Cytomegalovirus

68. What are the different external factors which reduce the life span of RBC?

A. Burns
B. Parasites
C. Drugs
D. All of the above

69. Which of the following mechanisms is not used in case of drug-induced haemolytic anaemia?

A. Drug elimination
B. Drug-absorption
C. Immune complex
D. Autoantibody

70. What are the different methods of treatment for haemolytic anaemia?

A. Blood and marrow stem cell transplant
B. Blood transfusion
C. Surgery
D. All of the above

71. The causative agent of tuberculosis is __________

A. Protozoa B. Virus
C. Bacterium D. Malnutrition

72. The following drug combination used in the treatment of tuberculosis __________

A. Isoniazid, Rifampicin
B. Streptomycin, Pyrazinamide
C. Both A and B
D. None of the above

73. The BCG vaccine is administered for immunity against __________

A. Hepatitis B. Malaria
C. Tuberculosis D. Jaundice

74. The pneumonia is __________

A. Advanced bronchitis
B. A lung infection
C. A severe chest cold
D. An unusual result of hepatitis

75. The symptoms of pneumonia are __________

A. Jaundice and peeling skin
B. Cough, fever, and chills are symptoms of pneumonia
C. Rash, painful joints, and itching skin
D. All of the above

76. The most common cause of UTI is __________

A. *Staphylococcus aureus* (*S. aureus*)
B. Chlamydia
C. Mycoplasma
D. *Escherichia coli* (*E. coli*)

77. What are the signs and symptoms of an UTI in adults?

A. Milky/cloudy urine
B. Frequent urge to urinate
C. Pain during urination
D. All of the above

78. Hepatitis C virus is from which of the following family?

A. Flaviviridae
B. Coronaviridae
C. Hepadnaviridae
D. Caliciviridae

79. The highest incident of gonorrhoea usually happens in which age group?

A. 09–15 B. 15–24
C. 15–35 D. 30–45

80. Gonorrhoea is caused by which microorganism?

A. Ventral pallidum
B. *Treponema pallidum*
C. *Neisseria gonorrhoeae*
D. *P. vivax*

81. Which of the following disease is an STD?

A. Syphilis B. Gonorrhoea
C. Leprosy D. Both A and B

82. The causative agent of syphilis is __________

A. *Treponema pallidum*
B. *Entamoeba histolytica*
C. *Neisseria gonorrhoeae*
D. Plasmodium

83. Syphilis is often called __________

A. The great terminator
B. The invisible dictator
C. The terrorizing emperor
D. The great imitator

84. Experimental entities that are utilized for the study of syphilis are __________

A. Rabbits
B. Chimpanzees
C. Both A and B
D. None of the above

85. DOT stands for __________

A. Direct obese treatment
B. Direct observation treatment
C. Direct own treatment
D. Direct over treatment

86. The incubation period of malaria is __________

A. 2 to 3 days B. 1 to 5 days
C. 12 to 14 days D. 5 to 6 days

87. Jarisch-Herxheimer reaction is seen in syphilis with __________

A. Penicillin B. Chloroquine
C. Dapsone D. Quinine

88. Which of the following is a symptom of AIDS?

A. Tiredness
B. Fever
C. Swollen lymph nodes
D. All of the above

89. **The first ever instance of AIDS was reported in ______**

A. Russia
B. USA
C. France
D. None of the above

90. **HIV can also spread through ____________.**

A. Kissing
B. Sharing water
C. Breathing in infected droplets
D. Sharing needles

91. **DOTS is a pharmacological treatment of which disease?**

A. Tuberculosis
B. Pneumonia
C. Malaria
D. Syphilis

92. **Which amongst the following is not a first line drug for treatment of tuberculosis?**

A. Ethambutol
B. Isoniazid
C. Rifampin
D. Capreomycin

93. **Trimethoprim/sulphathiazole is used in treatment of which infectious disease?**

A. HIV
B. Urinary tract infection
C. Gonorrhoea
D. Opportunistic infections

94. **Which amongst the following is not a malaria parasite?**

A. *P. falciparum*
B. *P. vivax*
C. *P. nesseria*
D. *P. ovale*

95. **Which amongst the following is the recent world pandemic?**

A. Candidiasis
B. Covid-19
C. Toxoplasmosis
D. HSV-1

96. **Diagnosis of tuberculosis is done by __________**

A. Petroff's method
B. Emulator and antiformin method
C. Concentration method
D. All of the above

97. **Number of variables included in the Pneumonia Severity Index (PSI) is?**

A. 26
B. 8
C. 15
D. 20

98. **Hospital-acquired pneumonia (HAP) is defined as pneumonia occurring how many hours after hospital admission?**

A. At least 48 hours
B. At least 12 hours
C. At least 24 hours
D. At least 36 hours

99. **STD stands __________**

A. Sexually tinea diseases
B. Sexually terminal diseases
C. Sexually transmitted diseases
D. Sexually transition diseases

100. **The incubation period of SARS-CoV-2 is __________.**

A. 1 to 2 days
B. 1 to 6 days
C. 1 to 14 days
D. 1 to 7 days

Answer Key

1 D	2 A	3 C	4 B	5 C	6 C	7 A	8 D	9 C	10 B
11 A	12 A	13 B	14 A	15 B	16 C	17 B	18 C	19 D	20 B
21 C	22 D	23 C	24 B	25 C	26 D	27 B	28 C	29 D	30 C
31 C	32 D	33 C	34 D	35 B	36 A	37 B	38 D	39 A	40 D
41 B	42 B	43 D	44 D	45 A	46 C	47 C	48 D	49 B	50 B
51 C	52 B	53 B	54 C	55 A	56 D	57 B	58 D	59 C	60 A
61 B	62 C	63 B	64 D	65 A	66 B	67 B	68 D	69 B	70 D
71 C	72 C	73 C	74 B	75 B	76 D	77 D	78 A	79 B	80 C
81 D	82 A	83 D	84 C	85 B	86 C	87 A	88 D	89 B	90 D
91 A	92 D	93 B	94 C	95 B	96 D	97 D	98 A	99 C	100 C

CHAPTER 9

Musculoskeletal Disorders
Rheumatoid Arthritis, Osteoarthritis

1. __________ **means inflammation of joint.**
   A. Nephritis **B.** Arthritis
   C. Otitis **D.** Glossitis

2. **Which among the following is an autoimmune disease?**
   A. Peptic ulcer
   B. Rheumatoid arthritis
   C. Angina pectoris
   D. Epilepsy

3. **Rheumatoid arthritis is __________ disorder.**
   A. Acute
   B. Chronic
   C. Both A and B
   D. None of the above

4. **ACPA stands for __________**
   A. Anti-cholesteryl protein antigen
   B. Anti-cholesteryl protein antibody
   C. Anti-citrullinated protein antibody
   D. Anti-citrullinated protein antigen

5. **Rheumatoid arthritis and osteoarthritis are _______**
   A. Neuronal disorders
   B. Musculoskeletal disorders
   C. Renal disorders
   D. Connective disorders

6. **ACPA is associated with __________**
   A. Peptic ulcer B. Ulcerative colitis
   C. Crohn's disease D. Rheumatoid arthritis

7. **Initiation of rheumatoid arthritis seems to result from production of __________**
   A. ASCA **B.** ACPA
   C. PANCA **D.** IgM

8. **Which of the following drugs is used in osteoarthritis?**
   A. Piroxicam
   B. Paracetamol
   C. Duloxetine
   D. Aceclofenac

9. **DMARD full form is __________**
   A. Drug modifying autoimmune disease
   B. Disease model antirheumatic drug
   C. Disease modifying antirheumatic drug
   D. Derivative of mono autoreceptor drug

10. **Which of the following disease modifying antirheumatic drugs (DMARDs) is the drug of first choice?**
    A. Gold compounds
    B. Methotrexate
    C. D-penicillamine
    D. None of the above

11. **Osteoarthritis is primary disease of __________**
    A. Bone **B.** Cartilage
    C. Muscle **D.** Blood

12. **Osteoarthritis where there is no identifiable underlying cause is __________**
    A. Rheumatoid arthritis
    B. Idiopathic osteoarthritis
    C. Secondary osteoarthritis
    D. Arthritis

13. __________ **are mainly affected in osteoarthritis.**
    A. Bones
    B. Cartilages
    C. Blood vessels
    D. Lymph vessels

14. The NSAID used in rheumatoid arthritis is _______

A. Analgin
B. Indomethacin
C. Paracetamol
D. Caffeine

15. Which of the following is a clinical manifestation of rheumatoid arthritis?

A. Myalgia
B. Low-grade fever
C. Splenomegaly
D. All of the above

16. __________ is frequently described as 'wear and tear' condition.

A. Osteoarthritis
B. Rheumatoid arthritis
C. Nephritis
D. Otitis

17. The sudden appearance or worsening of rheumatoid arthritis symptom is referred to as __________

A. Flush
B. Wheal
C. Flare
D. Edema

18. DJD stands for __________

A. Deep joint disorder
B. Degenerative joint disorder
C. Defective joint disorder
D. Deceptive joint disorder

19. Rheumatoid arthritis is characterized by __________

A. Multisystem extra-articular manifestations
B. Symmetric synovitis
C. Joint erosion
D. All of the above

20. Osteoarthritis affecting the distal interphalangeal joints is known as __________

A. Bouchard's nodes
B. Richard's nodes
C. Heberden's nodes
D. Both A and B

Answer Key

1 B	2 B	3 B	4 C	5 B	6 D	7 B	8 C	9 C	10 B
11 B	12 B	13 B	14 B	15 D	16 A	17 C	18 B	19 D	20 C

CHAPTER 10

Dermatology

Psoriasis, Scabies, Eczema (Dermatitis)

1. **The psoriasis is ___________**
   - **A.** A type of skin cancer
   - **B.** A chronic autoimmune disease that appears on the skin
   - **C.** A fungal skin infection
   - **D.** A rash caused by insect bites

2. **Koebner's response is an etiological factor for ______**
   - **A.** Scabies **B.** Eczema
   - **C.** Psoriasis **D.** None of the above

3. **The following class of a drug can be used to relieve pruritus in eczema ___________**
   - **A.** Corticosteroid B. Antihistamines
   - **C.** Methotrexate D. Calcineurin inhibitor

4. **The life cycle of mite is ___________ days.**
   - **A.** 10 **B.** 30
   - **C.** 40 **D.** 20

5. **The psoriasis is treated by ___________**
   - **A.** Immune system treatment
   - **B.** Topical medicines
   - **C.** Phototherapy
   - **D.** All of the above

6. **The most common symptom of a scabies infestation is ___________**
   - **A.** Formation of skin crust
   - **B.** Rash
   - **C.** Itching
   - **D.** Both A and B

7. **Auspitz sign is associated with ___________**
   - **A.** Covid-19 **B.** Syphilis
   - **C.** Gonorrhoea **D.** Psoriasis

8. **Most severe form of scabies is ___________**
   - **A.** Genital scabies
   - **B.** Norwegian scabies
   - **C.** Nebular scabies
   - **D.** Animal scabies

9. **Oral medication used in the treatment of scabies is ___________**
   - **A.** Albendazole **B.** Mebendazole
   - **C.** Ivermectin **D.** Ketoconazole

10. **Which is the most common symptom of a scabies infestation?**
    - **A.** Rash
    - **B.** Itching
    - **C.** Formation of skin crust
    - **D.** Both A and B

11. **The pathogen of scabies is ___________**
    - **A.** *Plasmodium vivax*
    - **B.** *Sarcoptes scabiei*
    - **C.** *E. coli*
    - **D.** *Staphylococcus aureus*

12. **First line treatment for scabies is ___________**
    - **A.** Ivermectin **B.** Permethrin
    - **C.** Lindane **D.** Corticosteroids

13. **The organism which cause scabies is ___________**
    - **A.** Bacteria **B.** Mite
    - **C.** Mouse **D.** Fungus

14. **The term eczema is synonymous with the term ______**
    - **A.** Scabies
    - **B.** Allergy
    - **C.** Dermatitis
    - **D.** Psoriasis

15. Scabies is a skin disease caused by __________

A. Fungi
B. Mosquito
C. Mite
D. Flea

16. Which one of the following genes is associated with eczema?

A. BRCA
B. Filaggrin
C. BlaOXA-2
D. FOXP2

17. The main symptom of dermatitis is __________

A. Black skin
B. Itchy skin
C. Excoriated skin
D. Oozing

18. Atopic dermatitis is also often called __________

A. Pimples
B. Acne
C. Eczema
D. Psoriasis

19. Mites that cause human scabies are found which of the following primary lesions occurring on the skin?

A. In papules
B. At the edge of vesicles
C. In burrows
D. All of the above

20. __________ is a condition in which tiny, fluid-filled blisters appear on the palms and fingers.

A. Contact dermatitis
B. Stasis dermatitis
C. Dyshidrotic eczema
D. Seborrheic dermatitis

Answer Key

1 B	2 C	3 B	4 B	5 D	6 C	7 D	8 B	9 C	10 D
11 B	12 B	13 B	14 C	15 C	16 B	17 B	18 C	19 C	20 C

CHAPTER

11

Psychiatric Disorders

Depression, Anxiety, Psychosis

1. **An inability to feel pleasure in normally pleasurable activities is ___________**
   A. Alzheimer's disease
   B. Psychosis
   C. Anhedonia
   D. Melancholia

2. **Schizophrenia is a psychic disorder characterized by ___________**
   A. Sound mind B. Split of mind
   C. Moderate mind D. Soft mind

3. **OCD stands for ___________**
   A. Obsessive compulsive disorder
   B. Obese compulsive disorder
   C. Optional compulsive disorder
   D. Optimum compulsive disorder

4. **Loss of interest in all the things is a symptom of ______**
   A. Epilepsy B. Angina
   C. Hypertension D. Depression

5. **The first line treatment for depression is ___________**
   A. TCAs B. SSRIs
   C. SNRIS D. MAOIS

6. **SAD stands for ___________**
   A. Seasonal adverse disorder
   B. Seasonal affective disorder
   C. Seasonal another disorder
   D. Seasonal anginal disorder

7. **Venlafaxine belongs to the class of antidepressant drugs ___________**
   A. SSRIs B. MAOIs
   C. TCAs D. SNRIs

8. **A major cause of depression in women is ___________**
   A. Jealousy B. Increased stress
   C. Sadness D. Competitiveness

9. **Which of these vitamins may help ease depressed moods?**
   A. Vitamin E B. Vitamin C
   C. Vitamin B-complex D. Vitamin A

10. **MAOIs stand for ___________**
    A. Mono amino oxidase inhibitor
    B. Mono aniline oxidase inhibitor
    C. Mono acetyl oxidase inhibitor
    D. Mono antioxidase inhibitor

11. **Depression is a ___________**
    A. Mental illness B. Anginal disorder
    C. Hypertension D. None of the above

12. **Which of the following is a symptom of depression?**
    A. Fatigue B. Feeling guilt
    C. Mood changes D. All of the above

13. **Depression mainly caused by impairment of neuro-transmitters like ___________**
    A. GABA B. Serotonin
    C. 5HT D. All of the above

14. **A ___________ is a condition where a person has an unshakeable belief in something untrue.**
    A. Delirium B. Delusion
    C. Hallucinations D. None of the above

15. **Decreased levels of monoamine neurotransmitters (serotonin, noradrenaline, dopamine) are believed to be the pathophysiological basis of ___________**
    A. Alzheimer's disease B. Parkinson's disease
    C. Insomnia D. Depression

16. **The following action of Chlorpromazine is not based on its anti-dopaminergic property ___________**
   A. Hypotensive B. Antipsychotic
   C. Hyperprolactinemia D. Antiemetic

17. **Which of the following is atypical antipsychotic drug?**
   A. Thiothixene B. Haloperidol
   C. Clozapine D. Thioridazine

18. **Which chronic illness increases risk of depression?**
   A. Neurological disorders B. Viral illness
   C. Carcinoma D. All of the above

19. **___________ is a phobia of enclosed places.**
   A. Microphobia B. Claustrophobia
   C. Agarophobia D. Acquaphobia

20. **Depression can occur at what ages?**
   A. 40 to 50 B. 20 to 30
   C. 30 to 40 D. All of the above

21. **Venlafaxine belongs to which drug class?**
   A. Aminoketone
   B. Serotonin/norepinephrine reuptake inhibitors
   C. Selective serotonin reuptake inhibitors
   D. Tetracycline

22. **___________ can arise after exposure to a terrible experience in which severe bodily injury happened or was threatened.**
   A. Social phobia
   B. Obsessive-compulsive disorder
   C. Post-traumatic stress disorder
   D. Panic disorder

23. **Psychosis mainly deals with ___________**
   A. Confused and disturbed thought
   B. Hallucinations
   C. Delusions
   D. All of the above

24. **The drug of choice in severe panic disorder is _______**
   A. Imipramine B. Venlafaxine
   C. Benzodiazepines D. None of the above

25. **Which of the following is a symptom of schizophrenia?**
   A. Alogia
   B. Hallucinations
   C. Syncope
   D. Affective flattening

26. **A phobia of heights is known as ___________**
   A. Microphobia B. Acrophobia
   C. Aquaphobia D. Hematophobia

27. **Obsessive compulsive disorder (OCD) can be successfully treated using ___________**
   A. Massage therapy
   B. Antipsychotic medication
   C. Antidepressant medication
   D. Cognitive behavioural therapy

28. **Which of the following come under the term disorganized speech in schizophrenia?**
   A. Word salads B. Derailment
   C. Loose associations D. All of the above

29. **Non-pharmacological management of anxiety includes ___________**
   A. Psychotherapy B. Stress management
   C. Sound sleep D. All of the above

30. **The following are psychic disorders *except* ___________**
   A. Dementia B. Psoriasis
   C. Schizophrenia D. Psychosis

Answer Key

1 C	2 B	3 A	4 D	5 B	6 B	7 D	8 B	9 C	10 A
11 A	12 D	13 D	14 B	15 D	16 B	17 A	18 D	19 B	20 D
21 B	22 C	23 D	24 C	25 B	26 B	27 D	28 A	29 D	30 B

CHAPTER 12

Ophthalmology
Conjunctivitis (Bacterial and Viral), Glaucoma

1. __________ means a science of eye.

A. Myology
B. Angiology
C. Ophthalmology
D. Cardiology

2. The increased intraocular pressure means the condition of __________

A. Epilepsy
B. Glaucoma
C. Depression
D. Amnesia

3. Eye pressure is measured with the help of __________

A. Stethoscope
B. Tonometer
C. Sonometer
D. Peak flow meter

4. Which of the following is not used in conjunctivitis?

A. Naphazoline
B. Nepafenac
C. Tobramycin
D. Pilocarpine

5. Which of the following can increase intra-ocular pressure (IOP)?

A. Polyphenol
B. Vitamin A
C. Caffeine
D. Zinc

6. The normal average intra-ocular pressure is _______

A. 4 to 5 mmHg
B. 6 to 8 mmHg
C. 10 to 21 mmHg
D. 30 to 50 mmHg

7. Sticky purulent green yellow discharge is seen in __________

A. Open-angle glaucoma
B. Bacterial conjunctivitis
C. Viral conjunctivitis
D. Close-angle glaucoma

8. Which of the following stabilizes the mast cell?

A. Ketorolac
B. Pilocarpine
C. Timolol
D. Cromolyn sodium

9. Which of the following shows major cardiac adverse effects when used in glaucoma?

A. Prostaglandins
B. Beta-blockers
C. Alpha-agonist
D. Carbonic anhydrase inhibitors

10. Conjunctivitis is caused when __________

A. The pupil becomes damaged
B. The iris becomes infected
C. The surface of the cornea is too flat
D. The conjunctiva becomes infected and inflamed

11. What is the conjunctiva?

A. The eyelid
B. Membrane that covers the sclera
C. A nerve in the eye
D. The coloured part of the eye

12. The normal eyelid blinking rate is __________

A. 8 times/minute
B. 10 times/minute
C. 15 times/minute
D. 20 times/minute

13. Which of these is not a symptom of conjunctivitis?

A. Cannot see far
B. Blurred vision
C. Tears
D. Redness of the eye

14. **What is the common name for conjunctivitis?**
    A. Chickenpox
    B. Pink eye
    C. Measles
    D. Mumps

15. **If the pressure inside your eye is higher than normal, you __________**
    A. May be at risk for glaucoma
    B. May have glaucoma
    C. Need eyeglasses
    D. Both A and B

16. **What are the symptoms of angle-closure glaucoma?**
    A. Blurred vision
    B. Pain
    C. A red eye
    D. All of the above

17. **The bacteria which can attack the normal corneal epithelium is __________**
    A. *Neisseria gonorrhoeae*
    B. *Streptococcus aureus*
    C. *Treponema pallidum*
    D. *Mycobacterium leprae*

18. **An example of an antiviral drug that can prevent a viral nucleic acid from being replicated is __________**
    A. Azidothymidine
    B. Acyclovir
    C. Amantadine
    D. Both A and B

19. **Chemosis is __________**
    A. A type of skin disease
    B. A sign of eye irritation
    C. An inflammation
    D. A fever

20. **Pharyngoconjunctival fever may be a symptom of _____**
    A. Viral conjunctivitis
    B. Gonococcal conjunctivitis
    C. Trachoma
    D. General bacterial conjunctivitis

Answer Key

1 C	2 B	3 B	4 D	5 C	6 C	7 B	8 D	9 B	10 D
11 B	12 C	13 A	14 B	15 D	16 D	17 A	18 D	19 B	20 A

CHAPTER 13

Anti-microbial Resistance

1. **Micro-organisms that develop antimicrobial resistance are sometimes referred to as ________**
   A. Infections B. Superbugs
   C. Trauma D. Lesion

2. **The most common method of bacteria responsible for drug resistance is ________**
   A. Conjugation
   B. Transduction
   C. Transformation
   D. Enzyme inactivation

3. **Which of the following is a mechanism of resistance to antimicrobial agents?**
   A. Decreased antibiotic penetration
   B. Antibiotic inactivation by bacterial enzymes
   C. Changes in target sites
   D. All of the above

4. **Which of the following is a reason of antimicrobial resistance?**
   A. Self medication
   B. Clinical misuse
   C. Poor adherence of dosage regimen
   D. All of the above

5. **GLASS stands for ________**
   A. Gross antimicrobial resistance and use surveillance system
   B. General antimicrobial resistance and use surveillance system
   C. Genetic antimicrobial resistance and use surveillance system
   D. Global antimicrobial resistance and use surveillance system

6. **The drug resistance to most antimalarial drugs and tetracycline is due to ________**
   A. Activity of efflux pump
   B. Activity of influx pumps
   C. Changes in target sites
   D. Absence of binding sites

7. **AMA stands for ________**
   A. Antimicrobial agents B. Antimonic agents
   C. Anti-myogenic agents D. None of the above

8. **Which is not a cause of antimicrobial resistance?**
   A. Mutation B. Hospital use
   C. Gene transfer D. Pollution

9. **MRSA stands for ________**
   A. Methicillin-resistant *S. aureus*
   B. Methyldopa-resistant *S. aureus*
   C. Metformin-resistant *S. aureus*
   D. Mutation-resistant *S. aureus*

10. **Antimicrobial resistance can be prevented and controlled by ________**
    A. Use of quality medicines
    B. Avoiding use of OTC medicines
    C. Avoiding overdose or misuse of drugs
    D. All of the above

Answer Key

1 B	2 A	3 D	4 D	5 D	6 A	7 A	8 D	9 A	10 D

CHAPTER 14

Women's Health

Polycystic Ovary Syndrome (PCOS), Dysmenorrhoea, Premenstrual Syndrome

1. __________ means painful menstruation.

A. Amenorrhoea
B. Dysmenorrhoea
C. Leucorrhoea
D. Galactorrhea

2. Hyperandrogenism is associated with __________

A. Diabetes mellitus
B. Polycystic ovary syndrome
C. Peptic ulcer
D. Psoriasis

3. PCOS means __________

A. Polyclinic ovary syndrome
B. Polycystic ovary syndrome
C. Polycystic obese syndrome
D. Polycystic obstruction syndrome

4. Rotterdam criteria is used to establish the clinical diagnosis of __________

A. Polycystic ovary syndrome
B. Psoriasis
C. Depression
D. Anxiety

5. Menorrhagia is a menstrual bleeding that lasts for more than __________

A. 2 days
B. 15 days
C. 7 days
D. 30 days

6. First-line treatment for hyperandrogenism and/or menstrual cycle abnormalities in PCOS patients who do not desire pregnancy is __________

A. Antiandrogen agents
B. Combined oral contraceptives
C. Letrozole
D. Medroxyprogesterone acetate

7. __________ is the prominent cause of infertility.

A. PCOS
B. PMS
C. PMDD
D. None of the above

8. The first-line therapy of PCOS for the patients who wish to become pregnant is __________

A. Letrozole
B. Cyproterone
C. Spironolactone
D. Finasteride

9. Symptoms of primary dysmenorrhea are mainly due to release of __________

A. Prostaglandins
B. Histamine
C. Serotonin
D. Epinephrine

10. The first line treatment in most women with primary dysmenorrhea is __________

A. Antiandrogens
B. Estrogen
C. NSAIDs
D. Opioid analgesics

11. ________ is the abnormal growth of hair on a woman's face and body.

A. Alopecia
B. Hirsutism
C. Cramp
D. Acne

12. Hormonal disproportion like estrogen surplus and progesterone deficiency is associated with the etiology of __________

A. Amenorrhea
B. PMS
C. Polycystic ovary syndrome
D. Depression

13. A more severe form of PMS is also known as _______

A. Baby blues
B. Premenstrual dysphoric disorder
C. Menstrual-related mood disorder
D. Luteal disorder

14. Which of these hormones is thought to play a role in PMS?

A. Estrogen
B. Serotonin
C. Progesterone
D. All of the above

15. Polycystic ovarian syndrome is the prominent cause of __________ for women in US.

A. Obesity
B. Infertility
C. Dyslipidaemia
D. Insulin resistance

16. Clinical manifestations of PCOS induce the following __________

A. Amenorrhea or irregular menses
B. Facial hair
C. Acne
D. All of the above

17. Age at which PCOS is commonly diagnosed?

A. Less than 13 years
B. More than 50 years
C. 18–44 years
D. None of the above

18. Women suffering from PCOS are at increased risk of developing __________

A. Endometrial cancer
B. Diabetes
C. Dyslipidemias
D. All of the above

19. The major reason for women with PCOS to suffer from infertility is

A. Abnormal menstrual cycles
B. Excess insulin level
C. Obesity
D. None of the above

20. Which of the following is not used in PCOS?

A. Contraceptives
B. Metformin
C. NSAIDs
D. Diuretic

Answer Key

1 B	2 B	3 B	4 A	5 C	6 B	7 A	8 B	9 A	10 C
11 B	12 B	13 B	14 D	15 B	16 D	17 B	18 D	19 A	20 C

Section X

Hospital and Clinical Pharmacy

1. Hospital Pharmacy
2. Different Committees in the Hospital
3. Supply Chain and Inventory Control
4. Drug Distribution
5. Compounding in Hospitals
6. Radiopharmaceuticals
7. Application of Computers in Hospital Pharmacy Practice, Electronic Health Records, Softwares used in Hospital Pharmacy
8. Clinical Pharmacy
9. Clinical Laboratory Tests
10. Poisoning
11. Pharmacovigilance
12. Medication Errors
13. Drug Interactions

Syllabus (As Per ER 2020) Hospital and Clinical Pharmacy

Chapter	Topics
1	**Hospital Pharmacy** ■ Definition, scope, national and international scenario ■ Organizational structure ■ Professional responsibilities, Qualification and experience requirements, job specifications, work load requirements and inter-professional relationships ■ Good Pharmacy Practice (GPP) in hospital ■ Hospital Pharmacy Standards (FIP Basel Statements, AHSP) ■ Introduction to NAQS guidelines and NABH Accreditation and Role of Pharmacists
2	**Different Committees in the Hospital** ■ Pharmacy and Therapeutics Committee: Objectives, Composition, and functions ■ Hospital Formulary: Definition, procedure for development and use of hospital formulary ■ Infection Control Committee: Role of Pharmacist in preventing Antimicrobial Resistance
3	**Supply Chain and Inventory Control** ■ Preparation of Drug lists: High Risk drugs, Emergency drugs, Schedule H1 drugs, NDPS drugs, reserved antibiotics ■ Procedures of Drug Purchases: Drug selection, short term, long term, and tender/e-tender process, quotations, etc. ■ Inventory control techniques: Economic Order Quantity, Reorder Quantity Level, Inventory Turnover etc. ■ Inventory Management of Central Drug Store: Storage conditions, Methods of storage, Distribution, Maintaining Cold Chain, Devices used for cold storage (Refrigerator, ILR, Walk-in-Cold rooms) ■ FEFO, FIFO methods ■ Expiry drug removal and handling, and disposal. Disposal of Narcotics, cytotoxic drugs ■ Documentation: Purchase and inventory
4	**Drug Distribution** ■ Drug distribution (inpatients and outpatients) – Definition, advantages and disadvantages of individual prescription order method, Floor Stock Method, Unit Dose Drug Distribution Method, Drug Basket Method. ■ Distribution of drugs to ICCU/ICU/NICU/Emergency wards. ■ Automated drug dispensing systems and devices ■ Distribution of Narcotic and Psychotropic substances and their storage
5	■ **Compounding in Hospitals.** Bulk compounding, IV admixture services and incompatibilities, Total parenteral nutrition.
6	**Radio Pharmaceuticals:** Storage, dispensing and disposal of radiopharmaceuticals
7	**Application of computers in Hospital Pharmacy Practice, Electronic health records, Softwares used in hospital pharmacy**
8	**Clinical Pharmacy:** Definition, scope, and development - in India and other countries Technical definitions, common terminologies used in clinical settings and their significance such as Paediatrics, Geriatric, Anti-natal Care, Post-natal Care, etc. Daily activities of clinical pharmacists: Definition, goal, and procedure of: ■ Ward round participation ■ Treatment Chart Review ■ Adverse drug reaction monitoring ■ Drug information and poisons information ■ Medication history ■ Patient counselling ■ Interprofessional collaboration **Pharmaceutical Care:** Definition, classification of drug related problems. Principles and procedure to provide pharmaceutical care. Medication Therapy Management, Home Medication Review

Contd...

9	**Clinical Laboratory Tests used in the Evaluation of Disease States:** Significance and interpretation of test results ■ Haematological, Liver function, Renal function, Thyroid function tests ■ Tests associated with cardiac disorders ■ Fluid and electrolyte balance ■ Pulmonary Function Tests
10	**Poisoning:** Types of poisoning: Clinical manifestations and Antidotes **Drugs and Poison Information Centre and their services:** Definition, Requirements, Information resources with examples, and their advantages and disadvantages.
11	**Pharmacovigilance** ■ Definition, aim and scope ■ Overview of Pharmacovigilance
12	**Medication Errors:** ■ Definition, types, consequences, and strategies to minimize medication errors, LASA drugs and Tallman lettering as per ISMP **Drug Interactions:** ■ Definition, types, clinical significance of drug interactions

CHAPTER 1

Hospital Pharmacy

1. **The functions of hospitals are _________**
   - A. Training to the patients and medical practitioner
   - B. Prevention of diseases
   - C. Diagnosis of diseases
   - D. All of the above

2. **Hospital pharmacy is a _________ department in the hospital.**
   - A. Treatment department
   - B. Diagnostic department
   - C. Administration department
   - D. Supportive department

3. **Hospital pharmacy should be located ___________**
   - A. Near to the outpatient department
   - B. Near to the wards
   - C. Near to the inpatient department
   - D. Near to the gate of the hospital

4. **Which of the following is an objective of hospital pharmacy?**
   - A. To act as profit centre of the hospital
   - B. To implement decision of PTC
   - C. To participate in research work
   - D. All of the above

5. **ASHP stands for ________**
   - A. Asian Society of Hospital Pharmacy
   - B. American Society of Health-System Pharmacy
   - C. American Society of Hospital Pharmacy
   - D. Asian Society of Hospital Pharmacy Practice

6. **The head of the hospital pharmacy should be M Pharm in _________ with adequate abilities like administrative ability, technical ability.**
   - A. Biochemistry
   - B. Pharmaceutical chemistry
   - C. Pharmacology
   - D. Pharmacognosy

7. **The practice of pharmacy that responds to the needs of the people who use the pharmacist's services to provide optimal, evidence-based care is known as ___________**
   - A. GPP
   - B. GMP
   - C. GLP
   - D. None of the above

8. **The objectives of PTC is ___________**
   - A. Drug safety and ADR monitoring
   - B. Advisory
   - C. Education
   - D. All of the above

9. **NQAS stands for ___________**
   - A. National Quality Available Standards
   - B. National Quality Assurance Standards
   - C. Natural Quality Assurance Standards
   - D. All of the above

10. **The hospital accreditation program was started in the year ___________**
    - A. 1997
    - B. 2022
    - C. 2015
    - D. 2005

11. **For dispensing medicines, the required minimum qualification of hospital pharmacist is ___________**
    - A. M Pharm
    - B. D Pharm
    - C. B Pharm
    - D. None of the above

12. **GLP stands for ___________**
    - A. Good Labour Practices
    - B. Good Laboratory Practices
    - C. Good Licensing Practices
    - D. All of the above

13. The head of the hospital pharmacy should have the following abilities __________

A. Ability to develop manufacturing section
B. Academic ability
C. Administrative ability
D. All of the above

14. Voluntary or involuntary removal of a drug product by the manufacturer, usually pertaining to a particular shipment or lot number is called __________

A. Recall **B.** Code cart
C. IVPB **D.** Discard

15. The number of pharmacists required for a 280-bed size hospital is __________

A. 05 **B.** 10
C. 08 **D.** 03

16. The following are all quality indicators of pharmacy given by the NABH for the accreditation of hospital, *except* __________

A. Going out of stocks
B. Incidence of dispensing errors
C. Wastage of drugs
D. Salary on the time for interns

17. Number of beds in medium size hospitals are __________

A. Less than 1000 **B.** 500–1000
C. Less than 500 **D.** 100–500

18. Which of the following functions is performed by the hospital?

A. Control of population
B. Sanitization
C. Immunization
D. Salivation

19. District level civil hospitals come under __________

A. Private ownership **B.** Public ownership
C. Both A and B **D.** None of the above

20. The number of pharmacist required for 50-bed size hospital is __________

A. 3 **B.** 5
C. 8 **D.** 10

21. Hospital pharmacist supplies, stores, dispense the right medicine at right time at minimum cost under the supervision of __________

A. Physician
B. Head nurse
C. Qualified register pharmacist
D. None of the above

22. The number of pharmacists required for 300-bed hospital are __________

A. 15 pharmacists
B. 10 pharmacists
C. 12 pharmacists
D. 12–15 pharmacists

23. The FIP Basel Statements can be split into __________ areas

A. 5 **B.** 2
C. 6 **D.** 4

24. Which of the following is not a patient centered standards given by NABH for hospital accreditation?

A. Continuous Quality Improvement (CQI)
B. Care of Patients (COP)
C. Management of Medication (MOM)
D. Hospital Infection Control (HIC)

25. The hospital pharmacy must be located on __________

A. Third floor of the hospital
B. Ground floor of the hospital
C. Outside the hospital
D. Every floor of the hospital

26. Which record need to be maintained by hospital pharmacist?

A. Expiry date record
B. Indent and receipt voucher
C. Drug inspection record
D. All of the above

27. The responsibility of __________ is to manage the pharmacy department of a hospital.

A. Chief pharmacists
B. Junior pharmacist
C. Senior pharmacist
D. Managing director of pharmacy

28. NABH is responsible for __________ of hospitals.

A. Affiliation
B. Approval
C. Controlling
D. All of the above

29. The minimum area of pharmacy required for any hospital is __________

A. 300 sq.ft. **B.** 250 sq.ft.
C. 200 sq.ft. **D.** 350 sq.ft.

30. The Pharmacy Council of India published Pharmacy Practice Regulations in the year __________

A. 2012 A. 2002
C. 2015 **D.** 2016

31. Prescription is dispensed by ___________ only.
- **A.** Physician
- **B.** Pharmacist
- **C.** Doctor
- **D.** All of the above

32. GPP stands for ___________
- **A.** Goal pharmacy practice
- **B.** Good manufacturing practice
- **C.** Good pharmacy practice
- **D.** None of the above

33. A prescription for Schedule II and Schedule III controlled drug is valid for ___________
- **A.** 14 days
- **B.** 10 days
- **C.** 12 days
- **D.** None of the above

34. ___________ means International Pharmaceutical Federation.
- **A.** NABH
- **B.** ASHP
- **C.** FIP
- **D.** All of the above

35. The patient care services are also called ___________
- **A.** Administrative services
- **B.** Nursing services
- **C.** Public health services
- **D.** Allied health services

36. Accreditation programs of NABH include ___________
- **A.** Eye care organizations
- **B.** Small healthcare organizations
- **C.** Primary health centres
- **D.** All of the above

37. For 200 beds hospital, number of pharmacists required are ___________
- **A.** 05
- **B.** 08
- **C.** 10
- **D.** 15

38. DIS stands for ___________
- **A.** Drug Implementation Services
- **B.** Drug Including Syndromes
- **C.** Drug Information Services
- **D.** Drug Incorporation Services

39. The administrative services of the hospital include ___________
- **A.** Personnel
- **B.** Finance
- **C.** Both A and B
- **D.** None of the above

40. ___________ is an administrator of the hospital.
- **A.** Nurse
- **B.** Pharmacist
- **C.** Apprentice Master
- **D.** Dean

Answer Key

1 D	2 D	3 A	4 D	5 B	6 C	7 A	8 D	9 B	10 D
11 B	12 B	13 D	14 A	15 B	16 D	17 B	18 C	19 B	20 A
21 C	22 B	23 C	24 A	25 B	26 D	27 A	28 D	29 B	30 C
31 B	32 C	33 A	34 C	35 B	36 D	37 B	38 C	39 C	40 D

CHAPTER

2

Different Committees in the Hospital

1. **The pharmacy and therapeutics committee plays dual role of __________ and __________**
   A. Procurement of drug, dispensing of drug
   B. Advisory, education
   C. Selection, training
   D. Selection of drug, dispensing of drug

2. **The Secretary of PTC is __________**
   A. Pharmacist
   B. Administrator
   C. Physician
   D. Nurse

3. **The pharmacist who is member of PTC, works as __________ of PTC**
   A. Member Secretary
   B. Chairman
   C. Joint Secretary
   D. Head of PTC

4. **The hospital formulary consists of list of __________ in hospital.**
   A. Patients
   B. Instruments
   C. Drugs
   D. Staff

5. **The continually revised compilation of pharmaceuticals and medicines used in hospitals by medical staff and some important ancillary information that reflects the current clinical judgment of medical staff is known as __________**
   A. Hospital Form
   B. Hospital Formulary
   C. Hospital Federation
   D. Hospital File

6. **________ is a secretary of infection control committee.**
   A. Infection control nurse
   B. Infection control pharmacist
   C. Infection control physician
   D. Infection control compounder

7. **The __________ is responsible for oversight of all medications used in the hospital.**
   A. Hospital administration B. PTC
   C. Dean of hospital D. Pharmacist

8. **__________ is not under the purview of the PTC.**
   A. Laboratory testing
   B. Medication safety
   C. Antibiotic/infectious disease
   D. Purchasing policy

9. **The rationale for completing a drug use evaluation is to __________**
   A. Educate the nursing staff on appropriate medication administration
   B. Validate drug use is safe and appropriate
   C. Determine the most common prescribers of a specific drug
   D. None of the above

10. **In case of adverse drug reaction, nurse should report to the __________.**
    A. Adverse drug reporting center
    B. Head of the hospital
    C. Chairman of PTC
    D. Drug controller

11. **Hospital formulary is a __________**
    A. List of all items in the hospital
    B. List of selected drugs or preparation in hospital

C. List of all investigational drugs or preparations that are used by medical staff
D. None of the above

12. Drug utilization review by the PTC, does not consider one of the following __________
A. Prescribing
B. Selling
C. Dispensing
D. Administering

13. Following are the functions of the PTC, *except* ______
A. Procurement of drugs from the venders
B. Frames the policy for the hospital
C. Evaluate drug safety
D. Prevent adverse drug reaction

14. Who will take the daily measures to control hospital infection?
A. Head of the hospital
B. Infection control center
C. Infection control team
D. Infection control committee

15. The full form of HICC __________
A. Hospital infection control center
B. Hospital information and counselling center
C. Hospital industry control center
D. Hospital infection control team center

16. The hospital organization forms a committee regarding therapeutic use of drug is called the __________
A. Pharmacy and Theory Committee
B. Pharmacy and Therapeutic Committee
C. Pharmacy and Therapeutic Cell
D. None of the above

17. Primary purpose of the Pharmacy and Therapeutic Committee is to act as __________
A. An advisory and educational body
B. Nursing care
C. Diagnostic care
D. None of the above

18. ICC stands for __________
A. Infection Control Committee
B. Internal Control Committee
C. Inspection Control Committee
D. All of the above

19. The Member Secretary of ICC is __________
A. Store Officer
B. Head of the Institute
C. Senior Microbiologist
D. Infection Control Nurse

20. The following elements of the hospital formulary system are used to manage drug costs __________
A. Drug therapy guideline B. Therapeutic interchange
C. Generic substitution D. All of the above

Answer Key

1 B	2 A	3 A	4 C	5 B	6 A	7 B	8 A	9 B	10 C
11 C	12 B	13 A	14 C	15 A	16 B	17 A	18 A	19 D	20 D

CHAPTER 3

Supply Chain and Inventory Control

1. The purpose of supply chain management is _______

A. Integrating supply and demand management
B. Provide customer satisfaction
C. Improve quality of a product
D. Increase production

2. ___________ is the activity required by the organization to deliver goods or services to the consumers.

A. Cold chain
B. Supply chain
C. Moulded chain
D. Hybrid chain

3. ___________ is a time taken between placing an order and receipt of drugs to the department.

A. Over time B. Night time
C. Lead time D. Day time

4. EOQ stands for ___________

A. Economic Open Quality
B. Economic Order Quantity
C. Equipment Order Quantity
D. Essential Order Quantity

5. Logistics is the part of a supply chain involved with the forward and reverse flow of ___________

A. Cash B. Goods
C. Services D. All of the above

6. Due to small change in customer demands, inventory oscillations become progressively larger looking through the supply chain. This is known as _______

A. Reverse supply chain
B. Bullwhip effect
C. Net chain analysis
D. Reverse logistics

7. Following are the essential narcotic drugs *except* _____

A. Codeine B. Carbamazepine
C. Dihydrocodeinone D. Fentanyl

8. ____________ number of copies of purchase order are prepared.

A. 7 B. 6
C. 9 D. 8

9. ___________ is in written form evidence of agreement between the buyer and supplier.

A. Reorder B. Purchase order
C. Sale order D. Account order

10. Vitamins are stored in ___________

A. Cool temperature B. Freezer
C. Room temperature D. Cold temperature

11. ILR means ___________

A. Integrated light refrigerator
B. Intensive lined refrigerator
C. Ice light refrigerator
D. Ice-lined refrigerators

12. Which of the following disposal methods is used for cytotoxic drugs?

A. Directly to landfill
B. Low and medium temperature incineration
C. High temperature incineration
D. Disposal to sewers and water courses

13. The issuing of purchase order is role of ___________

A. Physician
B. Nurse
C. Purchase officer
D. Inventory control officer

14. **Which of the following is not a procurement method?**
    A. Open tender
    B. ABC analysis
    C. E-tender
    D. Direct purchase

15. **Drugs with a narrow therapeutic index is an example of __________**
    A. High-risk medicines
    B. Reserve drugs
    C. Narcotic drugs
    D. None of the above

16. **Which of the following is not an emergency use medicine?**
    A. Oxygen B. Paracetamol
    C. Heparin D. Atropine

17. **The example of NDPS is __________**
    A. Paracetamol B. Atropine
    C. Morphine D. Aspirin

18. **How many reserve antibiotics are there?**
    A. 21 B. 22
    C. 23 D. 32

19. **The long-form of FIFO and FEFO is __________**
    A. First In First Out, First Expiry First Out
    B. First In First On, First Expiry First On
    C. Fast In First Out, Fast Expiry First Out
    D. None of the above

20. **The drugs having therapeutic index less than 1 are categorized as __________**
    A. Schedule H drugs
    B. High risk drugs
    C. Schedule H1 drugs
    D. Emergency drugs

21. **Any drug capable of affecting the mind, emotions, and behaviour is __________**
    A. Psychotropic drugs
    B. Natural drug
    C. Preventative drug
    D. All of the above

22. **Which one of the following is not a key element of cold chain?**
    A. Procedure B. Personnel
    C. Transportation D. Equipment

23. **The full form of VED analysis __________**
    A. Vital, Efficient, Desirable
    B. Vital, Efficient, Desirable
    C. Viable, Essential, Desirable
    D. Vital, Essential, Desirable

24. **In ABC analysis A items are __________**
    A. 10% quantity of drug with neither high cost nor cheap, 10% consumption
    B. 10% quantity of drug with low cost, 70% consumption
    C. 10% quantity of drug with high cost, 70% consumption
    D. 70% quantity of drug with high cost, 10% consumption

25. **Sewer is the technique of disposal of drugs used for __________**
    A. Anticonvulsants
    B. Antibiotics
    C. Narcotics
    D. Concentrated IV fluids

26. **Mixing of crushed expired drugs with water, lime and cement then send it to landfill, this process is known as __________**
    A. Physical incineration
    B. Landfill
    C. Waste inertization
    D. Waste encapsulation

27. **Cold storage temperature is __________**
    A. –25°C to –10°C B. –5 to 2°C
    C. 2 to 8° C D. 8°C to 25°C

28. **All of the following are methods of inventory control, *except* __________**
    A. Graphical method
    B. Visual method
    C. Perpetual method
    D. Barcoding method

29. **Medicines that fulfil the medicinal demand of public in the country and available at reasonable cost at every healthcare sector is known as __________**
    A. General purpose medicine
    B. Emergency medicine
    C. Essential medicine
    D. Schedule H1 medicine

30. **Idiosyncrasy is __________**
    A. Type B ADRs B. Type D ADRs
    C. Type A ADRs D. Type C ADRs

31. **The process of acquiring supplies through purchase agents, distributors or from private or public suppliers is called __________**
    A. Procurement B. Tender
    C. Notice D. Inventory control

32. **Which of the following drugs is not needed to be TDM?**
    A. Gentamicin B. Carbamazepine
    C. Penicillin D. Digoxin

33. Grey baby syndrome occurs in newborn with ______

A. Erythromycin
B. Penicillin
C. Tetracycline
D. Chloramphenicol

34. All of the following are used for cold storage, *except* ______

A. Ice-lined refrigerator
B. Iced bag packs
C. Domestic refrigerator
D. Deep freezer

35. The drugs that have heightened risk of causing significant patient harm are known as ______

A. Emergency drugs
B. High-risk drugs
C. Treatment drug
D. NDPS drugs

36. According to IP cool means any temperature ranging between ______

A. 2°C and 8°C
B. 30°C and 40°C
C. 8°C and 25°C
D. Above 40°C

37. The time taken by the equipment to raise the inside cabinet temperature from its cut-off temperature to the maximum temperature limit of its recommended range is known as ______

A. Holding temperature
B. Holdover time
C. Refrigeration time
D. Freeze time

38. ______ is the level of stock of any item at which next purchase procedure is started.

A. Minimum stock level
B. Maximum stock level
C. Reorder level
D. Safety level

39. ______ is based on the cost, quantity and consumption of items.

A. VED analysis
B. ABC analysis
C. Input–output ratio
D. EOQ method

40. ______ is a written offer to supply materials at a given fixed price within a prescribed period and under specific conditions.

A. Tender
B. Quotation
C. Account
D. Share

Answer Key

1 A	2 B	3 C	4 B	5 D	6 B	7 B	8 A	9 B	10 D
11 D	12 C	13 C	14 B	15 A	16 B	17 C	18 B	19 A	20 B
21 A	22 C	23 D	24 C	25 D	26 C	27 C	28 A	29 C	30 A
31 A	32 C	33 D	34 B	35 B	36 C	37 B	38 C	39 B	40 B

CHAPTER 4

Drug Distribution

1. **The system in which there is a main pharmacy and it has subpharmacies under it is called ___________**
   A. Satellite pharmacy
   B. Floor stock system
   C. Unit dose dispensing system
   D. Bed side pharmacy
2. **The selection of charge drug for distribution is carried out by ___________**
   A. Governing body of hospital B. Hospital administrator
   C. PTC D. Chief pharmacist
3. **ICU stands for ___________**
   A. Intensive Colour Unit
   B. Intensive Colony Unit
   C. Intensive Care Unit
   D. International Care Unit
4. **The sale/purchase records of NDPS drugs shall be maintained for minimum ___________ years.**
   A. 01 B. 02
   C. 03 D. 04
5. **The patients, who require hospitalization are as _____**
   A. Referred patients B. Inpatients
   C. Outpatients D. None of the above
6. **The types of floor stock system of distribution of medicines are ___________**
   A. Centralized and decentralized
   B. Charge and noncharge floor stock drugs
   C. Simple and complex
   D. None of the above
7. **CSSD stands for ___________**
   A. Central Sterile Supply Department
   B. Center Sterile Social Dispensing
   C. Central Sterile Supply Dispensed
   D. None of the above
8. **_________ is a patient who occupies space in a hospital.**
   A. Operational patient
   B. Outpatient
   C. Inpatient
   D. None of the above
9. **A prescription for Schedule II and Schedule III controlled drugs is valid for ___________**
   A. 10 days B. Infinite
   C. 12 days D. 14 days
10. **The drugs under this schedule have a high potential for abuse but are accepted for medical use are included in ___________**
    A. Schedule 1 B. Schedule 4
    C. Schedule 2 D. Schedule 3
11. **UDDS stands for ___________**
    A. Unique Drug Distribution System
    B. Unit Drug Distribution System
    C. United Dose Dispensing System
    D. Useful Drug Distribution System
12. **___________ formulates procedures for distribution of drugs to different ICUs and emergency ward.**
    A. Medicine Department B. PTC
    C. Pharmacist D. Administrator
13. **Which of the following is the part of hospital formulary?**
    A. Information on hospital policies
    B. Drug products listing
    C. Special information
    D. All of the above

14. __________ serves as a link between the medical staff and hospital pharmacist.
 A. Patient
 B. Modern dispensing aspects
 C. Pharmacy therapeutic
 D. None of the above

15. All of the following are secondary source of information *except* __________
 A. Research papers B. Formulary
 C. Pharmacopoeia D. Textbooks

16. OPD stands for __________
 A. Outpatient Demand
 B. Out passive Department
 C. Out portion Department
 D. Outpatient Department

17. __________ are mainly used in the operations.
 A. Acrylate adhesive
 B. Rubber adhesive taps
 C. Both A and B
 D. None of the above

18. The hospital formulary consists of list of __________ in hospital.
 A. Patients B. Instruments
 C. Drugs D. Staff

19. ICCU __________
 A. Intensive Causal Care Unit
 B. Intensive Coronary Care Unit
 C. Intensive Common Care Unit
 D. Intensive Care Career Care

20. __________ means those patients who are not admitted in the hospital or who are not confined to bed.
 A. Inpatients B. Ambulatory patients
 C. Both A and B D. None of the above

21. While prescribing medicines, the physician must write __________ name of drug.
 A. Non-proprietary B. Proprietary
 C. Both A and B D. None of the above

22. The needs of the hospital formulary system are increasing nowadays because of __________
 A. Competition in marketing practice
 B. Increase in number of new drug in market
 C. Increased influence of advertising
 D. All of the above

23. NDPS stands for __________
 A. Natural and Psychotropic Substances
 B. Narcotic Drugs and Psychotropic Substances
 C. Narcotic and Physiological Substances
 D. None of the above

24. The substantial patient care and financial benefits can be greatly increased by using __________
 A. Branded drugs B. Non-branded drugs
 C. Generic drugs D. None of the above

25. The items provided by CSSD include all *except* _____
 A. Gloves B. Syringe
 C. Catheter D. Blood

26. NICU stands for __________
 A. Normal Intensive Care Unit
 B. Neonatal Intensive Care Unit
 C. Natural Intensive Care Unit
 D. Nominal Intensive Care Unit

27. The patients, who come to the hospital for general symptoms like fever, cough, and cold are known as _______
 A. Ambulatory outpatient B. Emergency outpatients
 C. General outpatient D. Referred outpatient

28. Noncharge floor stock drugs use dispensing by _____
 A. Mobile dispensing unit B. Drug basket method
 C. Both A and B D. None of the above

29. A single unit package is one which contains one complete pharmaceutical dosage form is __________
 A. Tablet B. Pill
 C. Capsule D. All of the above

30. Which among the following prepares requisition for narcotic drugs?
 A. Patient B. Nurse
 C. Doctor D. Pharmacist

Answer Key

1 A	2 C	3 C	4 C	5 B	6 B	7 A	8 C	9 D	10 C
11 B	12 C	13 D	14 B	15 C	16 D	17 B	18 C	19 B	20 B
21 C	22 D	23 B	24 C	25 D	26 B	27 C	28 C	29 D	30 B

CHAPTER 5

Compounding in Hospitals

1. **Prescription is dispensed by the __________**
   A. Pharmacist B. Doctor
   C. Physician D. Patient

2. **Clinical pharmacist educates ________ for reducing medication errors.**
   A. Administrator B. Pharmacist
   C. Patient D. Nurse

3. **Which of the following carbohydrate is used in TPN as source of energy?**
   A. Fructose B. Dextrose
   C. Galactose D. None of the above

4. **TPN means __________**
   A. Total Pure Nutrition
   B. Total Protein Nutrition
   C. Total Parenteral Nutrition
   D. Total Particular Nutrition

5. **The emergency services are available for _________ hours**
   A. 8 B. 24
   C. 12 D. 20

6. **When two or more drugs are administered concurrently resulting in undesirable pharmacological activity is __________**
   A. Therapeutic incompatibility
   B. Physical incompatibility
   C. Chemical incompatibility
   D. None of the above

7. **Patient who occupies space in hospital is __________**
   A. Outpatient
   B. Inpatient
   C. Operational patient
   D. None of the above

8. **CSD stands for __________**
   A. Central social dispensing
   B. Central supply dispensed
   C. Central sterile department
   D. None of the above

9. **The complications associated with use of TPN are __________**
   A. Liver toxicity
   B. Electrolyte imbalance
   C. Hyperglycaemia
   D. All of the above

10. **__________ deals with majority care for daily personal health needs**
    A. Primary care
    B. Secondary care
    C. Operational patient
    D. None of these

11. **____________ services are provided for immediate medical attention or in case of an accident**
    A. Primary care
    B. Secondary care
    C. Emergency care
    D. Referral care

12. **Dispensing of controlled drug is according to _______**
    A. Narcotic and Psychotropic Substance Act 1984
    B. Narcotic and Psychotropic Substance Act 1985
    C. Narcotic and Psychotropic Substance Act 1986
    D. None of above

13. Prepared solution of TPN should be stored at ______

A. Room temperature
B. Cool condition
C. Refrigerator
D. Any condition

14. Incompatibility generally occurs between ________

A. Two drugs
B. Drugs and materials of IV containers
C. Drugs and unsuitable diluents
D. All of the above

15. The mixing of menthol and camphor __________ type of problem?

A. Quality
B. Dosage form
C. Stability
D. Incompatibility

16. The advantages of IV admixtures is __________

A. No risk of incompatibilities compliance
B. Well-trained pharmacist is required
C. Quick onset of action
D. Environmental control is required

17. TPN is administered by __________ route.

A. IV B. IM
C. SC D. Oral

18. Which of the following is not an aspect of compounding?

A. Therapeutic
B. Pharmaceutical
C. Clinical
D. Administrative

19. TPN is also known as __________

A. Protein energy malnutrition
B. IV nutrition feeding
C. Balanced diet
D. Rehydration

20. __________ is used for IV admixtures.

A. Lactated Ringer B. Basic Ringer
C. Acidic Ringer D. Hartmann's Ringer

Answer Key

1 A	2 D	3 B	4 C	5 B	6 A	7 B	8 C	9 D	10 A
11 C	12 B	13 C	14 D	15 C	16 C	17 A	18 A	19 B	20 D

CHAPTER 6.

Radiopharmaceuticals

1. **The compounds or substances which exhibit radioactivity and which are used as medicine for various purposes are called __________**
   A. Nutraceuticals
   B. Pharmaceuticals
   C. Biopharmaceuticals
   D. Radiopharmaceuticals

2. **Radiopharmaceuticals should emit __________**
   A. Gamma particles
   B. Alpha particles
   C. Beta particles
   D. None of the above

3. **Radiopharmaceuticals should have a __________ half life.**
   A. Medium B. Short
   C. Long D. Faster

4. **Radioactivity is the spontaneous and continuous emission of __________ radiation from substances.**
   A. Alpha
   B. Beta
   C. Gamma
   D. All of the above

5. **Usually radiopharmaceuticals are stored at ________**
   A. 2° to 8°C
   B. 25°C
   C. 0ºC
   D. 20°C

6. **__________ is used in liver scanning.**
   A. Xenon-133 gas (Xe-133)
   B. Sodium Rose Bengal (I-131)
   C. Carbon-11
   D. Tritium

7. **Which radioactive nuclide used in thyroid conditions?**
   A. I-131 B. Cr-51
   C. Fe-59 D. Co-57

8. **__________ substances should never be touched with hand but handled with forceps.**
   A. Phytopharmaceuticals
   B. Pharmaceuticals
   C. Nutraceuticals
   D. Radiopharmaceuticals

9. **GRP stands for __________**
   A. Good radiology process
   B. Good reference practice
   C. Good radiation practices
   D. None of the above

10. **The use of Xenon-133 gas (Xe-133)**
    A. Pulmonary scan
    B. Liver scan
    C. Brain scan
    D. All of the above

11. **__________ reduce the bulk of waste.**
    A. Land filling
    B. Segregation
    C. Incineration
    D. Chlorination

12. **Which of the following is not used to produce radioisotopes?**
    A. Gamma cameras
    B. Cyclotrons
    C. Radioisotope generators
    D. Nuclear reactors

13. The radioactivity is measured in terms of__________

A. Curie

B. Microcurie

C. Millicurie

D. All of the above

14. What is detected during Positron Emission Tomography (PET)?

A. Positrons

B. Photons

C. Electrons

D. Neutrons

15. Gamma rays are electromagnetic radiations with a wavelength __________

A. Much larger than those of light

B. Much shorter than those of light

C. Equal to light

D. None of the above

16. The correct statement regarding the storage and handling of radioactive material is __________

A. Radioactive materials are never touched with a hand

B. Sufficient protective clothing must be while handling

C. Kept in a suitable labelled container

D. All of the above

17. Which of the following isotopes has the shortest half life?

A. Fluorine-18

B. Carbon-11

C. Tritium

D. Carbon-14

18. __________ is used in pernicious anaemia.

A. Cobalt

B. Cyanocobalamin

C. Iodine

D. None of above

19. Which method is used for the disposal of radiopharmaceutical waste?

A. Hold for decay

B. Dump to sanitary sewer

C. Incineration

D. All of the above

20. __________ radiation has high penetration power?

A. Alpha

B. Beta

C. Gamma

D. UV

21. Which of the following is used for relieving arthritis pain in synovial joints?

A. Yttrium-90

B. Strontium-89

C. Erbium-169

D. All of the above

22. Which of the following is used in diagnosis of pernicious anaemia?

A. Cyanocobalamin

B. Calcium

C. Iodine

D. Gold

23. Short half-life radioactive waste is the material with half-life of __________

A. Less than one year

B. Less than six months

C. Less than three months

D. Less than one month

24. Which of the following is not a type of gas-filled detector?

A. Proportional counter

B. Ionization chamber

C. GM Counter

D. Semiconductor detector

25. Which of the following detection methods is not commonly used to detect isotopically labelled drug metabolites?

A. Infra-red spectroscopy

B. Mass spectrometry

C. Nuclear magnetic resonance spectroscopy

D. Scintillation counting

26. According to level of activity radioactive waste can be __________

A. High level waste

B. Low level waste

C. Medium level waste

D. All of the above

27. The hospital radioactive waste is mostly composed of __________

A. High level waste

B. Low level waste

C. Medium level waste

D. All of the above

28. Gold-198 is used in the treatment of __________

A. Rheumatoid arthritis B. Pernicious anemia

C. Detection of tumors D. Thyroid functioning

29. ________ is used for the measurement of radioactivity.

A. GM counter

B. Laminar flow counter

C. Stainless steel counter

D. Electric counter

30. The following is a method of disposal of radioactivity ________

A. Delay and decay

B. Incineration

C. Concentrate and buried

D. All of the above

Answer Key

1 D	2 A	3 B	4 D	5 A	6 B	7 A	8 D	9 C	10 A
11 C	12 A	13 D	14 B	15 B	16 D	17 B	18 B	19 D	20 C
21 D	22 A	23 D	24 C	25 B	26 D	27 B	28 A	29 A	30 D

CHAPTER 7

Application of Computers in Hospital Pharmacy Practice, Electronic Health Records, Softwares used in Hospital Pharmacy

1. **Computer generated prescriptions created by health-care provider are __________**
   A. Orders
   B. E-prescriptions
   C. Prescriptions
   D. All of the above

2. **The word computer comes from the word "compute", which means to __________**
   A. Add
   B. Mix
   C. Calculate
   D. None of the above

3. **______________ software is used for screening drug interactions in patients.**
   A. SUMEX
   B. NONLIN
   C. QUAR
   D. Micromedex

4. **__________ is meant to reduce the risks associated with traditional prescription script writing.**
   A. E-prescribing
   B. BCMA
   C. Automated dispensing
   D. Mobile technology

5. **EHR stands for __________**
   A. Electronic Home Record
   B. Elective Health Record
   C. Electronic Health Record
   D. Early Health Record

6. **The following is a benefit of pharmacy operation softwares.**
   A. Medical billing
   B. Hospital management
   C. Therapeutic drug monitoring
   D. All of the above

7. **In __________ inventory levels are manually checked.**
   A. Biologic inventory control system
   B. Periodic inventory control system
   C. Perpetual inventory control system
   D. Systemic inventory control system

8. **The following is an online databases available ______**
   A. MICROMEDEX
   B. MEDLINE
   C. MEDLARS
   D. All of the above

9. **NLM stands for __________**
   A. Native Library of Medicine
   B. National Library of Medicine
   C. Northern Library of Medicine
   D. Nominal Library of Medicine

10. **The Managerial Report includes __________**
    A. Preparation of daily sales report
    B. Preparation of prescription label
    C. Building a patient profile
    D. None of the above

11. **DAWN stands for __________**
    A. Drug Access Warning Network
    B. Drug Acute Warning Network
    C. Drug Abuse Warning Network
    D. Drug Against Warning Network

12. **The database produced by the American Society of Hospital Services is __________**
    A. Medicine
    B. International Pharmaceutical Abstracts
    C. Biosis
    D. MDB

13. **The whole hospital is controlled using __________**
    A. Medical management software
    B. Hospital pharmacy software
    C. Hospital management software
    D. Electronic patient record software

14. **EHR system performs following functions, *except* __________**
    A. Organize problem lists
    B. Maintain patient inventories
    C. Control patient demographics
    D. Maintain patient records

15. **__________ computer program is made for screening of interactions.**
    A. MEDIINE
    B. METAPHOR
    C. MEDLARS
    D. Medcem

16. **____________ database is used in drug information centre.**
    A. C
    B. Pascal
    C. MEDLINE
    D. Microcem

17. **___________ is useful for tracking and monitoring diseases.**
    A. EHR
    B. DIC
    C. DIB
    D. TDM

18. **MAR stands for __________**
    A. Minimum Administration Record
    B. Medication Administration Record
    C. Medium Administration Record
    D. Mean Administration Record

19. **A hardware device that is capable of executing a sequence of instruction is called __________**
    A. ALU
    B. CU
    C. Processor
    D. CPU

20. **AMA stands for __________**
    A. American Medical Association
    B. American Monopoly Association
    C. American Medication Annexure
    D. American Medicine Addendum

21. **Which type of telemedicine software eliminates the need of healthcare professional meeting to the patient?**
    A. Main telemedicine
    B. Remote control
    C. Store and forward telemedicine software
    D. Interactive telemedicine services in real time

22. **The patient profile is prepared in ______________ function.**
    A. Professional
    B. Clerical
    C. Managerial
    D. Personal

23. **__________ is a balance between not ordering too much and avoiding out-of-stock situation.**
    A. Data management
    B. Drug inventory control
    C. Software management
    D. TDM

24. **MEDLAR stands for __________**
    A. Medical Literature Analysis and Retrieval
    B. Medical Literature Automatic and Retrieval System
    C. Medical List Analysis and Retrieval System
    D. None of the above

25. **The medication monitoring is done with respect to __________**
    A. Volume of drug distribution
    B. Drug clearance
    C. Drug–laboratory and drug–disease interactions
    D. All of the above

26. **Which one of the following is not a storage device?**
    A. Pen drive
    B. CD
    C. Em drive
    D. Hard drive

27. **__________ provides information on drugs and their identification, poison, emergency drugs**
    A. Pubmed
    B. Goggle scholar
    C. Micromedex
    D. None of the above

28. **TDM stands for __________**
    A. Therapeutic Drug Monitoring
    B. Thesis of Drug Monitoring
    C. Theory of Drug Monitoring
    D. Telepathic Drug Monitoring

29. _______ software is used in drug information retrieval.

A. Mechanics

B. MEDLARS

C. DDD

D. Microcem

30. The following is a role of computers in drug store.

A. Maintenance of record

B. Storage of prescription

C. Preparation of purchase order

D. All of the above

Answer Key

1 B	2 C	3 D	4 A	5 C	6 D	7 B	8 D	9 B	10 A
11 C	12 B	13 C	14 B	15 B	16 C	17 A	18 B	19 C	20 A
21 C	22 A	23 B	24 A	25 D	26 C	27 C	28 A	29 B	30 D

CHAPTER

8

Clinical Pharmacy

1. The __________ is the heart of the patient counselling session.

A. Preparing for the session
B. Counselling content
C. Opening the session
D. Closing the session

2. The branch of pharmacy science, concerned with patient-oriented services and includes not only the dispensing of required medication but to advice the patient on safe and effective use of medicines is __________

A. Pharmacy
B. Hospital pharmacy
C. Clinical pharmacy
D. None of the above

3. _____________ is the responsible provision of drug therapy for the purpose of achieving definite outcomes that improves patient's quality of life.

A. Healthcare
B. Pharmaceutical care
C. Management care
D. Social care

4. __________ is a major role of clinical pharmacist.

A. Pre-marketing surveillance
B. Patient counselling
C. Post-marketing surveillance
D. Preclinical study

5. The following is medication related problems related to prescription is __________

A. Adverse drug reaction
B. Overusage of medicines
C. Improper drug selection
D. Untreated indications

6. _____________ helps to motivate the patient to take medicine for improvement of health status.

A. Pharmacovigilance
B. Patient counselling
C. Drug–drug interaction
D. Pharmacotherapy

7. Who is credited "Father of Clinical Pharmacy or Pharmacy Practice"?

A. Professor Heber W Youngken
B. Dr Eugene White
C. Prof L Wait
D. None of the above

8. Ward round participation involves _____________

A. Chief rounds
B. Pre-ward rounds
C. Resident rounds
D. All of the above

9. Pharmacovigilance is term related to ___________

A. OTC
B. ADR
C. MTM
D. WHO

10. The following is a drug related problem __________

A. Non-compliance
B. Use of wrong drug
C. New drug therapy
D. All of the above

11. Which of the following is the method of pharmacovigilance?

A. Sentinel site
B. Induced reporting
C. Active surveillance
D. Online reporting

12. Type of comparative observational studies is _______

A. Randomized controlled trials
B. Qualitative studies
C. Cohort studies
D. Test controlled studies

13. The location of Drug Information Centre should be near to the __________ department.

A. Inpatient
B. Pharmacy
C. Operation theatre
D. Store

14. The loss of urine, especially at night while sleeping, is known as __________

A. Pyelonephritis
B. Diabetes insipidus
C. Enuresis
D. Cystitis

15. Hora somni means __________

A. In the morning
B. At bedtime
C. In afternoon
D. In the evening

16. All are the effects of home medication review *except* __________

A. Evaluation of disposing of medicines
B. Minimize cost of healthcare
C. Assurance about the effects of medicines
D. Routine set according to patient life

17. The term paediatrics is __________

A. Related to elders
B. Related to children
C. Related to adult
D. Related to the foetus

18. Barriers to Home Medicines Review in India are _____

A. Faith in pharmacist
B. Salary to pharmacist
C. New concept
D. All of the above

19. Anorexia means __________

A. Agents that cause dilation of the pupil.
B. Loss of appetite
C. Agents that increase the secretion of saliva
D. Increase in acidity

20. __________ is a passive surveillance method.

A. Drug event monitoring
B. Registries
C. Spontaneous reports
D. Sentinel site

21. Advice must be given to patients while using MAO inhibitors is __________

A. Avoid cheese, alcoholic beverages and liver or yeast extract
B. Do not drive vehicle
C. Do not work with dangerous machinery
D. This laxative may colour the urine and faeces pink

22. The necrosis means __________

A. An agent that enhances the flow of bile into the intestine
B. Death of cells or tissues
C. Agent that helps to expel the gases from GI tract
D. An agent that produces evacuation of gallbladder

23. The English translation of Charta is __________

A. A lozenge
B. A powder
C. Every 4 hours
D. A drop

24. __________ is a branch of medicine that deals with the problems and diseases of old age and the medical care and treatment of aging people.

A. Postnatal care
B. Geriatric
C. Anti-natal care
D. All of the above

25. Drug therapy monitoring, also known as __________

A. Patient monitoring
B. Therapeutic drug monitoring
C. Both A and B
D. None of the above

26. All are principal elements of pharmaceutical care, *except* __________

A. Patient specific outcomes
B. Patient care
C. GPs consult
D. Medication use

27. __________ colour form is used to report ADR.

A. Blue
B. Yellow
C. Red
D. Brown

28. Which one of the following is not true for medication therapy management?

A. Pharmacist centred approach
B. A group of services
C. Individualistic outcomes set for patient
D. Responsibility of healthcare providers

29. All of the following are the needs for Home Medication Review *except* __________

A. Patients diseased condition
B. Polypharmacy
C. Cost of medicines
D. Patient compliance

30. The English meaning of Collyrium is __________

A. At bedtime
B. Before breakfast
C. When the pain is severe
D. An eye lotion

Answer Key

1 B	2 C	3 B	4 B	5 C	6 B	7 B	8 D	9 B	10 D
11 C	12 C	13 B	14 C	15 B	16 A	17 B	18 D	19 B	20 C
21 A	22 B	23 B	24 B	25 B	26 C	27 B	28 A	29 D	30 D

CHAPTER

9

Clinical Laboratory Tests

1. **Physical examination of urine includes __________**
   A. Odour
   B. Volume
   C. Colour
   D. All of the above

2. **Positive direct van den Bergh's reaction indicates presence of __________**
   A. Bile salts
   B. Conjugated bilirubin
   C. Unconjugated bilirubin
   D. Urobilinogen

3. **The normal value of haemoglobin in adult male is __________**
   A. 16 to 18 grams per decilitre
   B. 10 to 12 grams per decilitre
   C. 9 to 10 grams per decilitre
   D. 13.2 to 16.6 grams per decilitre

4. **__________ tests measures GFR accurately.**
   A. Inulin clearance
   B. Creatinine clearance
   C. Urea clearance
   D. None of the above

5. **The normal range of creatinine in females is ________**
   A. 150–200 ml/minute
   B. 100–120 ml/minute
   C. 95–105 ml/minute
   D. 100–150 ml/minute

6. **What tests are used to diagnose cardiovascular system disorders?**
   A. CCTA
   B. ECG
   C. MRI
   D. All of the above

7. **Conjugated hyperbilirubinemia with raised alkaline phosphatase levels are found in __________**
   A. Haemolytic jaundice
   B. Viral hepatitis
   C. Obstructive jaundice
   D. Neonatal physiological jaundice

8. **Inulin clearance is used to assess __________**
   A. Diluting ability of tubules
   B. Renal threshold
   C. Concentrating ability of tubules
   D. GFR

9. **__________ has protective effect against myocardial infarction.**
   A. HDL
   B. LDL
   C. VLDL
   D. Chylomicrons

10. **Failure of concentrating capacity of urine is assessed by measurement of __________**
    A. Creatinine clearance test
    B. Inulin clearance test
    C. Fluid deprivation test
    D. Acid load test

11. **Absence of urobilinogen in urine occurs in __________**
    A. Hepatic jaundice
    B. Obstructive jaundice
    C. Haemolytic jaundice
    D. All of the above

12. **Modified Gmelin's test is used for the detection of ___________**

    A. Proteins   B. Carbohydrates
    C. Bile pigments   D. Sugars

13. **All of the following are the cardiac markers, *except* ___________**

    A. Troponin
    B. Alkaline phosphatase
    C. Myoglobin
    D. CK-MB

14. **Average value of RBC in adult female is ___________ per cubic mm of blood.**

    A. 4.4–5.0 million
    B. 4.8–7.3 million
    C. 4–10 million
    D. 3–4 million

15. **___________ is a pulmonary function test.**

    A. Glucometry
    B. Spirometry
    C. Spleenometry
    D. Urinometry

16. **The indication of a low RBC count ___________**

    A. Calcium deficiency
    B. Vitamin B_6 deficiency
    C. Protein deficiency
    D. None of the above

17. **Which enzymes are measured in the liver function test?**

    A. SGPT   B. SGOT
    C. Both A and B   D. None of the above

18. **In haemolytic jaundice ___________**

    A. Bilirubin is excreted in urine
    B. Urinary urobilinogen excretion is increased
    C. Serum conjugated bilirubin is increased
    D. Serum alkaline phosphatase is increased

19. **___________ is good cholesterol.**

    A. VLDL
    B. LDL
    C. HDL
    D. All of the above

20. **In obstructive jaundice ___________ enzyme is diagnostically important.**

    A. Alkaline phosphatase
    B. Acid phosphatase
    C. Lactate dehydrogenase
    D. Creatine phosphokinase

21. **___________ is an instrument used for measuring changes in volume within an organ or whole body.**

    A. Kymograph
    B. Plethysmograph
    C. Electrocardiograph
    D. Eco-cardiograph

22. **Which of the following tests are done to check liver function?**

    A. Alkaline phosphatase (ALP)
    B. Alanine transaminase (ALT)
    C. Aspartate transaminase (AST)
    D. All of the above

23. **The laboratory phone report communication should be ___________**

    A. Accurate with no ambiguity
    B. Accurate message delivered by both parties
    C. Precise and accurate
    D. Quick and accurate

24. **What level of glucose indicates that patient is pre-diabetic in the fasting glucose test?**

    A. 200 mg/dL and higher
    B. 100–125 mg/dL
    C. 140–199 mg/dL
    D. All of the above

25. **A complete blood count (CBC) measures the size, number, and maturity of the different ________ cells.**

    A. Neuron
    B. Blood
    C. Liver
    D. None of the above

26. **The volume of plasma that would be completely cleared of creatinine per minute is ___________**

    A. Blood clearance
    B. Creatinine clearance
    C. Renal clearance
    D. All of the above

27. **The total solute concentration expressed as milli-osmols per litre is known as ___________**

    A. Isotonicity
    B. Osmolality
    C. Both A and B
    D. None of the above

28. Fouchet's test is used for the detection of __________

A. Glucose
B. Proteins
C. Bile pigments
D. Pus

29. The normal value of blood pressure is __________

A. 120 to 140 mm Hg
B. 120 to 80 mm Hg
C. 80 to 100 mm Hg
D. 140 to 180 mm Hg

30. In polyuria, the volume of urine excreted per day is more than __________

A. 500 ml
B. 600 ml
C. 1000 ml
D. 2500 ml

Answer Key

1 D	2 B	3 D	4 A	5 C	6 D	7 C	8 D	9 A	10 C
11 B	12 C	13 B	14 A	15 B	16 B	17 C	18 B	19 C	20 A
21 B	22 D	23 A	24 B	25 B	26 B	27 B	28 C	29 C	30 D

CHAPTER 10

Poisoning

1. **The Greek word for poison is ___________**
   A. Pharmacology
   B. Pharmaton
   C. Pharmakon
   D. Pharmacy

2. **PIC stands for ___________**
   A. Poison Intake Cell
   B. Poison Information Centre
   C. Poison Information Council
   D. None of the above

3. **The requirements for PIC are ___________**
   A. Communication equipment
   B. Appropriate location
   C. Educated specialized staff
   D. All of the above

4. **Antidote in Morphine poisoning is ___________**
   A. Dimercaprol B. Codeine
   C. Naloxone D. EDTA

5. **In acute poisoning ___________**
   A. Symptoms appear suddenly for short duration
   B. Symptoms appear for longer duration
   C. Both A and B
   D. None of the above

6. **BAL means ___________**
   A. Belgium anti-Lewisite
   B. British anti-Lewisite
   C. Boston anti-Lewisite
   D. Boronia anti-Lewisite

7. **Corrosive poison ___________**
   A. Produces ulceration of tissues
   B. Is highly active irritant
   C. Produces inflammation of tissues
   D. All of the above

8. **When type of poison is not known, then _____________ is used.**
   A. Acidic antidote
   B. Alkaline antidote
   C. Universal antidote
   D. Neutral antidote

9. **EDTA stands for _________________**
   A. Ethylene diamine tri acetic acid
   B. Ethylene diamine tetra acetic acid
   C. Ethyl diamine tetra acetic acid
   D. Ethylene trihydroxy tetra acetic acid

10. **What are the general principles for the treatment of poisoning?**
    A. Administration of known antidote
    B. Identification of poison
    C. Stabilization of patient
    D. All of the above

11. **___________ is an antidote used in mercury poisoning.**
    A. EDTA
    B. BAL
    C. Penicillamine
    D. Charcoal powder

12. **Uncontrollable muscle twitches, pinpoint pupils, and convulsions are the symptoms of ___________**
    A. Severe poisoning
    B. Mild poisoning
    C. Moderate poisoning
    D. All of the above

13. **DDT means __________**
    A. Dibromo-diphenyl-trichloroethane
    B. Dichloro-diphenyl-trichloroethane
    C. Difluoro-diphenyl-trichloroethane
    D. Diiodo-diphenyl-trichloroethane

14. **Naloxone is systemic antidote for ______ poisoning.**
    A. Iron B. Barbiturate
    C. Narcotics D. Methanol

15. **Opium is a __________ type of poison.**
    A. Animal poison
    B. Corrosive poison
    C. Irritant
    D. Neurotic

16. **____________ is a toxic substances is more likely to cause sickness in infants and elderly adults.**
    A. Bleach
    B. Lead
    C. Carbon monoxide
    D. Bee venom

17. **The antidote for iron poisoning is __________**
    A. Desferrioxime
    B. EDTA
    C. Dimercaprol
    D. Charcoal powder

18. **The risk for accidental poisoning with medicine can be reduced by __________**
    A. Carefully read the labels on your medicine
    B. Always turn on the light when taking medicine
    C. Clean out your medicine cabinet regularly
    D. All of the above

19. **__________ is also known as Dimercaprol.**
    A. EDTA B. DDT
    C. BAL D. DDS

20. **What information should you have ready when you call a Poison Control Centre?**
    A. Name of the product taken
    B. Time the poisoning occurred
    C. Age of your child
    D. All of the above

Answer Key

1 C	2 B	3 D	4 C	5 A	6 B	7 D	8 C	9 B	10 D
11 C	12 A	13 B	14 C	15 D	16 B	17 A	18 D	19 C	20 D

CHAPTER

11

Pharmacovigilance

1. **___________ is the science and activities relating to the detection, assessment, understanding and prevention of adverse effects or any other drug-related problems.**
   A. Project management
   B. Clinical research
   C. Pharmacovigilance
   D. Clinical data management

2. **Pharmacovigilance continue throughout ___________**
   A. Pre-marketing surveillance
   B. Post-marketing surveillance
   C. Pre- and post-marketing surveillance
   D. None of the above

3. **Pharmacovigilance ___________**
   A. Discourage effective drug use
   B. Increase economic burden on healthcare system
   C. Improve public health
   D. Neglect patients safety

4. **National Pharmacovigilance Program (NPP) was initiated in 2004 under the guidance of the _______**
   A. UNISCO **B.** CDSCO
   C. UMC **D.** DIC

5. **Pharmacovigilance programme of India was started by Govt of India on ___________**
   A. 14 July 2010
   B. 10 July 2010
   C. 14 July 2012
   D. 10 June 2012

6. **The Uppsala Monitoring Centre is located in which of the following countries?**
   A. Sweden **B.** China
   C. Japan **D.** India

7. **The Pharmacovigilance Programme of India, coordinated by the Indian Pharmacopeia Commission, is situated in ___________**
   A. Mumbai **B.** Ghaziabad
   C. Calcutta **D.** Jaipur

8. **Who is responsible for the WHO international drug monitoring programme?**
   A. WHO Drug Dictionary
   B. PVPI
   C. Uppsala Monitoring Centre
   D. Contract Research Organization

9. **The full form of MedDRA is ___________**
   A. Medical Directory for Regulations of Affairs
   B. Medical Dictionary for Regulatory Activities
   C. Medical Directory for Regulatory Affairs
   D. Medical Dictionary for Regulations and Actions

10. **One of the databases is open access database from the following ___________**
    A. Micromedex
    B. AfriTox
    C. PubChem
    D. Poisindex

11. **CROS stands for ___________**
    A. Contract Risk Organizations
    B. Contract Research Organizations
    C. Controlled Research Organizations
    D. Controlled Risk Organization

12. **The International Centre for Monitoring of Adverse Drug Reaction by WHO was established in ________**
    A. Sweden **B.** Geneva
    C. Japan **D.** China

13. **Adverse drug reaction is __________**
   A. Efficacy of drug
   B. Mechanism of drug
   C. Wanted effect of drug
   D. Unwanted effect of drug

14. **__________ manages the international database of ADRs reports received from National Centres.**
   A. CDSCO
   B. UNISCO
   C. Uppsala Monitoring Centre
   D. Medication Monitoring Centre

15. **NDA stands for __________**
   A. New drug application
   B. Non-drug application
   C. New device application
   D. New dose application

16. **The legislative requirement of pharmacovigilance in India comes under Schedule __________ of the Drugs and Cosmetics Act 1945.**
   A. O B. Y
   C. C D. H

17. **The information exchange between WHO and National Centre mainly through __________**
   A. Vigimed B. Google
   C. Both A and B D. None of the above

18. **UMC stands for __________**
   A. Union Monitoring Centre
   B. Uppsala Monitoring Centre
   C. Upper Monitoring Centre
   D. Urugave Monitoring Centre

19. **The function of ADRs monitoring centres is __________**
   A. Monitoring benefits/risk of medicine
   B. Monitoring spontaneous report
   C. Post-marketing surveillance of medicine
   D. All of the above

20. **__________ is a vigorous search of data with specific inputs of parameter to identify an important observation with probable relation of ADR and drug.**
   A. Drug monitoring
   B. Drug mining
   C. Drug analysis
   D. Drug evaluation

Answer Key

1 C	2 B	3 C	4 B	5 B	6 A	7 B	8 C	9 B	10 C
11 B	12 B	13 C	14 C	15 A	16 B	17 A	18 B	19 D	20 B

CHAPTER 12

Medication Errors

1. ___________ is a type of medication error in a prescription for a client with known allergy or tolerance.
   A. Prescription error B. Transcription error
   C. Dispensing error D. Administration error

2. ___________ is an error preventing strategy used to reduce the risk of look-alike medicine name errors.
   A. Alphabetical lettering B. Capital lettering
   C. Tall man lettering D. Lower case lettering

3. What type of medication error is misunderstanding of intended order?
   A. Prescription error B. Dispensing error
   C. Administration error D. Transcription error

4. The term tall man lettering, coined by the _________
   A. Institute of Safe Medication Practice
   B. Food and Drug Administration
   C. World Health Organization
   D. United States Food and Drug Administration

5. A medication error is a failure in the treatment process that leads to potential harm to the __________
   A. Nurses B. Pharmacists
   C. Physicians D. Patients

6. The cause of medication errors is ___________
   A. Incorrect preparation
   B. Expired product
   C. Incorrect duration
   D. All of the above

7. LASA stands for ___________
   A. Look-alike, sound-alike
   B. Look and sound alike
   C. Like and same agents
   D. Look and sound the same

8. _______________ is a type of medication error, i.e. an incorrect drug or dose sent to the unit.
   A. Documentation error
   B. Transcription error
   C. Dispensing error
   D. Administration error

9. Chlorpromazine vs. chlorpropamide is an example of ___________
   A. Drug classification
   B. Drug use
   C. Drug interaction
   D. Tall man lettering system

10. ASHP stands for ___________
    A. American Society for Hospital Pharmacists
    B. Asian Society for Hospital Pharmacists
    C. Administrative Society for Hospital Pharmacists
    D. Amazon Society for Hospital Pharmacists

11. The sources of medication errors are ___________
    A. Unclear labelling of drugs
    B. Incomplete delivery of drugs
    C. Misidentification of patient
    D. All of the above

12. The license of a physician may be cancelled due to ___________
    A. Checking of patient
    B. Medication error
    C. Prescribing
    D. None of the above

13. The medication error caused due to failure to adhere to prescribed medications is known as __________

A. Prescription error
B. Dispensing error
C. Compliance error
D. Compounding error

14. The preventive measures can be taken to reduce medication errors are __________

A. Correction of any doubts
B. Use of tall man lettering system
C. Double-reading the prescription
D. All of the above

15. vinCRIStine and vinBLAStine are examples of_______

A. Drug interaction
B. Tall man lettering system
C. Drug use
D. Drug classification

16. The most common type of medication error is_______

A. Wrong patient
B. Wrong drug
C. Wrong route of administration
D. Administering improper dose

17. ISMP stands for__________

A. Input of Safe Medication Practice
B. Institute of Safe Medication Practice
C. Incidence of Safe Medication Practice
D. Interference of Safe Medication Practice

18. The failure to administer an ordered dose is_______

A. Prescribing Errors
B. Wrong Time Errors
C. Monitoring Errors
D. Omission Errors

19. LASA drugs are look-alike, ______________-alike medicines.

A. Symptom
B. Seen
C. Sound
D. None of the above

20. Medication error can be caused due to __________

A. Documenting
B. Transcribing
C. Ordering/prescribing
D. All of the above

Answer Key

1 A	2 C	3 D	4 A	5 D	6 D	7 A	8 C	9 D	10 A
11 D	12 B	13 C	14 D	15 B	16 D	17 B	18 D	19 C	20 D

CHAPTER 13

Drug Interactions

1. **An alteration of effects of one drug by prior or concurrent administration of another drug is called ___________.**
   - **A.** Food interaction
   - **B.** Drug interaction
   - **C.** Food–food interaction
   - **D.** Tachyphylaxis

2. **________ causes pharmacodynamic drug interaction.**
   - **A.** Gastric motility changes
   - **B.** Stimulation of metabolism
   - **C.** Alteration of pH of GIT
   - **D.** Interactions at receptor site

3. **___________ should not be administered along with cheese, chocolate, banana, etc.**
   - **A.** Carbonic anhydrase inhibitors
   - **B.** MAO inhibitors
   - **C.** ACE inhibitors
   - **D.** COMT inhibitors

4. **Displacement of Tolbutamide or Warfarin by effective competitors like non-steroidal anti-inflammatory agents is an example of ___________.**
   - **A.** Interaction due to condition of patient
   - **B.** Interaction due to pharmacodynamics
   - **C.** Interaction due to pharmacokinetics
   - **D.** Interaction due to food

5. **Reduced tetracycline activity due to intake of calcium is ___________.**
   - **A.** Interaction due to condition of patient
   - **B.** Interaction due to pharmacodynamics
   - **C.** Interaction due to pharmacokinetics
   - **D.** Interaction due to food

6. **Folate deficiency maybe caused due to interaction of folic acid with ___________.**
   - **A.** Tetracycline
   - **B.** Phenytoin
   - **C.** Paracetamol
   - **D.** Aspirin

7. **Interactions at receptor sites cause ___________ drug interactions.**
   - **A.** Pharmaceutical
   - **B.** Pharmacokinetic
   - **C.** Pharmacodynamic
   - **D.** All of the above

8. **Which of the following are causes of drug interactions? ___________**
   - **A.** Patients non-compliance
   - **B.** Availability of potent drugs
   - **C.** Hepatic or renal disease
   - **D.** All of the above

9. **The comparison of bioavailability between two dosage forms is referred to as ___________.**
   - **A.** Bioavailability
   - **B.** Biopharmaceutics
   - **C.** Biological
   - **D.** Bioequivalence

10. **Tetracyclines should not be given with ___________.**
    - **A.** Juices
    - **B.** Milk or antacids
    - **C.** Honey
    - **D.** Fruits

Answer Key

1 B	2 D	3 B	4 D	5 C	6 B	7 C	8 D	9 D	10 B

Section XI

Pharmacy Law and Ethics

1. General Principles of Law, History and Various Acts Related to Drugs and Pharmacy Profession
2. The Pharmacy Act 1948 and Rules
   - Pharmacy Practice Regulations 2015
3. Drugs and Cosmetics Act 1940 and Rules 1945 and New Amendments
   - Import of Drugs
   - Manufacture of Drugs
   - Study of Schedule
   - Sale of Drugs
   - Drugs Prohibited for Manufacture and Sale in India
   - Administration of the Act and Rules
4. Narcotic Drugs and Psychotropic Substances Act 1985 and Rules
5. The Drugs and Magic Remedies (Objectionable Advertisements) Act, 1954
6. The Prevention of Cruelty to Animals Act 1960
7. The Poisons Act 1919
8. Food Safety and Standards Authority of India Act and Rules
9. National Pharmaceutical Pricing Authority
10. Code of Pharmaceutical Ethics

11. Medical Termination of Pregnancy Act 1971
12. Central Drugs Standards Control Organization (CDSCO) and Indian Pharmacopoeia Commission (IPC)
13. Good Regulatory Practices (GRPs)
14. Introduction to BCS System of Classification
15. Blood Bank: Basic Requirements and Functions
16. Clinical Establishment Act and Rules
17. Biomedical Waste Management Rules 2016
18. Bioethics
19. The Consumer Protection Act 1986
20. Introduction to the Disaster Management Act
21. Medical Devices

Syllabus (As Per ER 2020) Pharmacy Law and Ethics

Chapter	Topics
1	**General Principles of Law, History and various Acts related to Drugs and Pharmacy Profession**
2	**Pharmacy Act 1948 and Rules:** Objectives, Definitions, Pharmacy Council of India; its constitution and functions, Education Regulations, State and Joint State Pharmacy Councils, Registration of Pharmacists, Offences and Penalties. **Pharmacy Practice Regulations 2015**
3	**Drugs and Cosmetics Act 1940 and Rules 1945 and New Amendments:** Objectives, Definitions, Legal definitions of schedules to the Act and Rules **Import of Drugs:** Classes of drugs and cosmetics prohibited from import, import under license or permit. **Manufacture of Drugs:** Prohibition of manufacture and sale of certain drugs, Conditions for grant of license and conditions of license for manufacture of drugs, manufacture of drugs for test, examination and analysis, manufacture of new drug, loan license and repacking license. **Study of Schedule** C and C1, G, H, H1, K, P, M, N, and X. **Sale of Drugs:** Wholesale, Retail sale and Restricted license, Records to be kept in a pharmacy. **Drugs Prohibited for Manufacture and Sale in India** **Administration of the Act and Rules:** Drugs Technical Advisory Board, Central Drugs Laboratory, Drugs Consultative Committee, Government analysts, licensing authorities, controlling authorities, Drug Inspectors.
4	**Narcotic Drugs and Psychotropic Substances Act 1985 and Rules:** Objectives, Definitions, Authorities and Officers, Prohibition, Control and Regulation, Offences and Penalties.
5	**Drugs and Magic Remedies (Objectionable Advertisements) Act 1954:** Objectives, Definitions, Prohibition of certain advertisements, Classes of Exempted advertisements, Offences and Penalties.
6	**Prevention of Cruelty to Animals Act 1960:** Objectives, Definitions, CPCSEA—brief overview, Institutional Animal Ethics Committee, Breeding and Stocking of Animals, Performance of Experiments, Transfer and Acquisition of animals for experiment, Records, Power to suspend or revoke registration, Offences and Penalties
7	**Poisons Act 1919:** Introduction, objective, definition, possession, possession for sales and sale of any poison, import of poisons
8	**FSSAI (Food Safety and Standards Authority of India) Act and Rules:** Brief overview and aspects related to manufacture, storage, sale, and labelling of food supplements.
9	**National Pharmaceutical Pricing Authority:** Drugs Price Control Order (DPCO)—2013. Objectives, Definitions, Sale prices of bulk drugs, Retail price of formulations, Retail price and ceiling price of scheduled formulations, Pharmaceutical Policy 2002, National List of Essential Medicines (NLEM)
10	**Code of Pharmaceutical Ethics:** Definition, ethical principles, ethical problem solving, registration, code of ethics for Pharmacist in relation to his job, trade, medical profession and his profession, Pharmacist's oath.
11	**Medical Termination of Pregnancy Act and Rules:** Basic understanding, salient features, and Amendments
12	**Role of all the Government Pharma Regulator Bodies:** Central Drugs Standards Control Organization (CDSCO), Indian Pharmacopoeia Commission (IPC)
13	**Good Regulatory Practices** (documentation, licenses, renewals, e-governance) in community pharmacy, hospital pharmacy, pharma manufacturing, wholesale business, inspections, import, export of drugs and medical devices

Contd...

14	**Introduction to BCS System of Classification:** Basic concepts of Clinical Trials, ANDA, NDA, new drug development, New Drugs and Clinical Trials Rules, 2019. Brand v/s Generic, Trade name concept, Introduction to Patent Law and Intellectual Property Rights, Emergency use Authorization
15	**Blood Bank:** Basic requirements and functions
16	**Clinical Establishment Act and Rules:** Aspects related to Pharmacy
17	**Biomedical Waste Management Rules 2016:** Basic aspects, and aspects related to pharma manufacture to disposal of pharma / medical waste at homes, pharmacies, and hospitals.
18	**Bioethics:** Basic concepts, history and principles. brief overview of ICMR's National Ethical Guidelines for Biomedical and Health Research involving human
19	**Introduction to the Consumer Protection Act**
20	**Introduction to the Disaster Management Act**
21	**Medical Devices:** Categorization, basic aspects related to manufacture and sale

CHAPTER 1

General Principles of Law, History and Various Acts Related to Drugs and Pharmacy Profession

1. **Government appointed a 'Drug Enquiry Committee' under the Chairmanship of _________ in 1931.**
   A. Prof TK Gajjar
   B. Acharya Prafulla Chandra Ray
   C. Lt Col RN Chopra
   D. None of the above
2. **The first Pharmacy class was started in _________ at _________.**
   A. 1947, Rajputana University
   B. 1950, Sagar University
   C. 1932, Banaras Hindu University
   D. 1860, Madras Medical College
3. **For the first time in India, a chemist shop was opened in about 1811 by _________.**
   A. Dr Ghosh B. Mr Bathgate
   C. Mr Gajjar D. Mr Mukharji
4. **_________ was framed for regulation of the pharmacy profession.**
   A. NDPS Act 1985
   B. Drug Price Control Order
   C. The Pharmacy Act 1948
   D. Drugs and Magic Remedies Act
5. **The Pharmaceutical Society of India was established in _________.**
   A. 1847 B. 1923
   C. 1925 D. 1864
6. **_________ is the father of medicine.**
   A. Hippocrates B. Dioscorides
   C. Galen D. None of the above
7. **Import of Drugs Bill was introduced in _________ in Legislative Assembly.**
   A. 1957 B. 1927
   C. 1937 D. 1947
8. **Bengal Chemical and Pharmaceutical works, was started in Calcutta in 1901 by _____________.**
   A. Mr Chakrawarti
   B. Acharya Prafulla Chandra Ray
   C. RN Chopra
   D. Mr Ghosh
9. **Jurisprudence is the study of ______________**
   A. Health education
   B. Public health
   C. Fundamental legal principles
   D. Maternity health
10. **The law framed for regulation of the framework for fair pricing is _________.**
    A. Drugs and Magic Remedies Act
    B. Drug price control order
    C. Pharmacy Act
    D. NDPS Act 1985

Answer Key

1 C	2 D	3 B	4 C	5 B	6 A	7 C	8 B	9 C	10 B

CHAPTER

2

The Pharmacy Act 1948 and Rules

1. **The main object of the Pharmacy Act, 1948 is to _____.**
   A. Prevent suffering on animals
   B. Control the advertisement of drugs
   C. Regulate the profession of pharmacy
   D. Regulate the sale of narcotic drugs

2. **A person whose name is for the time being entered in the register of the State in which he is for the time being residing or carrying on his profession or business of pharmacy is called ________.**
   A. Repatriate
   B. Registered pharmacist
   C. Displaced person
   D. None of the above

3. **________ has the power to constitute State Pharmacy Council.**
   A. PCI
   B. Central Government
   C. Central Council
   D. State Government

4. **First register is prepared by ________.**
   A. Registration Tribunal
   B. Central Government
   C. Registrar of State Pharmacy Council
   D. PCI

5. **The registration of pharmacist is done by the State PCI under _________ of the Pharmacy Act 1948.**
   A. Section 10 B. Section 19
   C. Section 8 D. Section 6

6. **For registration of pharmacist in state, the Pharmacy Act provide for constitution of ________.**
   A. Registrar of Central Pharmacy Council
   B. Registrar of State Pharmacy Council
   C. Registrar of co-operative society
   D. None of the above

7. **Central register of pharmacist is maintained by _____.**
   A. PCI
   B. Central government
   C. AICTE
   D. State government

8. **Total area required for retail and wholesale drug store together is ________.**
   A. 20 sqm B. 40 sqm
   C. 15 sqm D. 60 sqm

9. **Pharmacy Act was established in ________.**
   A. 1995 B. 1948
   C. 1940 D. 1919

10. **In State Pharmacy Council all of the following are ex-officio members *except* ________.**
    A. Chief Administrator medical officer of state
    B. The officer in charge of Drugs Control Organization
    C. Government Analyst
    D. President of India

11. **The PCI was constituted under ___________ of the Pharmacy Act 1948.**
    A. Section I
    B. Section II
    C. Section III
    D. Section IV

12. **The State Pharmacy Council should have the following number of elected members ________.**
    A. Seven B. Six
    C. Five D. Nine

13. **The Education Regulation (ER) is published in official gazette by ________.**
    A. President, Pharmacy Council of India
    B. Ministry of Education
    C. Central Government
    D. Drug Controller

14. **The education regulations (ER) were laid down by ________.**
    A. PCI B. DCC
    C. DTAB D. State PCI

15. **Who is responsible for evolving educational standard and regulations for the course in pharmacy through education regulations?**
    A. Indian Patent Act B. Education Act
    C. Pharmacy Act D. D and C Act

16. **The Registration Tribunal for first register consists of ________ persons.**
    A. 02 B. 03
    C. 04 D. 05

17. **Following are the ex-officio members of PCI *except* ________________.**
    A. Director of Central Drug Laboratory
    B. Drug Inspector
    C. Director of General of Health Services
    D. Drug Controller of India

18. **University Grants Commission is established under ________ of UGC Act, 1956.**
    A. Section 3A B. Section 6
    C. Section 4 D. Section 10

19. **The PCI is constituted by ________.**
    A. State government
    B. Central government
    C. Joint state government
    D. None of the above

20. **Pharmacy Act, 1948 provides for the constitution of central council under ______________ by central government.**
    A. Section 4
    B. Section 3
    C. Section 3 of Chapter 1
    D. Section 4 of Chapter 1

21. **The order of executive committee directing removal of a name from register should be confirmed by ______________.**
    A. Central Government
    B. State Government
    C. State Pharmacy Council
    D. Central Pharmacy Council

22. **Education regulation prepared under subject to provision of ________ of Pharmacy Act, 1948.**
    A. Section 3A
    B. Section 3
    C. Section 4
    D. Section 10

23. **For the preparation of Central Register each state council is required to supply ________ copies of its register to central council after 1st April of each year along with amendment if any for updating the central register.**
    A. 07 B. 05
    C. 06 D. 11

24. **In elected member of PCI six members elected by______.**
    A. AICTE
    B. Central Council
    C. UGC
    D. All of the above

25. **How many members are elected among themselves by registered pharmacy of state?**
    A. Six B. Three
    C. Four D. Five

26. **The following is register of pharmacists maintained as per Pharmacy Act 1948.**
    A. Subsequent register
    B. First register
    C. Central register
    D. All of the above

27. **Nominated or elected members in "State Pharmacy Council" hold office for a term of ________ .**
    A. 5 years
    B. 3 years
    C. 4 years
    D. 6 years

28. **Who among the following is not a member of the Pharmacy Council of India?**
    A. The Director General Health Sciences
    B. The Director, Central Research Institute
    C. The Drugs Control of India
    D. The Director, Central Drugs Laboratory

29. **Joint State Pharmacy Council is constituted under Section ________ of Pharmacy Act.**
    A. 19 B. 10
    C. 12 D. 20

30. A person who has attained his __________ years residing or carrying on his profession or business of pharmacy and has been paid the prescribed fees for registration shall be eligible registration on first registration.

A. 18 B. 21
C. 15 D. 25

31. The prescribed renewal fees should be paid before of every __________ year.

A. 25th March B. 14th April
C. 31st December D. 1st January

32. Joint State Pharmacy Council are constituted for __________.

A. 1 year B. Indefinite years
C. 2 years D. 5 years

33. __________ of pharmacist is essential for maintaining the standards of pharmacy profession.

A. Qualification
B. Registration
C. Licence
D. Registrar of State Pharmacy Council

34. Central Council means __________.

A. Pharmacy Council of India constituted under Section 3
B. State Pharmacy Council constituted under Section 20
C. State Pharmacy Council constituted under Section 19
D. Pharmacy Council of India constituted under Section 15A

35. In India, the Pharmacy Council of India was firstly constituted in the year __________.

A. 1951 B. 1948
C. 1949 D. 1950

36. The PCI inspectors report to the __________ after inspection.

A. Joint state council B. Central council
C. State council D. Central government

37. History of Pharmacy Act was studied in __________.

A. Chapter I B. Chapter IV
C. Chapter III D. Chapter II

38. Upon entry of the name of person in the register, the "Registrar" is required to issue to him a __________.

A. Application form B. Certificate
C. Receipt D. Prize

39. PCI is reconstituted after every __________.

A. 1 year B. 5 years
C. 2 years D. 4 years

40. The minimum age limit for registration as pharmacist is __________.

A. 20 years B. 19 years
C. 18 years D. 21 years

41. Education institutions providing pharmacy education are approved by the __________.

A. Pharmacy Council of India
B. Central government
C. Drug Controller of India
D. None of the above

42. __________ is maintained by Central Council.

A. Tribunal register
B. Subsequent register
C. Central register
D. First register

43. Which authority approves courses of study and examination for the purpose of qualifying for registration as pharmacist?

A. SPC B. University
C. AICTE D. PCI

44. President and Vice President of central council shall hold office for a term of __________ from the date of nomination of election.

A. 5 B. 3
C. 2 D. 4

45. Pharmacy Council of India also known as __________.

A. State Council B. Central Council
C. Medical Council D. None of the above

46. Registered pharmacist is the person who should be __________.

A. Qualified B. Pharmacy
B. Qualified Diploma Pharmacy
C. Having his name entered in the state, register of pharmacists
D. All of the above

47. Education Regulation is published in __________.

A. Rajya Sabha Assembly
B. Official Gazette
C. Parliament
D. Lok Sabha Assembly

48. A State Council may appoint a registrar who may act as __________.

A. Executive member B. Secretary
C. Treasurer D. Vice President

49. Minimum training required to be a pharmacist is ____________.

A. 550 hours in 3 months
B. 500 hours in 3 months
C. 300 hours in 3 months
D. 750 hours in 3 months

50. The Pharmacy Council of India is required to maintain a register containing the name of _________.

A. Offences of pharmacy
B. Nominated member of central council
C. All Registered pharmacists
D. Elected member of state

Answer Key

1 C	2 B	3 D	4 A	5 B	6 B	7 A	8 C	9 B	10 D
11 C	12 B	13 C	14 A	15 C	16 B	17 B	18 C	19 B	20 C
21 C	22 D	23 B	24 C	25 D	26 D	27 A	28 B	29 D	30 A
31 C	32 B	33 B	34 A	35 C	36 B	37 A	38 B	39 B	40 C
41 A	42 C	43 D	44 A	45 B	46 C	47 B	48 C	49 B	50 C

CHAPTER

3

Drugs and Cosmetics Act 1940 and Rules 1945 and New Amendments

1. The Drug and Cosmetics Act has been divided into _________ parts.

A. 15 B. 18
C. 16 D. 24

2. Blood Bank comes under the Schedule _________.

A. B B. D
C. G D. F

3. Cosmetics mean any article intended to _________.

A. Alter the appearance of human body
B. Affect the structure of the human body
C. Destruct vermin of insects
D. All of the above

4. The members of DTAB hold the office for a period of _____________.

A. 7 years B. 3 years
C. 1 year D. 5 years

5. Central Drug Laboratory is located at _________.

A. Hyderabad
B. Mumbai
C. Lucknow
D. Kolkata

6. Schedule C is related to _____________.

A. List of allopathic product
B. List of biological and immunological product
C. List of homeopathy product
D. List of ayurvedic product

7. List of minimum equipments required for efficient running of pharmacy is given in Schedule _______.

A. N B. F
C. M D. J

8. Good manufacturing practices for Ayurvedic, Siddha and all Unani medicines comes under ___________.

A. Schedule M
B. Schedule T
C. Schedule S
D. Schedule U

9. The drugs which are imported under the names of other drugs are called ________.

A. Adulterated drugs
B. Spurious drugs
C. Misbranded drugs
D. None of the above

10. Drug Inspector is appointed under Section _________ of the Act.

A. 41 of IPC B. 42 of IPC
C. 36 of IPC D. 21 of IPC

11. The drug samples taken by drug inspector for analysis are sent to __________.

A. Manufacturer
B. Government Analyst
C. Testing Laboratories
D. Chemical Analyst

12. The Schedule for life period of drug is ___________.

A. Schedule S
B. Schedule Q
C. Schedule P
D. Schedule R

13. The DCC is constituted under _________ of the D and C Act 1940.

A. Section 6 B. Section 7
C. Section 8 D. Section 9

14. Particulars to be shown in the manufacturing records, records of raw materials, analytical records of drugs is specified in ___________.

A. Schedule S B. Schedule P
C. Schedule Y D. Schedule U

15. Schedule J is related to ____________.

A. Standards for umbilical tapes
B. List of disease which cannot be cured
C. Blood and blood products
D. Drugs marketed under generic name

16. As per D and C Act "Schedule FF" is related with ___________.

A. Ophthalmic preparation
B. Parenteral preparation
C. Ointment formulation
D. Skin cosmetic preparation

17. Insulin injection comes under __________.

A. Schedule A B. Schedule B
C. Schedule C D. Schedule E

18. Which of the following is prohibited to be imported?

A. Toilet preparations
B. Misbranded drugs
C. Ayurvedic drugs
D. Schedule 'C' drugs

19. Standard for mechanical contraceptive comes under Schedule ________ as per D and C Act

A. X B. S
C. R D. O

20. Pack size of drug is covered under __________.

A. Schedule P
B. Schedule R
C. Schedule O
D. Schedule P1

21. Aspirin sodium comes under ____________.

A. Schedule W B. Schedule G
C. Schedule H D. Schedule J

22. DTAB and DCC are purely ________ bodies.

A. Analytical
B. Advisory
C. Professional
D. Cooperative

23. Example of Schedule G drug is ___________.

A. Barbital B. Metformin
C. Enalapril D. Cefuroxime

24. List of drugs which should be used by patient under medical supervision is covered under ________ as per D & C Act.

A. Schedule H
B. Schedule 1
C. Schedule G
D. Schedule J

25. Which form number required for licence for retail sale of schedule C and C1 drug?

A. 20 B. 19
C. 22 D. 21

26. Biological and biotechnological products are included in Schedule __________.

A. C and C1 B. A
C. B D. X

27. ________ means the licensed premises for the sale of drugs which do not require the services of qualified persons.

A. Pharmacy
B. Chemist and Druggist
C. Drug store
D. All of the above

28. Requirements and guidelines for permission to import and/or manufacture of New Drug for sale or to undertake clinical trials comes under ________.

A. Schedule A
B. Schedule Y
C. Schedule T
D. Schedule W

29. DTAB has _________ ex-officio members.

A. Eight B. Five
C. Six D. Four

30. Schedule __________ of Drugs and Cosmetics Act includes requirements and guidelines on clinical trials for import and manufacturing of new drugs.

A. V B. W
C. X D. Y

31. Biologicals are tested at which of the following centres?

A. Kasauli B. Mumbai
C. Hyderabad D. Delhi

32. Which of the following Schedule of Drugs and Cosmetics Rules 1945 deals with objectionable advertisements?

A. Schedule C
B. Schedule F
C. Schedule H
D. Schedule J

33. Medical stores are inspected by drug inspector for at least _____________.

A. Thrice in a year B. Once a year
C. Twice in a year D. Quarterly in a year

34. In relation to Ayurvedic, Siddha or Unani drug Government analyst appointed under _________.

A. Section 33-E B. Section 33-G
C. Section 33-F D. Section 33-H

35. Minimum area of the shop to obtain a wholesale licence to sell and stock drugs shall be _________.

A. Fifteen square metres
B. Five square metres
C. Ten square metres
D. Twenty square metres

36. Who among the following is the Chairman of Drug Technical Advisory Board?

A. The Drugs Controller of India
B. The Director General of Health Services
C. The President of Pharmacy Council of India
D. The President of Medical Council of India

37. The penalty for using Government Analyst report for advertising is _________.

A. ₹100 B. ₹50
C. ₹200 D. ₹500

38. The licence of import of drug is obtained in application to _____________.

A. PCI
B. DCC
C. Drug Controller of India
D. DTAB

39. The schedules to the Drugs and Cosmetics Act are _____________.

A. 1 to 25 B. A to Y
C. First and Second D. A and B only

40. Which of the following drug products will have NRx on its label?

A. Antidiabetic
B. Antihypertensive drug
C. Antimicrobial drug
D. Narcotic analgesic

41. License to sell, stock or exhibit or offer for sale, or distribute by wholesale drugs specified in Schedule C and C1 is __________.

A. 20 B B. 21 B
C. 20 A D. 22 A

42. __________ are provided for the analysis of drugs and cosmetics.

A. Control Laboratory
B. State Drug Laboratory,
C. Central Drug Laboratory
D. Both A and B

43. As per Schedule M the permitted limit of solid content in water for injection is ___________.

A. 1 ppm B. 10 ppm
C. 100 ppm D. 0.1 ppm

44. Biological and microbiological tests are carried out at _________________.

A. Central Drugs Laboratory, Kolkata
B. Central Research Institute, Kasauli
C. National Institute of Biologicals, Noida
D. Central Drugs Research Institute, Lucknow

45. Application to manufacture cosmetics made to the licensing authority in _________.

A. Form 32 A
B. Form 12
C. Form 31
D. Form 31A

46. Dettol comes under _____________.

A. Schedule N
B. Schedule O
C. Schedule Q
D. Schedule X

47. Requirement of factory for manufacture of medical devices is dealt under _____________.

A. Schedule M1
B. Schedule R1
C. Schedule M2
D. Schedule M3

48. Barbiturates are _________ drug.

A. Schedule H
B. Schedule X
C. Schedule C
D. Schedule Y

49. ____________ has the power to fix the ceiling price of scheduled formulations.

A. State Government
B. Central Government
C. Lok Sabha
D. Rajya Sabha

50. Under Section 21 of the Indian penal code all Drug Inspectors are _________.

A. Officer-in-charge Drug Control
B. Qualified person
C. Competent Person
D. Public servants

51. Private testing laboratory for carrying out tests on drugs requires _________.

A. Form 32 B. Form 36
C. Form 31 D. Form 30

52. A cosmetic preparation containing hexachlorophene or mercury compounds are _________ from import.

A. Prohibited
B. Exempted
C. Allowed
D. Provided Special Provision

53. In relation to a Ayurvedic, Siddha or Unani drug an inspector appointed by central or state government under _________.

A. Section 33-E
B. Section 33-G
C. Section 33-F
D. Section 33-H

54. Drug for examination test of analysis can be imported under the license in Form

A. 10 B. 12
C. 11 D. 13

55. Specify the form number required for license for retail sale of schedule C and C1 _________.

A. 22 B. 21
C. 19 D. 18

56. As per Supreme Court, the Drugs and Cosmetics Act as statute of _________.

A. Life saving B. Social
C. Moral D. Economic

57. The Schedule in D and C Act that deals with the standard for disinfection fluid is _________.

A. Schedule M
B. Schedule B
C. Schedule F
D. Schedule O

58. One of the following is needed for the cosmetic manufacture _________.

A. Form 24 B. Form 36
C. Form 32 D. Form 20

59. Schedule M is related to _________.

A. Pack sizes of drug
B. GMP
C. Curable disease
D. List of diseases and ailments which drug cannot claim

60. Injection syringes and needle are covered under ____.

A. Schedule X
B. Schedule A
C. Schedule B
D. Schedule C

61. Kala jadu or Kavach comes under _________.

A. Schedule P
B. Schedule J
C. Schedule K
D. Schedule L

62. Indian Veterinary Research Institute is situated at _________.

A. Kolkata
B. Lucknow
C. Izatnagar
D. Ghazipur

63. Schedule F(ii) prescribes the standards for _________

A. Surgical dressings
B. Ophthalmic preparations
C. Cosmetics
D. Umbilical taps

64. Schedule M (i) prescribes the requirements of factory premises, plant, equipment, etc. for the manufacture of _________.

A. Drugs
B. Homoeopathic medicine
C. Cosmetics
D. Medical devices

65. Drugs marketed under the generic names only are specified in _________.

A. Schedule T
B. Schedule V
C. Schedule Y
D. Schedule W

66. Standards of patent and proprietary medicine is specified in _________.

A. Schedule T
B. Schedule M
C. Schedule V
D. Schedule Q

67. Schedule B is related with ________.

A. Forms

B. Fees for analysis

C. GMP

D. Pharmacy

68. List of permitted coal tar colours for use in cosmetics is specified in ________.

A. Schedule T

B. Schedule X

C. Schedule Q

D. Schedule S

69. ________ is used to issue licence for wholesale of drugs other than specified in Schedule C, C1 and X.

A. Form 20A

B. Form 20B

C. Form 15A

D. From 15B

70. ___________ drugs are manufactured in accordance with the formulae described in the first schedule.

A. Allopathic

B. Standard quality

C. Homoeopathic

D. Ayurvedic, Siddha and Unani

Answer Key

1 B	2 C	3 A	4 B	5 D	6 B	7 A	8 B	9 B	10 D
11 B	12 C	13 B	14 D	15 B	16 A	17 C	18 B	19 C	20 D
21 C	22 B	23 B	24 C	25 D	26 A	27 C	28 B	29 A	30 D
31 A	32 D	33 B	34 C	35 A	36 B	37 D	38 C	39 C	40 D
41 B	42 D	43 B	44 B	45 C	46 B	47 D	48 B	49 B	50 D
51 B	52 A	53 B	54 C	55 B	56 A	57 D	58 D	59 B	60 D
61 B	62 C	63 A	64 B	65 D	66 C	67 B	68 C	69 B	70 D

CHAPTER 4

Narcotic Drugs and Psychotropic Substances Act 1985 and Rules

1. **The Narcotic Drugs and Psychotropic Substances Act was passed in year _______________.**
   A. 1955 B. 1965
   C. 1975 D. 1985

2. **As per Narcotic Drugs and Psychotropic Substances Act, the Ganja means ________________.**
   A. Flowering and fruiting tops of *Cannabis sativa*
   B. Flowering and fruiting tops, leaves and seeds of *Cannabis sativa*
   C. Roots of *Cannabis sativa*
   D. All parts of *Cannabis sativa*

3. **____________ Act was passed to fight against the fast increasing use of addictive materials.**
   A. DMR B. NDPS
   C. MTP D. Poison Act 1919

4. **The following is example of narcotic drug _______.**
   A. Opium B. Coca
   C. Hemp D. All of the above

5. **Diacetyl morphine is also known as _____________.**
   A. Hemp B. Cannabis
   C. Charas D. Heroin

6. **The Narcotic Drugs and Psychotropic Substances consultative committee consists of ___________.**
   A. 20 members B. 30 members
   C. 40 members D. 50 members

7. **___________ means the plant of any species of genus Erythroxylon.**
   A. Cannabis
   B. Coca plant
   C. Poppy straw
   D. Opium poppy

8. **Coca derivatives include ______________.**
   A. Ecgonine B. Cocaine
   C. Both A and B D. None of the above

9. **Opium derivatives include _______________.**
   A. Medicinal opium
   B. Phenanthrene alkaloids such as Morphine, Codeine, Thebaine and their salts
   C. Diacetyl Morphine and its salts
   D. All of the above

10. **Punishment for illegal possession of small quantities of cocaine, morphine, diacetyl morphine, etc for personal consumption is ______________.**
    A. Imprisonment up to 1 year or fine or both
    B. Imprisonment up to 5 years or fine or both
    C. Imprisonment up to 1 year or fine
    D. Imprisonment up to 5 years or fine

11. **Under the provisions of NDPS Act, the Government may appoint ____________.**
    A. Police commission B. Narcotic commission
    C. Political commission D. State commission

12. **_________ means the opium manipulated to make it suitable for smoking and the residue left after it has been smoked.**
    A. Coca B. Charas
    C. Prepared Opium D. Hemp

13. **NDPS consultative committee has been formed by ___________.**
    A. State Government
    B. Central Government
    C. Inter-state Government
    D. Non-government

14. The Narcotic Drugs and Psychotropic Substances Act 1985, come into force on ____________.
A. 01 April 1986
B. 01 March 1986
C. 14 November 1985
D. 23 April 1985

15. _________ resin is obtained from Indian hemp plant.
A. Charas B. Bhang
C. Opium D. Codeine

16. Prevention of illicit traffic in Narcotic and Psychotropic Drug Act was come in __________.
A. 1986 B. 1987
C. 1988 D. 1990

17. As per narcotic drugs, controlled substance means ________________.
A. Drug notified in central government gazette
B. Drug banned by state
C. Drug includes in controlled price list
D. Drug dispensed by RMP

18. Geneva Convention was held on Narcotic Drugs in ______________.
A. March 1962 B. March 1972
C. March 1983 D. March 1993

19. Coca derivatives include __________.
A. Preparation containing less than 0.1% cocaine
B. Preparation containing less than 0.2% cocaine
C. Preparation containing more than 0.1% cocaine
D. Preparation containing more than 0.2% cocaine

20. *Cannabis sativa* yields ______________.
A. Opium B. Medicinal opium
C. Morphine D. Hemp

21. Charas is obtained from the _____________.
A. Coca plant B. Opium poppy
C. Opium D. Indian hemp plant

22. Coca, opium and hemp come under ___________.
A. Insecticide Act B. Poisons Act
C. Dangerous Drug Act D. Spurious Drug Act

23. The price of opium is fixed by ____________.
A. State Government B. Central Government
C. Non-government D. None of the above

24. The percentage content of morphine in opium is ___________.
A. Less than 0.2% B. More than 0.02%
C. More than 0.2% D. Less than 0.02%

25. Licence for cultivation of opium poppy is granted by ________________.
A. District Opium Officer B. District Police Officer
C. District Commissioner D. Collector

26. Plant of the species of Papaver, from which opium or any phenanthrene alkaloid can be extracted, is called ________________.
A. Opium poppy B. Coca
C. Heroin D. *Cannabis sativa*

27. ________ means the plant *Papaver somniferum*.
A. Opium poppy B. Coca
C. Hemp D. All of the above

28. Government opium factory is situated at ________.
A. Ghazipur B. Lucknow
C. Srinagar D. Calcutta

29. A person who has dependence on any narcotic drug or psychotropic substance is known as ________.
A. Guardian B. Minor
C. Addict D. None of the above

30. Opium derivatives include all the following *except* _____________.
A. Prepared of opium B. Medicinal opium
C. Heroin D. Charas

Answer Key

1 D	2 A	3 B	4 D	5 D	6 A	7 B	8 C	9 D	10 A
11 B	12 C	13 B	14 C	15 A	16 C	17 A	18 B	19 D	20 D
21 D	22 C	23 B	24 C	25 A	26 A	27 A	28 A	29 C	30 D

CHAPTER 5

The Drugs and Magic Remedies (Objectionable Advertisements) Act, 1954

1. **Any announcement made orally or by means of producing or transmitting light, sound or smoke, is known as _________.**
   A. Advertisement B. Order
   C. Commitment D. Resolution

2. **Advertisement of the report of Government analyst is ________.**
   A. Permitted B. Prohibited
   C. Exempted D. None of the above

3. **Taking part in the publication of advertisement means _________.**
   A. Advertising any notice
   B. Advertising magic remedy
   C. Printing and publication of the advertisement in any country
   D. None of the above

4. **Drugs and Magic Remedies (Objectionable Advertisements) Act was passed in _________.**
   A. 1945 B. 1954
   C. 1985 D. 1991

5. **Talisman, Mantra and Kavacha comes under _____.**
   A. Adulterated drug B. Misbranded drug
   C. Magic remedies D. Spurious drug

6. **Magic remedy which is claimed to have miraculous powers to cure, diagnose, prevent or mitigate a disease in humans or animal include _________.**
   A. Amulet B. Any talisman
   C. Mantra D. All of the above

7. **Advertisement of prescription drugs are meant for _________.**
   A. Manufacturer B. Patients
   C. Retailers D. Physician

8. **Advertisement of drug claiming to cure a disease mentioned in Schedule J is _________.**
   A. Prohibited
   B. Permitted
   C. Exempted
   D. None of the above

9. **Advertisement claiming to cure blindness is an example of _________.**
   A. Regular Advertisement
   B. Permitted Advertisement
   C. Exempted Advertisement
   D. Prohibited Advertisement

10. **List of diseases and ailments that a drug should not claim to prevent or cure is given in Schedule ________.**
    A. A B. J
    C. E D. F

11. **Display signboard or notices by a registered medical practitioner on his premises falls under _________.**
    A. Regular Advertisement
    B. Banned Advertisement
    C. Exempted Advertisement
    D. Prohibited Advertisement

12. **Advertisement means any _________ circular, label, wrapper or any other document made orally or by transmitting _________ sound or smoke.**
    A. Paper, Light B. Notice, Like
    C. Notice, Light D. Paper, Like

13. **Which one of the following is exempted advertisement?**
    A. Advertisement made for the treatment of diabetes
    B. Advertisement made by any person
    C. Advertisement made by the Government
    D. None of the above

14. The Act provides regulations for objectionable advertisement is ________.

A. Drug and Magic Remedies Act
B. Poisons Act
C. Medicinal and Toilet Preparations Act
D. Pharmacy Act

15. Which of the following disease is not listed in the Schedule of Drugs and Magic Remedies Act 1954?

A. Deafness B. Diarrhoea
C. Cataract D. Blindness

16. The advertisement claiming to cure blindness is an example of which advertisement?

A. Prohibited B. Permitted
C. Exempted D. None of the above

17. Which of the following is the example of magic remedies?

A. Kavacha B. Talisman
C. Mantra D. All of the above

18. Power of search, entry and seizure as per rules of Drugs and Magic Remedies (Objectionable Advertisements) Act 1954 is authorized by ________.

A. Government analyst
B. Central Government
C. State Government
D. Drug Inspector

19. Cure for cancer in an example of the following advertisements.

A. Bonafide B. Prohibited
C. Permitted D. Exempted

20. Advertisement of drugs claiming cure of disease mentioned in Schedule-J is ________.

A. Exempted
B. Granted
C. Prohibited
D. None of the above

Answer Key

1 A	2 B	3 C	4 B	5 C	6 D	7 D	8 A	9 D	10 B
11 C	12 C	13 C	14 A	15 B	16 A	17 D	18 D	19 B	20 C

CHAPTER 6

The Prevention of Cruelty to Animals Act 1960

1. ___________ **means the infliction of unnecessary pain or suffering on the animals.**
   A. Death B. Cruelty
   C. Monitoring D. All of the above

2. **According to the Prevention of Cruelty to Animals Act, 1960, animal means any living creature** ***except*** ___________.
   A. Microorganisms B. Birds
   C. Animals D. Human beings

3. **The chairman of Animal Welfare Board of India is appointed by** ___________.
   A. Pharmacy Council of India B. Central Government
   C. State Government D. None of the above

4. **How many members from Indian Council of Medical Research (ICMR) are nominated in Animal Welfare Board of India by the Central Government?**
   A. 6 B. 2
   C. 4 D. 3

5. **The experiments on the animals are done for** _______.
   A. Advancement in medical, pharmaceutical, and biological field
   B. Checking out the disease in animals
   C. Checking animal efficiency
   D. None of the above

6. **Animal Welfare Board is established by** _______.
   A. State Government B. Central Government
   C. State Council D. Central Council

7. **CPCSEA head office is situated in** ___________.
   A. Kolkata B. Chennai
   C. New Delhi D. Mumbai

8. **Full form of IAEC is** ___________.
   A. Institutional animal entitled committee
   B. Institutional animal ethical committee
   C. Institutional animal ethics corporation
   D. None of the above

9. **When was the Prevention of Cruelty to Animals Act passed?**
   A. 1955 B. 1961
   C. 1651 D. 1960

10. **Who of the following is the member of IAEC?**
    A. Biological scientist B. Veterinarian
    C. Socially aware member D. All of the above

11. **For performing animal studies permission has to take from** ___________.
    A. State Government B. IAEC
    C. Central Government D. None of the above

12. **The cruelty of animal includes** _________.
    A. Keeping in a small cage B. Not giving food
    C. Causing pain D. All of the above

13. **For treating animal cruelty how much fine has to be imposed for first conviction?**
    A. ₹ 150 B. ₹ 50
    C. ₹ 100 D. ₹ 200

14. **CPCSEA is a statutory committee established under** ___________.
    A. NDPS Act
    B. Drugs and Magic Remedies Act
    C. The Prevention of Cruelty to Animals Act, 1960
    D. MTP Act 1954

15. **The objective of IAEC under this Act is ________.**
   A. To protect the animal
   B. To prevent the unnecessary pain to animal
   C. To stop the use of animal
   D. None of the above

16. **In phooka or doom dev, ________ or any substance is introduced into female organ of milch animal with the intention of drawing off any secretion of ________.**
   A. Water, milk
   B. Air, water
   C. Water and saliva
   D. Air, milk

17. **Animal Welfare Board of India constituted under the Prevention of Cruelty to Animal Act started in ________.**
   A. Chennai B. New Delhi
   C. Mumbai D. Kolkata

18. **Supreme Court banned Jalli-kattu under which of the following Act?**
   A. Environment Prevention Act
   B. Prevention of Animal Cruelty Act 1960
   C. Drugs and Magic Remedies Act
   D. None of the above

19. **Committee for the purpose of control and supervision of experiment on animals (CPCSEA)—head office is situated in ________.**
   A. Kolkata B. New Delhi
   C. Mumbai D. Chennai

20. **For the registration of breeders, the permission has to be taken from ________.**
   A. CPCSEA
   B. IAEC
   C. IBSC
   D. Central Government

Answer Key

1 B	2 D	3 B	4 B	5 A	6 B	7 C	8 B	9 D	10 D
11 B	12 D	13 B	14 C	15 B	16 D	17 A	18 B	19 B	20 A

CHAPTER 7

The Poisons Act 1919

1. **The main objective of Poisons Act was ________.**
   - **A.** To achieve adequate supply
   - **B.** To regulate and control of import, possession and sale of poisons
   - **C.** To achieve equal distribution
   - **D.** To import poisons

2. **According to Poison Act Central Government is authorized to ________.**
   - **A.** Regulate import of poisons
   - **B.** Regulate possession and sale of poisons
   - **C.** Both A and B
   - **D.** None of the above

3. **________ means all substances notified as poison under Poison Act 1919.**
   - **A.** Metabolite **B.** Poison
   - **C.** Waste **D.** All of the above

4. **The Poisons Act came into existence in ________.**
   - **A.** 1985 **B.** 1920
   - **C.** 1919 **D.** 1930

5. **According to Poisons Act 1919 State Government is authorized to ________.**
   - **A.** Regulate possession of poisons
   - **B.** Regulate possession for sale and sale of poisons
   - **C.** Regulate import of poisons
   - **D.** None of the above.

6. **The poisonous substances from the ________ are exempted from certain provisions of the Poison Act.**
   - **A.** List A
   - **B.** List B
   - **C.** List C
   - **D.** List D

7. **According to the Poison Act ________ is authorized to regulate import poison.**
   - **A.** State government
   - **B.** Poison rehabilitation bureau
   - **C.** Central government
   - **D.** None of the above

8. **List A Poisons include ________.**
   - **A.** Aconite
   - **B.** Cantharides
   - **C.** Belladona
   - **D.** All of the above

9. **Penalty for unlawful importation possession for sale of poisons for the first conviction is ________.**
   - **A.** Imprisonment up to 5 months and fine up to ₹ 100
   - **B.** Imprisonment up to 3 months and fine up to ₹ 500 or both
   - **C.** Imprisonment up to 2 months and fine up to ₹ 500
   - **D.** Imprisonment up to 5 months and fine up to ₹ 1000 or both

10. **Penalty for the import of poison without license is punishable with fine up to ________ on first conviction.**
    - **A.** ₹ 5000 **B.** ₹ 1000
    - **C.** ₹ 500 **D.** ₹ 2000

11. **Insecticide Act was passed in ________.**
    - **A.** 1968 **B.** 1978
    - **C.** 1988 **D.** 1998

12. **List B Poisons include ________.**
    - **A.** Chloroform
    - **B.** Carbolic acid
    - **C.** Zinc chloride
    - **D.** All of the above

13. The main objectives of the Poison Act are to ________.

A. Control sale of poison
B. Control the import of poison
C. Control the possession of poison
D. All of the above

14. Arsenic is categorized in ______ under Poison Act, 1919.

A. List B
B. List A
C. Both of the above
D. None of the above

15. The objective of The Poisons Act 1919 is all the following *except* ________ .

A. To control the manufacture of poison
B. To control the import of poison
C. To control the possession for sale of poison
D. To control the possession of poison

16. Who is empowered to issue a warrant for search of any place under the Poison Act?

A. Subdivisional magistrate
B. District magistrate
C. Commissioner police
D. All of the above

17. Which of the following is an example of List B poison?

A. Cyanide
B. Ergot
C. Oxalic acid
D. Ecgonine

18. ________ may regulate the possession and sale of any specified poison.

A. Poisons control authority
B. Central government
C. State government
D. Poison rehabilitation bureau

19. Belladonna comes under ________ of poison.

A. List A
B. List B
C. List C
D. List D

20. Which of the following are the powers of state government?

A. Granting licence
B. Deciding in whom to grant licence
C. Fixing maximum quantity of poison to be sold.
D. All of the above

Answer Key

1 B	2 A	3 B	4 C	5 B	6 B	7 C	8 D	9 B	10 C
11 A	12 D	13 D	14 B	15 A	16 D	17 C	18 C	19 A	20 D

CHAPTER 8

Food Safety and Standards Authority of India Act and Rules

1. **Full form of FSSAI is _________.**
   - **A.** Food Standards and Safety Authority of India
   - **B.** Food Safety and Standards Authority of India
   - **C.** Food Sample and Standards Authority of India
   - **D.** None of the above

2. **_________ means the Food Safety and Standards Authority of India established under Section 4 of the Act.**
   - **A.** Safety Authority
   - **B.** Cleaning Authority
   - **C.** Food Authority
   - **D.** Maintenance Authority

3. **The Food and Adulteration Act was passed in ______.**
   - **A.** 1954 **B.** 1964
   - **C.** 1974 **D.** 1984

4. **According to FSSAI, food analyst should analyse the samples and shall send four copies of report to _____________.**
   - **A.** Commissioner
   - **B.** Food Safety Officer
   - **C.** Assistant Commissioner
   - **D.** Designated Officer

5. **The Food Authority shall consist of a Chairperson and the following _________ number of members.**
   - **A.** 20 **B.** 22
   - **C.** 11 **D.** 10

6. **The Food Officer means an officer appointed under the FSSAI Act _________.**
   - **A.** Section 41 **B.** Section 30
   - **C.** Section 37 **D.** Section 40

7. **The Food Safety and Standards Authority of India (FSSAI) has issued a set of guidelines regarding the recall of _____________ from the market**
   - **A.** Unsafe food products
   - **B.** Unsafe labelling
   - **C.** Unsafe drinking water
   - **D.** Unsafe packaging

8. **FSSAI has issued an advisory banning the use of which material for wrapping and packaging of food items?**
   - **A.** Newspaper **B.** Plastic
   - **C.** Polythene **D.** None of the above

9. **According to FSSAI, Food Safety Officer should remain _________ part/parts of sample with him.**
   - **A.** 3 **B.** 5
   - **C.** 1 **D.** 2

10. **Food analyst means an analyst appointed under _________ of the FSSAI Act.**
    - **A.** Section 40 **B.** Section 43
    - **C.** Section 44 **D.** Section 45

11. **The vertical issues of FSSAI Act include _________.**
    - **A.** Genetically modified organisms and foods
    - **B.** Functional food
    - **C.** Food additives
    - **D.** Water, flavoured water and beverages

12. **Which the following are included in the specific requirements for the labelling of alcoholic beverages?**
    - **A.** Nutritional information
    - **B.** Health claims
    - **C.** Alcohol content declaration
    - **D.** Nutritional facts

13. The penalty for sub-standard food under Section 51 is _________.

A. 2 lakhs
B. 5 lakhs
C. 3 lakhs
D. 10 lakhs

14. The head office of Food Safety and Standards Authority of India is located at _________.

A. Ahmadabad
B. Delhi
C. Mumbai
D. Kolkata

15. The penalty for misleading advertisement or label under Section 53 is _________.

A. 10 lakhs
B. 2 lakhs
C. 3 lakhs
D. 5 lakhs

16. _________ has power to make rules under FSSAI.

A. FSSAI
B. Central Government
C. State Government
D. None of the above

17. The Chairperson and the members other than ex-officio members of FSSAI shall hold office for ___________ years

A. Three
B. One
C. Two
D. Four

18. According to FSSAI _________ shall be responsible for inspection of food business, drawing samples and sending them to food analyst for analysis.

A. Assistant Commissioner
B. Food Safety Officer
C. Designated Officer
D. Commissioner

19. _______________ means an article of food for which standards have not been specified but is not unsafe.

A. Proprietary or novel food
B. Organic food
C. GM food
D. None of the above

20. The punishment for food containing extraneous matter is _________.

A. 5 lakhs
B. 1 lakh
C. 2 lakhs
D. 3 lakhs

Answer Key

1 B	2 C	3 A	4 D	5 B	6 C	7 C	8 A	9 C	10 D
11 D	12 C	13 B	14 B	15 A	16 B	17 A	18 C	19 A	20 B

CHAPTER 9

National Pharmaceutical Pricing Authority

1. _________ is a government regulatory agency that controls the prices of pharmaceutical drugs in India.
   A. MAPE
   B. DPEA
   C. NPPA
   D. DPCO

2. DPEA stands for _________
   A. Drug Price Equalisation Account
   B. Drug Pending Equalisation Account
   C. Drug Poor Equalisation Account
   D. Drug Penal Equalisation Account

3. What is the purpose of DPCO?
   A. To prohibit certain kinds of advertisements
   B. To achieve adequate production
   C. Misleading or exaggerated statements or claims
   D. An offer to refund money paid

4. For production from basic stage post-tax return of _________ on net worth is considered.
   A. 8% B. 10%
   C. 18% D. 20%

5. The provisions of DPCO are implemented and enforced by _________
   A. MAPE
   B. DPEA
   C. NPPA
   D. None of the above

6. The first National List of Essential Medicine of India was prepared and released in _________
   A. 1976 B. 1986
   C. 1996 D. 2006

7. A manufacturer who starts production of scheduled bulk drug has to furnish details to government within _________
   A. 30 days B. 60 days
   C. 10 days D. 15 days

8. The main objective of _________ is to make sure that the essential drugs are available to all at a reasonable price.
   A. Excise Duty Act
   B. DMR Act
   C. DPCO Act
   D. D and C Act

9. The latest Drug Price Control Order was passed on _________
   A. 2013 B. 2012
   C. 2011 D. 2014

10. For calculation of price of bulk drugs, a return of 12% is allowed on _________ costing.
    A. Intermediate
    B. Long-term marginal
    C. Short-term marginal
    D. Periodic

11. DPCO 1987 was replaced by _________
    A. 2000 B. 1990
    C. 1995 D. 1997

12. Drug Price Control Order was passed with the aim to _________
    A. Make these available at fair price
    B. Achieve adequate production
    C. Secure or regulate equitable distribution
    D. All of the above

13. While fixing the price of bulk drugs government shall take into consideration post-tax return of ________

A. 14% B. 10%
C. 12% D. 20%

14. NLEM is a list of medicines prepared by the ________

A. Ministry of Health and Social Welfare
B. Ministry of Health and Family Welfare
C. Ministry of Home and Family Welfare
D. Ministry of Health and Formal Welfare

15. How many drugs are scheduled under DPCO 1955?

A. 76 B. 77
C. 74 D. 78

16. The main objective of which act is to make sure that the essential drugs are available to all at a reasonable price?

A. NDPS Act
B. DPCO Act
C. MTP Act
D. D and C Act

17. Who has the power to fix the ceiling price of scheduled formulations?

A. Rajya Sabha
B. State Government
C. Central Government
D. Lok Sabha

18. Loose quantities of any formulation cannot be sold at a price exceeding ________ pro rate of formulation.

A. 10% B. 2%
C. 5% D. 9%

19. Which of the following drugs is a scheduled bulk drug?

A. Amikacin
B. Alprazolam
C. Salbutamol
D. Codeine

20. MAPE shall not exceed ________ for indigenously manufactured scheduled formulation.

A. 20% B. 50%
C. 100% D. 70%

Answer Key

1 C	2 A	3 B	4 C	5 C	6 C	7 D	8 C	9 A	10 B
11 C	12 D	13 A	14 B	15 C	16 B	17 C	18 C	19 A	20 C

CHAPTER 10

Code of Pharmaceutical Ethics

1. **The code of ethics of pharmacy is developed by ______.**
   A. MCI B. PCI
   C. SPC D. IDMA

2. **_________ means a science of morals or "code of moral principles".**
   A. Law
   B. Ethics
   C. Morality
   D. Pharmaceutical ethics

3. **_________ is the rules of human conduct binding to all persons in the State or Nation.**
   A. Status
   B. Law
   C. Ethics
   D. Power

4. **What is the code of ethics for pharmacists?**
   A. Pharmacist in relation to his trade
   B. Pharmacist in relation to his job
   C. Pharmacist in relation to medical profession
   D. All of the above

5. **Pharmacist is a liaison between _________ .**
   A. Medical profession or physician and public
   B. Retailer and public to alone
   C. Industry and public
   D. Pharmacist and physician

6. **Which one of the following is the ethical in pharmacy profession?**
   A. Consumer first priority
   B. Public trust
   C. Quality use of medicine
   D. All of the above

7. **Clandestine arrangement is also known as _________.**
   A. Open agreement
   B. Family agreement
   C. Secret agreement
   D. Social agreement

8. **Fair trade practice is a part of ethics related to ______.**
   A. Pharmacist in relation to medical profession
   B. Pharmacist in relation to his job
   C. Pharmacist in relation to his trade
   D. Pharmacist in relation to his own profession

9. **Which of the following statement is true in case of ethics?**
   A. Ethics comes from within a person's moral values
   B. Ethics is a set of guidelines
   C. Ethics are rules of conduct
   D. All of the above

10. **Authoritative instruments that rule on society is ______.**
    A. Code B. Ethics
    C. Law D. None of the above

11. **Handling of prescription is a part of ethics related to _________.**
    A. Pharmacist in relation to his job
    B. Pharmacist in relation to his trade
    C. Pharmacist in relation to medical profession
    D. Pharmacist in relation to his own profession

12. **_________ deals with right or wrong.**
    A. Code
    B. Ethics
    C. Law
    D. None of the above

13. Pharmacist in relation to medical profession _______.
A. Liaison with public
B. Provide professional limitation
C. Provide clandestine arrangement
D. All of the above

14. _________ is a set of rules and regulations.
A. Code
B. Law
C. Ethics
D. None of the above

15. The pharmacist should keep in mind the following points while dealing with his trade _________.
A. Purchase of drugs
B. Price structure
C. Fair trade practice
D. All of the above

16. The Federal rules primarily relate to _________.
A. Practice site
B. Drug product
C. Pharmacy practice
D. All of the above

17. The pharmacist should keep in mind the following points while dealing with his medical profession.
A. Liasion with public
B. Limitation of professional activity
C. Cladenstine arrangement
D. All of the above

18. _________ deals with actions that are punishable.
A. Law
B. Code
C. Ethics
D. None of the above

19. Hawking of drugs is a part of ethics related to ______.
A. Pharmacist in relation to his own profession
B. Pharmacist in relation to his job
C. Pharmacist in relation to his trade
D. Pharmacist in relation to medical profession

20. Which of the following points should be considered by a pharmacist while dealing with his trade?
A. Purchase of drugs
B. Price structure
C. Fair trade price
D. All of the above

Answer Key

1 B	2 B	3 B	4 D	5 A	6 D	7 C	8 C	9 D	10 C
11 A	12 B	13 D	14 B	15 D	16 B	17 D	18 A	19 C	20 D

CHAPTER 11

Medical Termination of Pregnancy Act 1971

1. **Medical Termination of Pregnancy Act was passed in the year ________.**
   A. 1945 B. 1965
   C. 1971 D 1947

2. **Places permitted for termination of pregnancy may be examined by ________.**
   A. Chief Medical Officer
   B. Drug Inspector
   C. Registered Medical Practitioner
   D. None of the above

3. **Guardian is ________.**
   A. A person who is a minor
   B. A person who has care for minor or lunatic
   C. A person who is a lunatic
   D. None of the above

4. **MTP Act 1971 was passed to provide for the termination of pregnancies of women by __________ for bonafide medical reason and for the matter concerned therewith.**
   A. Registered pharmacists
   B. Registered nurses
   C. Registered medical practitioners
   D. Compounders

5. **________ is a person who has not attained majority under the provisions of Indian Majority Act, 1875.**
   A. Major B. Minor
   C. Youngster D. Lunatic

6. **RMP may terminate the pregnancy of women who are ________ of age or more with their written consent.**
   A. 17 years
   B. 15 years
   C. 18 years
   D. 16 years

7. **12-week pregnancy can be terminated with the consent of ________.**
   A. 3 Registered medical practitioner
   B. 1 Registered medical practitioner
   C. 2 Registered medical practitioner
   D. None of the above

8. **Lunatic means as specified under ________ of Indian Lunacy Act, 1912.**
   A. Section 8
   B. Section 7
   C. Section 4
   D. Section 3

9. **Places approved for termination of pregnancy may be inspected by ________.**
   A. Registered medical practitioner
   B. Drug Inspector
   C. Chief medical officer
   D. None of the above

10. **MTP stands for ________.**
    A. Menstrual termination of pregnancy
    B. Medical termination of pregnancy
    C. Medical test for pregnancy
    D. Menstrual test for pregnancy

11. **A 20-week pregnancy can be terminated with the consent of ________.**
    A. Two registered medical practitioners
    B. Doctor holding MBBS degree
    C. Doctor holding MD degree
    D. Gynaecologist

12. **Admission register means a register maintained as per ________ of the MTP Act 1971 and rules there under.**
A. Regulation IV
B. Regulation V
C. Regulation VI
D. Regulation III

13. **When the length of pregnancy exceeds from 12 to 20 weeks, the opinion of how many RMP is considered for termination of pregnancy?**
A. 4
B. 1
C. 2
D. 3

14. **A registered medical practitioner may terminate pregnancy if it is ________.**
A. Not more than 12 weeks old
B. Not less than 20 weeks old
C. Not more than 20 weeks old
D. None of the above

15. **Termination of pregnancy should be made only at ________.**
A. A place approved by district level committee
B. Hospital established and maintained by Government
C. Any place approved by the Government for this purpose
D. All of the above

16. **Minor is a person who has not attained majority under the provisions of ________.**
A. Indian Majority Act 1888
B. Indian Majority Act 1857
C. Indian Majority Act 1875
D. Indian Majority Act 1867

17. **Medical termination of pregnancy is safe up to ______.**
A. 12 weeks
B. 10 weeks
C. 18 weeks
D. 6 weeks

18. **Which period of pregnancy are the MTPs safest?**
A. Fourth trimester
B. First trimester
C. Second trimester
D. Third trimester

19. **Approved place means a place approved under ______ of the MTP Act, 1971 and rules thereunder.**
A. Rule II
B. Rule III
C. Rule IV
D. Rule V

20. **MTP Rules, 1975 provide for the maintenance of ____________.**
A. First register
B. Subsequent register
C. Central register
D. Admission Register

Answer Key

1 C	2 A	3 B	4 C	5 B	6 C	7 B	8 D	9 C	10 B
11 A	12 B	13 C	14 A	15 D	16 C	17 A	18 B	19 C	20 D

CHAPTER 12

Central Drugs Standards Control Organization (CDSCO) and Indian Pharmacopoeia Commission (IPC)

1. **The CDSCO is a _________ for drugs, cosmetics, medical and diagnostic devices and clinical trails.**
   - **A.** State Level Committee
   - **B.** National Regulatory Body
   - **C.** WHO Regulatory Bodies
   - **D.** None of the above

2. **The headquarter of CDSCO is located at _________.**
   - **A.** Kolkata
   - **B.** Mumbai
   - **C.** Delhi
   - **D.** Chennai

3. **The IPC has become fully operational from _________.**
   - **A.** 1 Jan. 2010
   - **B.** 1 Jan. 2011
   - **C.** 1 Jan. 2012
   - **D.** 1 Jan. 2009

4. **The _____________ create a set of standards of drugs in India.**
   - **A.** Indian Pharmaceutical Course
   - **B.** Indian Pharmacopoeia Commission
   - **C.** Indian Pharmacovigilance Course
   - **D.** Indian Pharmacy Course

5. **Who is the head of CDSCO?**
   - **A.** ADC
   - **B.** DDC
   - **C.** DCGI
   - **D.** DI

6. **The function of IPC is _________.**
   - **A.** Publishing of IP
   - **B.** Regulating standards of drugs
   - **C.** Providing IPRS
   - **D.** All of the above

7. **The CDSCO is responsible for _________.**
   - **A.** Laying down the Standards for Drugs
   - **B.** Approval of Drugs
   - **C.** Conduct of clinical trials
   - **D.** All of the above

8. **Full form of CDSCO is _________.**
   - **A.** Central Drugs Sell Corporation Office
   - **B.** Central Drug State Corporation Office
   - **C.** Central Drugs Standards Control Organization
   - **D.** None of the above

9. **AYUSH staff involved in the organization of CDSCO includes _________.**
   - **A.** ADC (Ayurveda/ Unani/ Siddha)
   - **B.** DDC (Ayurveda)
   - **C.** DDC (Homeopathy)
   - **D.** All of the above

10. **Indian Pharmacopoeia Commission headquarter is located at _________.**
    - **A.** Ghaziabad
    - **B.** Delhi
    - **C.** Mumbai
    - **D.** Hyderabad

11. **Indian Pharmaceutical Committee was appointed in _________.**
    - **A.** 1968
    - **B.** 1938
    - **C.** 1948
    - **D.** 1958

12. **The function of CDSCO is _________.**
    - **A.** Testing of new drug
    - **B.** Approval of new drug
    - **C.** Import Registration and Licensing
    - **D.** All of the above

13. **License for blood and blood products, IV fluids, vaccines and sera is granted by _________.**
    - **A.** CDSCO
    - **B.** FDCA
    - **C.** CDSCO and state regulators
    - **D.** IPC

14. What is the full form of IPC?

A. International Pharmacy Commission
B. Indian Pharmaceutical Company
C. Indian Pharmacopoeia Commission
D. Indian Pharmaceutical Commission

15. Indian Veterinary Research Institute (IVRI) is located at ________.

A. Delhi **B.** Ghaziabad
C. Noida **D.** Izatnagar

16. The 1st edition of Indian Pharmacopoeia was published in the year ________.

A. 1960 **B.** 1966
C. 1955 **D.** 1950

17. The sub-zonal office of CDSCO is located at ______.

A. Ghaziabad **B.** Bangalore
C. Ahmedabad **D.** Chennai

18. The chairman of Indian Pharmacopoeia Commission is ________.

A. The Drugs Controller General
B. Chairman-Scientific Body
C. The Secretary, Ministry of Health and Family Welfare
D. Directorate General of Health Services

19. The Drug Regulatory Authority in India is ________.

A. TGA
B. MHRA
C. USFDA
D. CDSCO

20. Major vision of CDSCO is ___________.

A. Remove impurities
B. Safety of public health
C. Efficacy of drug
D. Quality of drug

Answer Key

1 B	2 C	3 D	4 B	5 C	6 D	7 D	8 C	9 D	10 A
11 C	12 D	13 B	14 C	15 D	16 C	17 B	18 C	19 D	20 B

CHAPTER 13

Good Regulatory Practices

GRPs

1. **GRPs stand for ________.**
   A. Good Regulatory Policies
   B. Good Regulatory Practices
   C. Good Regulatory Principles
   D. Good Reframe Policy

2. **________ is internationally recognized processes, systems, tools and methods for improving the quality of regulations**
   A. CDSCO B. GDP
   C. GLP D. GRP

3. **The Pharmaceutical Industry always adopted good regulatory practices because ________.**
   A. It prevents ineffective medicine
   B. It prevents and mitigates adverse health effects
   C. It prevents poor quality
   D. All of the above

4. **________ is defined as actual practice of pharmacy in a hospital.**
   A. Hospital pharmacy B. Social pharmacy
   C. Community pharmacy D. Hospital

5. **________ is e-governance system to discharge various functions performed by CDSCO under Drugs and Cosmetics Act 1940.**
   A. e-commerce B. SUGAM
   C. Swayam D. e-Pharmacy

6. **________ is a registered pharmacist is involved in hospital pharmacy services ensuring distribution of safe, efficacious, and cost-effective medicaments to both inpatients and outpatients.**
   A. Clinical Pharmacist
   B. Hospital Pharmacist
   C. Community Pharmacist
   D. All of the above

7. **________ defined as the direct computer to computer transmission of electronic prescriptions from prescriber offices to community pharmacies.**
   A. e-Commerce B. e-filling
   C. e-pharmacy D. e-prescription

8. **Which authority issues license for permission to manufacture post-successful clinical trials?**
   A. UGC B. IPC
   C. DCGI D. AICTE

9. **The first guidelines for import or export of human biological samples was published by ________.**
   A. GDP B. ASHP
   C. CDSCO D. None of the above

10. **The National e-Governance plan (NeGP) was launched in ________.**
    A. 2008 B. 2006
    C. 2007 D. 2008

Answer Key

1 B	2 D	3 B	4 A	5 B	6 B	7 D	8 C	9 C	10 B

CHAPTER

14

Introduction to BCS System of Classification

1. Biopharmaceutical Classification System classifies the drugs into one of the ________ groups.

A. 1 B. 2

C. 3 D. 4

2. The BCS was first developed in 1995 by ________.

A. Samson et al

B. Amidol et al

C. Rudolph et al

D. Watson et al

3. ________ has notified the 'New Drugs and Clinical Trails" Rules, 2019.

A. Ministry of Health and Former Welfare

B. Ministry of Health and Family Welfare

C. Ministry of Health and Female Welfare

D. Ministry of Health and Food Welfare

4. A drug with high solubility is the one whose largest dosage strength is soluble in ________ ml of water over a pH range of 1–8.

A. 100 B. 200

C. 250 D. 300

5. ________ means ideas owned by a person or a firm.

A. Intangible property

B. Intellectual property

C. Real property

D. Tangible property

6. Drugs with high absorption number have ________ permeability.

A. High

B. Low

C. Both A and B

D. None of the above

7. Topography of integrated circuit is ________ type of invention.

A. Patentable

B. Semi-patentable

C. Non-patentable

D. None of the above

8. ________ refers to creation of mind inventions literacy and artistic works and symbols, names and images used in commerce.

A. Status

B. Image

C. Intellectual property

D. General property

9. The optimum dose for therapy and therapeutic window for new drug is determined by which phase of clinical trial?

A. Phase 1 B. Phase 4

C. Phase 2 D. Phase 3

10. IND is filed by Innovator Company to FDA at which stage?

A. Before Phase 0

B. After Phase III

C. Before Phase III

D. After Phase 0

11. The BCS is represented by 4 major classes and the drugs are classified based on three major factors governing bioavailability, namely ________.

A. Dissolution, Solubility, Dissolution Rate

B. Dissolution Rate, Solubility, Permeability

C. Dissolution, Solubility, Polymorphism

D. Solubility, Absorption, Distribution

12. The requirement and guidelines for conduct of clinical trials of new drug comes under ________.

A. Schedule T
B. Schedule V
C. Schedule Q
D. Schedule Y

13. The adverse drug effects and new indication of the drug can be studied in which phase of clinical trial?

A. Phase 4
B. Phase 0
C. Phase 2
D. Phase 1

14. TRIPS means ________.

A. Trade Research Aspects of Intellectual Property Rights
B. Trade Related Aspects of Intellectual Property Rights
C. Trade Revamping Aspects of Intellectual Property Rights
D. Trade Relevant Aspects of Intellectual Property Rights

15. The comparison of efficacy of new drug with already marketed standard drug was done in which phase of clinical trial?

A. Phase 1
B. Phase 2
C. Phase 4
D. Phase 3

16. ANDA is applicable to ________.

A. Branded drugs
B. Generic drugs
C. Patented drugs
D. All of the above

17. Patent Act is established in ________.

A. 1948
B. 1970
C. 1919
D. 1940

18. According to Biopharmaceutical Classification System, Class II drugs have ________.

A. Low Solubility/ Low Permeability
B. High Solubility/ High Permeability
C. Low Solubility/ High Permeability
D. High Solubility/ Low Permeability

19. Which BCS class shows high solubility and low permeability?

A. BCS Class IV
B. BCS Class III
C. BCS Class I
D. BCS Class II

20. According to Biopharmaceutical Classification System, Class IV drugs have ________.

A. Low Solubility/ Low Permeability
B. Low Solubility/ High Permeability
C. High Solubility/ High Permeability
D. High Solubility/ Low Permeability

21. As per Drugs and Cosmetics Act, the application for grant of permission to undertake clinical trial is given in which form?

A. Form 1
B. Form 21
C. Form 27
D. Form 44

22. ANDA is for ________.

A. Pre-clinical
B. Generic drug approval
C. Clinical trial
D. All of the above

23. A drug substance is considered to be highly permeable when the systemic bio-availability is ________.

A. 90% or more
B. 80% or more
C. 85% or more
D. 100% or more

24. Post-marketing surveillance comes under clinical trial ________.

A. Phase II
B. Phase I
C. Phase III
D. Phase V

25. How many people will be selected for phase III trial?

A. 300–3000 people
B. 200–300 people
C. Whole market will be under surveillance
D. 20–50 people

26. A drug substance is considered highly soluble when the highest strength is soluble in ________.

A. 550 ml
B. 450 ml
C. 250 ml
D. 350 ml

27. Drugs with low absorption number have ________ permeability.

A. Low
B. High
C. Both A and B
D. None of the above

28. At which stage IND is filed by Innovator Company to FDA?

A. After phase III
B. Before phase 0
C. Before phase III
D. After phase 0

29. Which of the clinical trial is called therapeutic confirmatory phase?

A. Phase 4 B. Phase 2
C. Phase 1 D. Phase 3

30. How many people will be selected for phase I trial?

A. Whole market will be under surveillance
B. 300–3000 people
C. 20–300 people
D. 20–50 people

31. NDA is for _________.

A. Approval from FDA pre-clinical trial
B. Approval from FDA for sale and marketing
C. Approval from FDA for clinical trial
D. All of the above

32. Which phase of the clinical trial is referred to as pharmacovigilance?

A. Phase 1 B. Phase 4
C. Phase 3 D. Phase 2

33. Which of the following cannot be patented in India?

A. A computer programs B. Scientific theory
C. Mathematical method D. All of the above

34. The optimum dose for the therapy is determined in ___________ of the clinical trial.

A. Phase 2 B. Phase 0
C. Phase 1 D. Phase 4

35. IND stands for _________.

A. International new drug
B. Investigational new drug
C. Insisted new drug
D. Inhibited new drug

36. _________ can be patented under Patent Act, 1970.

A. A computer programs
B. An Invention
C. Mathematical Method
D. An aesthetic creation

37. The Patent Act is established in _________ year.

A. 1948 B. 1945
C. 1970 D. 1919

38. A singer wishes to assign the rights to reproduce a video she has made of her concert comes under _________.

A. Copyrights
B. Industrial design
C. Trademark
D. Patent

39. How many people will be selected for phase II trial?

A. Whole market will be under surveillance
B. 20–300 people
C. 500–3000 people
D. 200–500 people

40. The optimum dose for the therapy is determined in which phase of the clinical trial?

A. Phase 0
B. Phase 4
C. Phase 1
D. Phase 2

41. Which of the following type of research trials do not involve human beings?

A. Human clinical trials
B. Preclinical trials
C. Clinical trials
D. None of the above

42. The life of a patented drug is _________.

A. 25 years B. 10 years
C. 20 years D. 15 years

43. NDA means _________.

A. New drug application
B. New dose application
C. National drug application
D. National development application

44. How long is patent valid in India?

A. 60 years
B. 30 years
C. 20 years
D. 40 years

45. Good clinical practice is seen in all *except*

A. Phase 2 trials
B. Pre-clinical trials
C. Phase 3 trials
D. Phase 4 trials

46. ANDA stands for _________

A. Associated new drug application
B. Abbreviated new dose application
C. Abbreviated new drug application
D. Associated national drug application

47. Patent is a _________

A. Real property
B. Transferable property
C. Negotiable property
D. Non-transferable property

48. IPRs means _________.
A. Integrated property rights
B. Internal property rights
C. Indian property rights
D. Intellectual property rights

49. NDCT stands for _________.
A. New Drugs and Combination Trials
B. New Drugs and Clinical Trials
C. New Drugs and Cohesive Trials
D. New Drugs and Company Trials

50. EUA means _________.
A. Emergency Unique Authorisation
B. Emergency Use Authorisation
C. Emergency Unit Authorisation
D. Emergency Under Authorisation

Answer Key

1 D	2 B	3 B	4 C	5 B	6 A	7 C	8 C	9 C	10 A
11 B	12 D	13 A	14 B	15 D	16 B	17 B	18 C	19 B	20 A
21 D	22 C	23 C	24 C	25 A	26 C	27 A	28 B	29 D	30 D
31 C	32 B	33 D	34 A	35 B	36 B	37 C	38 A	39 B	40 D
41 B	42 C	43 A	44 C	45 B	46 C	47 B	48 D	49 B	50 B

CHAPTER

15

Blood Bank: Basic Requirements and Functions

1. **A blood bank is ________.**
   A. Where blood is stored
   B. Where blood is collected.
   C. Where blood is separated into components.
   D. All of the above

2. **Who is the Pioneer/Father of the blood bank?**
   A. Sir Louis Braille
   B. Sir Alexander Godefroy
   C. Sir Charles Richard Drew
   D. Sir John Baggins

3. **The requirements of blood banks are given under ________ of the Drugs and Cosmetics Rules.**
   A. Schedule F part of XIIB
   B. Schedule F part of XIB
   C. Schedule F part of XB
   D. Schedule F part of IXB

4. **In sickle cell anaemia, red cell count is ________.**
   A. Normal
   B. Reduced
   C. Increased
   D. None of the above

5. **The lower limit of Hb in female blood donor is ______.**
   A. 14 gm/dl
   B. 10 gm/dl
   C. 12 gm/dl
   D. 13 gm/dl

6. **Government of India published the National Blood Policy in the year ________.**
   A. 2001 B. 2002
   C. 2000 D. 1999

7. **Fresh hold blood transfusion is done within how much time of collection?**
   A. 24 hours B. Immediately
   C. 1 hour D. 4 hours

8. **Massive blood transfusion is defined as ________.**
   A. Whole blood volume
   B. 350 ml in 5 min
   C. 50 ml in 5 min
   D. 1 litre in 5 min

9. **Red blood cells can be frozen and stored up to ______.**
   A. 7 years B. 3 years
   C. 5 years D. 8 years

10. **Advantage of blood donation to donor ________.**
    A. Decrease heart disease
    B. Free health check up
    C. Reduce iron in body
    D. All of the above

11. **Minimum haemoglobin value required for a donor to donate blood is ________ gm/dl.**
    A. 2.5 B. 10
    C. 9.5 D. 8.5

12. **How often we donate blood?**
    A. After 24 hours
    B. After 3 months
    C. After 3 hours
    D. After 6 months

13. **The interval between two blood donations should be ________.**
    A. 12 weeks B. 4 weeks
    C. 8 weeks D. 10 weeks

14. **What is the full form of NBTC?**
   A. National Blood Transfer Center
   B. National Blood Transfusion Council
   C. National Blood Transfer Council
   D. National Blood Transfusion Center

15. **During blood donation the removal of blood components is called _________.**
   A. Leukapheresis B. Cytopheresis
   C. Plasmapheresis D. Apheresis

16. **The disease cannot transmitted through transfusion of blood _________.**
   A. Cancer B. AIDS
   C. Hepatitis B D. Malaria

17. **Blood component products are _________.**
   A. Fresh frozen plasma B. Whole blood
   C. Platelets D. All of the above

18. **The process of formation of blood cell is called ______.**
   A. Haemopoiesis
   B. Mitosis
   C. Photosynthesis BOD
   D. Complement fixation

19. **What is the application form number for certificate of renewal of licence for manufacture of blood products?**
   A. 28 Y B. 26 I
   C. 27 Y D. 25 I

20. **First blood bank in India was established in ________.**
   A. Mumbai B. Delhi
   C. Kolkata D. Pune

21. **Which type of donor is avoided for donation?**
   A. Person who drink alcohol
   B. STD patient
   C. Dengue patient
   D. All of the above

22. **The minimum weight of blood donor should be______.**
   A. 60 kg B. 45 kg
   C. 50 kg D. 55 kg

23. **Which of the following investigations should be done immediately to best confirm a non-matched blood transfusion reaction?**
   A. Antibody in donor serum
   B. Antibody in patient's serum
   C. Indirect Coombs' test
   D. Direct Coombs' test

24. **License for blood storage centre is valid for ________.**
   A. 1 year B. 3 years
   C. 2 years D. 5 years

25. **Frozen RBCs can be stored up to _________.**
   A. 1 year B. 10 years
   C. 25 years D. 5 years

26. **Blood grouping is discovered by which of the following scientists in 1990?**
   A. Karl Landsteiner B. Charles Richard Drew
   C. Alexander S Weiner D. None of the above

27. **Maximum age for the first time blood donor is ______ years.**
   A. 45 B. 50
   C. 60 D. 40

28. **The blood bank unit shall have a minimum requirement floor area of _________.**
   A. 50 m^2 B. 100 m^2
   C. 40 m^2 D. 60 mv

29. **In dengue platelet count is _________.**
   A. Normal B. Reduced
   C. Increase D. None of the above

30. **Size of red blood cell is _________.**
   A. 2 µm B. 10 µm
   C. 7 µm D. 8 µm

Answer Key

1 D	2 C	3 A	4 B	5 C	6 D	7 A	8 D	9 B	10 D
11 A	12 B	13 A	14 B	15 D	16 A	17 D	18 A	19 B	20 C
21 D	22 C	23 D	24 C	25 B	26 A	27 C	28 B	29 B	30 C

CHAPTER 16

Clinical Establishment Act and Rules

1. **The Clinical Establishments Act was passed by Parliament of India on ____________.**
   A. 17th August 2014 B. 17th August 2010
   C. 17th July 2010 D. 17th August 2012

2. **Clinical Establishments (Registration and Regulation) Act was enacted in which year?**
   A. 2011 B. 2001
   C. 2010 D. 2020

3. **The chairperson of the Clinical Establishment Act is ____________.**
   A. Director General of Central Council
   B. Director General of Health Services
   C. Director General of Medical Council
   D. Director General of CDL

4. **National Council means National Council of Clinical Establishments established under ____________.**
   A. Section 10 B. Section 20
   C. Section 30 D. Section 40

5. **Which section mandates that no person shall run a clinical establishment unless it has been duly registered in accordance with the provisions of the Act?**
   A. 07 B. 10
   C. 04 D. 11

6. **The Clinical Establishment Act is enforced by ______.**
   A. Pharmacy Council of India
   B. State Government
   C. Central Government
   D. Medical Council of India

7. **Which type of Clinics are covered under the Clinical Establishment Act?**
   A. Private B. Government
   C. Both A and B D. None of the above

8. **What is the fine for running the Clinical Establishment without Registration under the Clinical Establishment Act?**
   A. ₹ 2000 B. ₹ 50,000
   C. ₹ 10,000 D. ₹ 20,000

9. **Who is the Chairperson of the State Council of Clinical Establishment under the Clinical Establishment Act?**
   A. Director General of Medical Council
   B. Director General of Health Services
   C. Secretary General of Health Services
   D. Director General of Central Council

10. **How many members are there in the National Council for Clinical Establishment?**
    A. 20 B. 25
    C. 15 D. 10

Answer Key

1 B	2 C	3 B	4 C	5 D	6 C	7 C	8 B	9 C	10 A

CHAPTER 17

Biomedical Waste Management Rules 2016

1. **Biomedical waste means _________.**
   A. Waste generated by nursing
   B. Waste generated by hospitals
   C. Waste generated by clinics
   D. All of the above

2. **The biomedical waste management rules are generated in _________.**
   A. 1998 B. 1901
   C. 1925 D. 2001

3. **___________ is a state-of- the-art technology for safe disposal of medical waste.**
   A. Sun drying
   B. Plasma pyrolysis
   C. Dumping
   D. None of the above

4. **How many categories are there for classification of biomedical waste?**
   A. 12 B. 08
   C. 09 D. 10

5. **In which colour bag collected bandage, cotton or any other things which is infected.**
   A. Yellow bags
   B. Red bags
   C. White bags
   D. Black bags

6. **The biomedical waste management rules are prescribed in _________ Schedule.**
   A. VII B. IX
   C. VI D. X

7. **The bags used for glass bottles and broken glass articles are _________.**
   A. Blue bags
   B. Yellow bags
   C. Red bags
   D. White bags

8. **As per government rule biomedical waste cannot be stored more than _________.**
   A. 36 to 48 hours B. 12 to 24 hours
   C. 24 to 48 hours D. 48 to 56 hours

9. **What is 3R Rule?**
   A. Regenerate-Rejoin-Reject
   B. Reduce-Reuse-Recycling
   C. Both A and B
   D. None of the above

10. **The simplest and most common method used in the cities is to collect and dump the waste in a ________.**
    A. Ocean
    B. Landfill
    C. River
    D. All of the above

11. **The following is a types of environmental and health hazard _________.**
    A. Biological B. Chemical
    C. Physical D. All of the above

12. **Which waste is collected in purple container?**
    A. Cytotoxic and cytostatic waste
    B. Syringes
    C. Hazardous waste
    D. None of the above

13. _________ is not a biomedical waste?
A. Microbiological waste B. Animal waste
C. Domestic waste D. Chemical waste

14. All of the following are methods of disposal of biomedical waste *except* _________.
A. Autoclaving
B. Chemical disinfecting
C. Incineration
D. Sieving

15. The paint, household cleaners, medical waste, and solvents belong to _________ waste.
A. Industrial B. Hazardous
C. Compost D. Municipal solid

16. Cytotoxic should be placed in _________.
A. Black container B. Red container
C. Yellow container D. Grey container

17. Which of the following is a method of disposal of hospital waste?
A. Incineration B. Microwave irradiation
C. Inertization D. All of the above

18. The anatomical waste should be placed in _________.
A. Black pail B. Yellow pail
C. Grey tote D. Red pail

19. Which of following item is categorized under white category of biomedical waste?
A. Waste tubes B. Expired medicine
C. Waste metal sharps D. Broken glass

20. Broken or contaminated glass is categorized in which category of biomedical waste?
A. White B. Blue
C. Yellow D. Red

21. _________ is categorised under red category of biomedical waste.
A. Waste tubes B. Discarded linen
C. Waste metal sharps D. Broken glass

22. _________ falls under non-hazardous waste?
A. Gases
B. Chemotherapy waste
C. Chemicals
D. Dextrose solution

23. The pills should be placed in _________.
A. Sharps container B. Yellow pail
C. Pharma pail D. Red pail

24. _________ can be produced from landfill waste.
A. Biogas
B. Natural gas
C. Liquefied petroleum gas
D. Any of the above

25. Which one of the following is not biomedical waste?
A. Animal waste
B. Domestic waste
C. Microbiological waste
D. Chemical waste

26. Which of the following should not be mixed with other waste to avoid contamination?
A. Vegetable oil B. Tarry residue
C. Oily sludge D. Animal waste

27. The blood product pack should be put in _________.
A. Red pail B. Yellow pail
C. White pail D. Sharps container

28. _____________ have the lowest chance of producing biomedical waste?
A. Agricultural lands B. Laboratories
C. Hospitals D. Clinics

29. _________ requires special treatment of bacteria.
A. Labelling of waste B. Transport of waste
C. Degradation of waste D. Packaging of waste

30. _________ is used to put a scalpel.
A. Sharps container B. Yellow pail
C. White pail D. Red pail

Answer Key

1 D	2 A	3 B	4 D	5 A	6 C	7 A	8 C	9 B	10 B
11 D	12 A	13 C	14 D	15 B	16 C	17 D	18 B	19 C	20 B
21 A	22 D	23 C	24 A	25 B	26 D	27 B	28 A	29 C	30 C

CHAPTER 18

Bioethics

1. **What are the common bioethical issues?**
   A. Organ donation B. Eugenics
   C. Euthanasia D. All of the above

2. **ICMR means _________.**
   A. Indian Cadre of Medical Research
   B. Indian Council of Medical Research
   C. Indian Component of Medical Research
   D. Indian Company of Medical Research

3. **The American biochemist _________coined the term bioethics in 1970.**
   A. James Franklin Childress
   B. Van Rensselaer Potter
   C. Tom Beauchamp
   D. None of the above

4. **The long form of IBC is _________.**
   A. International Biomedical Council
   B. International Bioethics Council
   C. International Bioethics Committee
   D. International Biomedical Committee

5. **The following principle is not relevant in autonomy?**
   A. Consent B. Confidentiality
   C. Self-determination D. Capacity

6. **What are the primary moral principles predominantly employed in bioethics?**
   A. Non-maleficence B. Autonomy
   C. Beneficence D. All of the above

7. **Which rules of conduct may be used to regulate our activities concerning the biological world?**
   A. Bioethics B. Bio-piracy
   C. Biosafety D. Bio-patents

8. **_________ standards are required to evaluate the morality of all human activities.**
   A. Social B. Ethical
   C. Pathological D. Psychological

9. **A moral rule to protect and defend the right of patient is mentioned under which principle of bioethics?**
   A. Principle of justice
   B. Principle of non-maleficence
   C. Principle of respect for autonomy
   D. Principle of beneficence

10. **Healthcare practitioner making sure the treatments given to a patient do not cause them any harm is an example of which of the following bioethics principle?**
    A. Autonomy B. Beneficence
    C. Non-maleficence D. Utility

Answer Key

1 D	2 B	3 B	4 C	5 B	6 D	7 A	8 B	9 D	10 C

CHAPTER

19

The Consumer Protection Act 1986

1. **In India, the Consumer Protection Act was initiated in the year ________.**

   A. 1947 B. 2019
   C. 1986 D. 2021

2. **The main objective of the consumer organization is to protect the interest of the ________.**

   A. Manufacturer
   B. Consumer
   C. Trader
   D. Producer

3. **The President of district commission is a ________.**

   A. District Judge
   B. High Court Judge
   C. Supreme Court Judge
   D. None of the above

4. **National Commission has ________ members.**

   A. 3 B. 1
   C. 4 D. 2

5. **The Consumer Protection Act is significant to ______.**

   A. Movable goods
   B. All goods and services
   C. Immovable goods
   D. Selected all goods and services

6. **________ is celebrated as World Consumer Day.**

   A. 1 January B. 10 April
   C. 15 March D. 28 February

7. **The Government has established ________ to settle the consumer dispute by compromise.**

   A. Consumer Organization
   B. District Commission
   C. Lok Adalat
   D. All of the above

8. **The District Commission entertains complaints of consumer for compensation which is less than ______.**

   A. 10 Lakh
   B. 10 Crore
   C. 1 lakh
   D. 1 Cr

9. **The following is consumer rights specified in the Consumer Protection Act, 1986.**

   A. Right to consumer education
   B. Right to safety
   C. Right to choose
   D. All of the above

10. **Rights of Consumer are protected under __________.**

    A. Consumer Protection Act, 1990
    B. Consumer Protection Act, 1986
    C. Consumer Protection Act, 1982
    D. Consumer Protection Act, 1991

11. **How many rights does a consumer have under the Consumer Protection Act?**

    A. 5 B. 8
    C. 6 D. 4

12. **According to the Consumer Protection Act, District Forum means ________.**

    A. Consumer Disputes Redressal Forum
    B. City Civil Court
    C. First Class Judicial Magistrate
    D. Munsif Court

13. What is the pecuniary jurisdiction of the state commission under the Consumer Protection Act?

A. Fifteen lakhs to one crore
B. Twenty lakhs to one crore
C. Twenty lakhs and above
D. No pecuniary jurisdiction

14. How much change in the amount to be deposited for filing an appeal?

A. 25% B. 20%
C. 50% D. 10%

15. Who is eligible to be appointed as a President of National Consumer Dispute Redressal Forum?

A. Judge of the Supreme Court
B. Judge of High Court
C. Chief Justice of High Court
D. Attorney General of India

16. Which of the following is a Consumer Protection Council?

A. District forum
B. The Central Consumer Protection Council
C. The State Consumer Protection Council
D. All of the above

17. A person aggrieved by any order passed by the Central Authority under Sections 20 and 21 may file an appeal to the National Commission within a period of________ days from the date of receipt of such order?

A. 45 days
B. 60 days
C. 30 days
D. 20 days

18. District Consumer Disputes Redressal Commission is established by

A. State Government
B. National Commission
C. Central Government
D. District Collector

19. Which Consumers Right is not guaranteed under Consumer Protection Act, 2019?

A. Right to be heard
B. Right to choose
C. Right to exploitation
D. Right to seek redressal

20. Who can make a complaint under this Act?

A. One or more consumers having the same interest
B. Consumer
C. Any recognized consumer association
D. All of the above

21. The order of National Commission can be challenged in Supreme Court within _________.

A. 30 days B. 10 days
C. 45 days D. 20 days

22. Who is the head of the Central Authority's Investigation Wing?

A. Magistrate
B. Police Officer
C. Director General
D. None of the above

23. Which of the following are Consumer Disputes Redressal Agencies?

A. State Commission
B. Panchayat Commission
C. Municipal Commission
D. None of the above

24. District Commission shall decide the admissibility of the complaint within _____________.

A. 45 days
B. 30 days
C. 07 days
D. 21 days

25. Where can the complaint are filed?

A. State Forum
B. Civil Court
C. District Forum
D. District Court

26. Under the Consumer Protection Act, the rights of a consumer do not include to be _________.

A. Informed
B. Safety
C. Choose
D. Presented

27. What are the powers of the Central Authority?

A. To protect the rights
B. To promote the rights
C. To enforce the rights
D. All of the above

28. On what grounds you cannot claim compensation from the product manufacturer _________.

A. Damaged by consumer
B. Manufacturing defect
C. Defect in design
D. Deviation from specification

29. Every document, record or article seized under Consumer Protection Act should be returned within _______________.

A. 10 days
B. 1 week
C. One month
D. 20 days

30. _______________ is the highest authority to settle the consumer dispute under act.

A. National Commission
B. District Commission
C. State Commission
D. All of the above

Answer Key

1 C	2 B	3 A	4 C	5 B	6 C	7 C	8 D	9 D	10 B
11 C	12 A	13 B	14 B	15 A	16 D	17 B	18 A	19 C	20 D
21 A	22 C	23 A	24 D	25 C	26 D	27 D	28 A	29 D	30 A

CHAPTER 20

Introduction to the Disaster Management Act

1. **National Institute of Disaster Management was introduced in _________.**
   A. August 14, 2001 B. August 14, 2004
   C. September 23, 2002 D. October 16, 2003
2. **The National Disaster Management Authority (NDMA) is headed by _________.**
   A. Chief Minister of States
   B. Governor of States
   C. Prime Minister of India
   D. President of India
3. **Head office of National Institute of Disaster Management is situated at_________.**
   A. Mumbai B. Kolkata
   C. New Delhi D. Manipur
4. **The State Disaster Management Authority is headed by _________.**
   A. Chief Secretary of the State
   B. Governor
   C. Chief Minister
   D. None of the above
5. **What is the full form of NDRF?**
   A. National Drainage Response Force
   B. National Disaster Response Force
   C. Natural Disasters Relief Factor
   D. National Disaster Relief Force
6. **The Disaster Management Act was made in _________.**
   A. 2009 B. 2006
   C. 2003 D. 2005
7. **Effective hazard management largely relies on ______.**
   A. Volcanoes B. Govt. agencies
   C. Emergency responses D. Pre-disaster planning
8. **Under which Ministry of Govt. of India does the National Disaster Management Authority function?**
   A. Ministry of Foreign Affairs
   B. Ministry of Environment
   C. Ministry of Home Affairs
   D. Ministry of Agriculture
9. **Who has the authority to select the vice-chairperson of SDMA?**
   A. Parliament B. Governor of the state
   C. Chief Minister D. State Legislature
10. **The full form of NDMA is _________.**
    A. National Drainage Management Authority
    B. National Disaster Management Area
    C. Natural Disasters Manmade Authority
    D. National Disaster Management Authority

Answer Key

1 B	2 C	3 C	4 C	5 B	6 D	7 D	8 C	9 C	10 D

CHAPTER

21

Medical Devices

1. **Medical device is used for which purpose?**
   A. Monitoring B. Diagnosis
   C. Prevention D. All of the above

2. **_________ is an instrument, apparatus, implements machine, implant, *in vitro* reagent or other similar article that is intended for use in the diagnosis, prevention and treatment of disease or other medical conditions.**
   A. Gadget B. Medical device
   C. Electronic device D. None of the above

3. **IMDRA means _________.**
   A. Indian Medical Drugs Regulation Act
   B. Indian Medical Dose Regulation Act
   C. Indian Medical Devices Regulation Act
   D. Indian Medical Diagnosis Regulation Act

4. **The lung ventilators are classified under which class of medical devices?**
   A. Class D B. Class B
   C. Class A D. Class C

5. **What are the categories of medical devices?**
   A. Active medical device
   B. Non-active medical device
   C. In *vitro* diagnostic medical device
   D. All of the above

6. **The high risk devices belong to which class of medical devices?**
   A. Class B B. Class D
   C. Class A D. Class C

7. **Which ministry has established medical devices rules in consultation with DTAB and GHTF?**
   A. CDSCO
   B. Ministry of Medical Devices
   C. Ministry of Health and Family Welfare
   D. Ministry of Family and Health Welfare

8. **Which of the class of medical devices are for low risk?**
   A. Class C B. Class A
   C. Class B D. All of the above

9. **The import of medical device licence is valid up to**
   A. 5 years B. 3 years
   C. 4 years D. 2 years

10. **The low risk devices belong to which class of medical devices?**
    A. Class D B. Class B
    C. Class A D. Class C

Answer Key

1 D	2 B	3 C	4 D	5 D	6 B	7 C	8 D	9 B	10 C